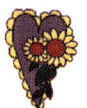

Paul White
4204 Deer Park Dr
Little Rock, AR 72223

Essential Malariology

Essential Malariology

Leonard Jan Bruce-Chwatt
CMG, OBE, MD, FRCP, MPH

Emeritus Professor of Tropical Hygiene
University of London
Member, Expert Advisory Panel on Malaria
World Health Organization
Formerly Director Ross Institute
London School of Hygiene and Tropical Medicine

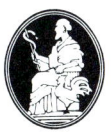

Distributed in the U.S. and Canada by
Springer Publishing Co., New York, N.Y.

William Heinemann Medical Books Ltd · London

William Heinemann Medical Books Ltd
23 Bedford Square
London WC1B 3HH

First published 1980
Copyright © L J Bruce-Chwatt 1980

ISBN 0 433 04520 5

Photoset in VIP Times at
D. P. Media Limited, Hitchin, Hertfordshire,
and printed in Great Britain by
The Camelot Press Ltd
Southampton

Contents

Acknowledgements		viii
Foreword		ix
Introduction		xi
1	Historical Outline	1
2	The Malaria Parasites	10
3	Clinical Course of Malaria	35
4	Pathology and Immunology of Human Malaria	52
5	Diagnostic Methods in Malaria	76
6	The Anopheles Vector	97
7	Epidemiology of Malaria	129
8	Chemotherapy and Chemoprophylaxis	169
9	Rationale and Technique of Malaria Control	209
10	Malaria Eradication	280
Selected References		294
Annex I	International non-proprietary names of antimalarial drugs and some synonyms or proprietary names	324
Annex II	Selected list of some common insecticides and their generic and other names	326
Annex III	Information on malaria risk	328

Annex IV Formulation of suspensions, emulsions, concentrates, and sprays for malaria control — 338

Annex V Conversion factors for metric and other units — 340

Index — 345

*To Joan
and in memory of
Dr Emilio Pampana*

Acknowledgements

I wish to acknowledge my debt of gratitude for the encouragement received from my wife whose interest and help allowed me to complete this book within the proposed time limit.

I am most grateful to my friend and mentor Dr Paul F. Russell, for his generous foreword as well as for his initial suggestion that a book on essential malariology may be needed at the present time.

Professor P. C. C. Garnham FRS has been my source of inspiration as a teacher and my fount of parasitological knowledge. I am greatly indebted to him for all his kindness.

During the long years of my work in Africa, the late Sir Samuel Manuwa, Kt., CMG, OBE, former Director General of Medical Services of the Federal Government of Nigeria, gave me his constant trust and great support.

The assistance and helpful comments received during the past few years from my friend and colleague Dr Tibor Lepeš, Director Malaria Action Programme of the World Health Organization in Geneva, have been much appreciated and are well remembered.

To Dr A. J. Duggan go my sincere thanks for all facilities so generously given at the Wellcome Museum of Medical Science, including the illustrations, most of which were selected from the rich collection of the Museum. The staff of the Museum and in particular Mrs Jacqui Carter, Miss Diana Godfrey, Mr Sam Land and Mr N. Haynes have shown me much kindness and great help. Mr Christopher Allen's skill in preparing a number of drawings was particularly appreciated.

Several line drawings and photographs were obtained from the World Health Organization's Headquarters in Geneva: I am greatly obliged to Dr A. Manuila, Director of Publications Division of WHO and to my good friend Dr James Haworth for the assistance received from them and through them from the WHO Division of Public Information. Thanks are due to the following publishers for permission to reproduce some figures: Blackwell Scientific Publications (Fig. 11); Baillière Tindall (Fig. 22), Oxford University Press (Figs 33 and 42); Superintendent of Documents, US Government Printing Office, Washington (Figs 31 and 32). The sources of other illustrations or tables are acknowledged in relevant captions. Finally, I offer my thanks to my publishers for their understanding and willing cooperation.

Leonard Jan Bruce-Chwatt

Foreword

Malariology – science and practice, has progressed importantly since last described in an authoritative text. Life histories of plasmodia and anophelines are better known, interactions with man more clearly understood, phenomena of immunity give more promise of helpful vaccines, wide spectra of drugs and insecticides have been explored, physical, chemical and biological control methods have been improved, and a most important concept of malaria eradication has had considerable success.

In 1955 the World Health Organization began a malaria eradication campaign that was strongly supported by the Pan American Health Organization, the United Nations Children's Fund, the US Public Health Service, the US Agency for International Development and its predecessors, and by many national health departments. Directly and indirectly this program resulted in the eradication of malaria from the United States, most of Europe, much of the Middle East, important areas in the Caribbean and South America. Two of the most malarious islands in the world, Taiwan and Mauritius, were completely freed from malaria. In India malaria incidence was reduced from millions of cases to an estimated 50 000 cases in 1961. In Sri Lanka (Ceylon) success seemed at hand.

But today malaria is tragically resurgent in Asia and in certain areas elsewhere. Estimates of malaria cases in India in 1977 were as high as 30 million! Malaria also returned to high incidence in Sri Lanka. Numerous failures to eradicate have occurred also in Central and South America. In fact, it seems reasonable to estimate that malaria incidence in the world today is as high as it was half a century ago.

Reasons for the present situation include increased costs of insecticides and labour, inability to obtain, or prohibition to use, DDT, and resistance of plasmodia or anophelines in localised areas to chemical weapons. Most importantly, adequate training of malariologists has been rare, and there has been a crippling decline in the attention devoted to malaria control by international, national, and philanthropic agencies. Other health problems have seemed more urgent or more interesting.

Very likely the demonstration of malaria's power of damaging human health and slowing down socio-economic advance will soon stimulate a revival of interest in malaria control.

In my opinion few men are so well prepared to write *Essential*

Malariology as is Prof. Bruce-Chwatt, whom I first met in 1950 in Lagos, where he was an energetic malariologist. During his brilliant career he has practiced this speciality in laboratory and field and at the director's desk, dealing with local and national areas and later with some international problems.

The author was for many years in the service of the Federal Government of Nigeria and of the World Health Organization. He then became Director of the Ross Institute and Professor of Tropical Hygiene at the London School of Tropical Medicine.

I welcome this concise and authoritative book, especially at a time when malaria is increasingly prevalent and neglected.

North Edgecomb, Maine, USA
July 1978

Paul F. Russell, MD, MPH
Formerly, Member Field Staff,
Rockefeller Foundation;
Chief Malariologist,
Allied Military Government, Italy;
Malaria Consultant to
Surgeon General, US Army and
to the World Health Organization.

Introduction

No one who has followed over the past five years the annual reports of the World Health Organization on the situation of malaria, can doubt that the former rapid progress of the eradication of this disease has now come to a halt and that the resurgence of the infection causes much concern. The number of confirmed cases of malaria reported to the WHO increased from 3.2 million in 1972 to 7.5 million in 1977, but this is only a small proportion of the total number of cases. Malaria continues to be a major problem of tropical developing countries and the recent years have seen the return of it to areas freed from the disease in the 1960s.

The causes of this setback to a unique international health endeavour have often been analysed and commented upon. Certainly technical factors such as resistance of insect vectors to insecticides played a major role in these reverses of fortune. Not less and probably more important were other, often imponderable factors. Inadequacy of planning, administrative shortcomings, financial stringency, shortage of personnel, poor training were equally responsible for the recent shift of strategy from malaria eradication to malaria control in countries not equipped for the undertaking of a complex and difficult programme of eradication.

One of the first steps needed for a realistic approach to the problem of malaria is to admit that we have not developed the technological means to control this disease in all circumstances. We have reduced the malaria morbidity and mortality over large areas of the world at the periphery of the natural geographical distribution of the disease but the core of endemic and epidemic malaria in the tropics remains.

The close relationship between disease and socio-economic advance of developing tropical countries has been abundantly proved. It is now clear that the successful implementation of malaria eradication requires a certain minimum level of basic health services. In countries where malaria is a serious impediment to general advance there is now a new drive for reduction of the burden of the disease to pave the way for speeding up the pace of socio-economic development, which may in the long run contribute to a future eradication of malaria.

One should beware of the error of considering malaria control as a poor man's malaria eradication. On the contrary, malaria control, because of its very flexibility, its adaptation to variable epidemiological conditions, its dependence on social, administrative, and even political conditions of the country or area concerned, presents new challenges and demands knowledgeable and determined leaders.

With the general recognition of the magnitude of our unfinished task came the understanding of pressing needs for further research into methods of malaria control and the return to the provision of adequate information on many essential aspects of parasitology, entomology, epidemiology, prevention, treatment and control of malaria. It is a fact that the older generation of malariologists has largely disappeared and the number of professional workers in tropical community health competent in the field of malaria control is woefully inadequate, while the need for them is steadily growing. In the context of factors related to the inadequacies of personnel and training, good leadership is an essential ingredient of success. Leadership is often an innate quality of an individual but it may be enhanced by judicious selection and proper training. The renewed concentration of both the national governments and international organisations on the provision of and assistance to training centres in malaria control is a good augury for the future.

The past progress of malaria eradication in advanced countries has engendered among many public health administrators, practising clinicians and the general public a false notion, that malaria is a vanishing, if not a vanished, disease. This undue optimism, largely based on the ignorance of the true situation, has often led to the neglect of recognising the infection brought into a non-endemic area of the temperate world by travellers arriving from the tropics. A number of tragic deaths due to missed diagnosis of malaria or to its wrong treatment have caused much concern among the medical profession. The need for more and easily available information on this subject has often been stressed.

The provision of concise and up-to-date description of clinical and public health aspects of human malaria is the purpose of this book. It attempts to present in a factual and readable form the principles and practice of prevention, diagnosis, treatment and control of malaria in individuals and in communities of both advanced and developing countries.

Its approach has been inspired by Dr Paul F. Russell's most successful primer, published a quarter a the century ago. Like Russell's *Malaria: Basic Principles briefly stated*, the present book does not intend to elaborate on all, often highly specialised and increasingly complex branches of applied science, which contribute to the sum total of the discipline of malariology. For this some of the older books, quoted in the references, are still unsurpassed, while much of the newer knowledge will be found in publications and other documents of the WHO, that form an admirable source and constant stream of authoritative information.

As a precept to this text which presents the essentials of the practical

Introduction

approach to an ancient disease, that still defies our ability to eradicate it, but which nevertheless can be substantially reduced, one could do no better than by quoting the following words:

> 'Malaria control is as simple as prescribing two tablets of chloroquine a week, and it is as complex as the distribution of residual DDT on the walls of 3 million houses in Brazil in one single year. It is as easy as releasing an aerosol spray and it is as technically difficult as the anti-anopheline engineering operations of the Tennessee Valley Authority. The old sayings: "Haste makes waste", and "Look before you leap" as well as "Nothing ventured nothing gained" all have basic implications as regards to malaria control schemes, but the greatest single danger lies in fetishes sometimes cherished by all sanitarians, who should keep their minds as cleanly functional as their spraying equipment. . . .
>
> 'One should cling tenaciously to sound general principles while departing freely from conventional methods in order to meet local needs. Obviously in view of the complex epidemiology of malaria and the multiple lines to its control those applying funds in this field have a special responsibility to comprehend the significance of what is being done and to determine if it can be done more effectively and cheaply' (Russell, 1952).

It is apposite and perhaps significant that the need for the present book arose at the time when we are about to commemorate in November 1980 the centenary of the discovery of the malaria parasite by Alphonse Laveran. The readers of *Essential Malariology* will be able to judge how much has been achieved since that date, but they may also realise what remains to be done to free the world from malaria.

Wellcome Museum of Medical Science
London NW 1

'Some of them will saye, seynge that I graunte that I have gathered this booke of so manye writers, that I offer unto you an heape of other mennis labours . . . To whom I aunswere, that if the honeye that the bees gather out of so manye floure of herbes, shrubbes, and trees, that are growing in other mennis medowes, feldes and closes maye justelye be called the bees' honeye . . . so maye I call it that I have learned and gathered of manye good autoures . . . my booke'.

William Turner
A New Herbal *(1551)*

Chapter 1

Historical Outline

It is assumed that the evolutionary history of mammalian plasmodia started with the adaptation of Coccidia of the intestinal epithelium to some tissues of the internal organs and then to the invasion of free cells in the blood. The next step was the possibility of transmission of the parasites from one animal to another by bloodsucking Arthropod vectors. The great antiquity of malarial infection is confirmed by the fact that about 100 parasite species similar to those of man are found in a wide range of vertebrates from reptiles or birds to higher apes. None of the parasites, except for those found in some monkeys, can be transmitted to man. This high host specificity indicates a long association between the human species and the four particular species of plasmodia that infect man.

Prehistoric man in the Old World was subject to malaria. It is probable that the disease originated in Africa which is believed to be the cradle of the human race. Fossil mosquitos were found in geological strata 30 million years old and there is no doubt that they have spread the infection through the warmer regions of the globe, long before the dawn of history. Malaria followed in the wake of human migrations to the Mediterranean shores, to Mesopotamia, the Indian peninsula and South-East Asia. How malaria established itself in the New World is subject to speculation as no reliable historical or other data exist on this point. It is possible that *Plasmodium vivax* and *P. malariae* were brought from South-East Asia by early trans-Pacific voyages, while *P. falciparum* is of post-Columbian origin, through the African slaves brought by the Spanish colonisers of Central America.

References to seasonal and intermittent fevers exist in the ancient Assyrian, Chinese and Indian religious and medical texts but their true identity with malaria is uncertain. These afflictions, usually ascribed to the punishment of gods or vengeance by evil spirits – were met only by incantations or sacrificial offerings. Hippocrates, who lived in Greece in the fifth century BC, was the earliest physician to discard superstition for logical observation of the relation between the appearance of the disease and the seasons of the year or the places where his patients lived. He was also the first to describe in detail the clinical picture of malaria and some complications of the disease. Galen and other Greek and Roman physicians have also left various references to malaria in the second century AD. Non-medical writers alluded to fevers that affected those who lived in marshy areas. Malaria or 'Roman fever' was common in the vicinity of Rome and cyclical epidemics of malaria continued in Greece, Italy, many parts of Europe and other continents through many centuries.

For nearly 1500 years no additional knowledge of the extent, cause or treatment of malaria was forthcoming. However, the awareness of the association of fevers with stagnant waters and swamps led to various methods of drainage practised by the Greeks and Romans already in the sixth century BC and continued, for the improvement of agricultural land and better health conditions, throughout the Middle Ages in Italy, France, Holland, England and elsewhere.

However, the main breakthrough in the long history of malaria was connected with the first real therapeutic advance. At the beginning of the seventeenth century came the discovery of the value of 'Peruvian bark' for treatment of fevers. The use of this remedy spread rapidly all over Europe and it soon became obvious that only certain fevers were easily cured by this drug. In the seventeenth century Morton and Sydenham in England and later Torti in Italy differentiated between the intermittent fevers and others that failed to respond to the drug, often known under the name of 'Jesuit's powder'.

These specific fevers known in England as 'agues' received in the eighteenth century the Italian name 'mal'aria', since it was then widely believed that their cause was related to the foul air common near marshy areas. The French term 'paludisme' indicating a close connection with swamps was introduced much later. In 1735 the tree producing the Peruvian bark was given, by Linnaeus, its scientific name of Cinchona but quinine, the active principle of it, was not isolated until 1820 by Pelletier and Caventou in France.

The most important events in the history of malaria took place towards the end of the nineteenth century, when the sciences of bacteriology and pathology were discovering the causes of infectious diseases, seeing the morbid changes in the organs and tissues and also perceived the role of insects in the transmission of some infections. It was in 1880 that Laveran, a French army surgeon in Algeria, first saw and described malaria parasites in the red blood cells of man. Soon after that Romanowsky in Russia developed a new method of staining the malaria parasites in blood films and this made further studies of plasmodia very much easier.

However, the way in which the disease was transmitted from man to man was still a mystery although a few early and inspired guesses pointed to the possible association between swamps, mosquitos and fevers.

Patrick Manson, a Scotsman who was practising medicine in China, showed in the 1880s that mosquitos were arthropod hosts of human filarial parasites found in the blood. Soon after that David Bruce demonstrated in Africa that tsetse flies can transmit the trypanosome, a blood parasite of horses and cattle, from one animal to another. This provided a new clue for considering mosquitos as possible vectors of malaria. But the final elucidation of the actual mode of transmission was not forthcoming until 1897 when Ronald Ross in Secunderabad (India) found a developing form of the malaria parasite in the body of a mosquito, that had previously fed on a patient with the plasmodia in his blood. The whole complex picture of the cycle of development of malaria parasites in man and in the female Anopheles mosquito became clear as a result of further studies by the Italians Amico Bignami, Giuseppe Bastianelli and especially Battista Grassi in 1898–99. A striking confirmation of the fact that malaria is transmitted by Anopheles mosquitos was based on the combined field experiment carried out by Patrick Manson and his colleagues near Rome and in London in 1900. This proved that protection from the bites of Anopheles prevents the occurrence of the infection; another experiment showed that Anopheles obviously infected in Italy and brought to England were capable of transmitting the disease by their bite.

During the twentieth century much research was devoted to malaria control. Larvicides in the form of oil or Paris green were introduced for preventing the breeding of mosquitos in various types of waters. Wider use of these and other methods of mosquito reduction demonstrated the practicability of controlling malaria and yellow fever in Cuba and the Panama Canal Zone, where two American campaigns brilliantly organised by General William Crawford Gorgas proved to be an outstanding success. This was followed in Malaya by Malcolm Watson who introduced the concept of 'naturalistic control' based on the knowledge of the breeding habits of species of Anopheles involved in the local transmission of the disease.

The ravages of malaria experienced during the First World War and the difficulties of securing cheap supplies of quinine stimulated a line of research in Germany aiming at the discovery of synthetic antimalarial drugs. This was brilliantly accomplished in 1924 by Schulemann's discovery of pamaquine. However, a much more valuable drug – atebrin (mepacrine) was prepared in 1930 by Kikuth, Mietzsch and Mauss. There can be no doubt that the availability of this compound played an immense role during the Second World War. Other valuable synthetic drugs developed by the Germans, the French, the Americans and the British followed in 1934 (chloroquine), 1945 (proguanil), 1946 (amodiaquine), 1950 (primaquine) and 1951 (pyrimethamine).

In the meantime another major discovery was to revolutionise the technique of malaria control by spraying insecticides against adult mosquitos. The possibility of the new method was foreshadowed in South Africa, where De Meillon's use of pyrethrum sprays greatly reduced the amount of malaria in rural areas.

At the beginning of the Second World War Paul Muller discovered in Switzerland the high insecticidal action of a synthetic compound, dichloro-diphenyl-trichloroethane, which was given the abbreviated name of DDT when samples of it were sent in 1942 to the United Kingdom. The value of this compound for control of flies and mosquitos was soon confirmed and in 1944 the first field tests were carried out in Italy. Other projects followed; in 1945 Venezuela and Guyana became the first countries where malaria control on a large scale was instituted.

Among other residual insecticides which were introduced soon after DDT, hexachlorocyclohexane (BHC or HCH) and dieldrin should be mentioned. Their general use for malaria control was less effective than first anticipated because of some unexpected difficulties related to the developing resistance of mosquitos.

The possibility of global extension of malaria control activities to bring about the final eradication of the disease was contemplated in the 1950s, when the results of the application of DDT in Venezuela, Italy, Greece, Guyana, Ceylon and the USA showed great promise.

In the meantime parasitological studies on the cycle of development of the malaria parasites continued although little progress had been made since 1900, when Grassi formulated the idea that there is a third, cryptic tissue phase following the inoculation of sporozoites by the bite of Anopheles. Raffaele in Italy was the first to demonstrate in 1934 the existence of this phase in bird malaria. This was soon followed by similar findings in other species of avian and monkey parasites. Then in 1948 the exo-erythrocytic stages first of monkey malaria (*P. cynomolgi*) then of human (*P. vivax*) malaria were discovered in the UK by Shortt and Garnham. This explained what happens to the parasite during the incubation period, how the relapses of malaria infection occur and gave new impetus to the chemotherapeutic research which was soon to develop new and powerful drugs.

The characteristics of DDT and other residual insecticides, namely their high potency against the mosquitos, low toxicity to man, ease of application in rural areas and relatively low cost, encouraged many health workers to press for malaria eradication. The examples of Greece and Italy, where in 1951 a temporary interruption of house spraying with DDT has not interfered with the elimination of the disease, confirmed the apparent practicability of malaria eradication, without necessarily eliminating the main Anopheles vector.

The concept of malaria eradication was adopted by the World Health Assembly in 1955 and two years later the World Health Organization launched the global campaign. Its results over the next fifteen years were excellent in Europe, North America, some parts of Asia, USSR, Australia and less good in tropical countries. The causes of this lack of progress are many and will be fully dealt with in the

Historical Outline

appropriate section of this book. In 1969 the World Health Organization revised the strategy of malaria eradication by stressing the need for greater involvement of general health services and for extension of research on new insecticides, improved surveillance, development of new antimalarial drugs and alternative methods of malaria control. This approach forms much of the present thinking with regard to malaria control in developing tropical countries.

However, during the past few years there has been a serious resurgence of malaria in several tropical countries where the eradication programmes appeared to advance satisfactorily. Moreover, the disease is now frequently imported into Europe, North America and other parts of the temperate world. The speed and constantly rising volume of international travel have created new conditions for massive influx of various communicable diseases into countries where these infections were unknown or from which they had disappeared.

The present concern with the problem of malaria is justified from the point of view of general practitioners and other clinicians in developed and in developing parts of the world. The specialist in community health is equally concerned since he recognises that there can be no complete safety from this disease and no satisfactory socio-economic advance of underprivileged countries as long as vast areas of the tropical world remain in the grip of the enormous accumulation of plasmodial infections.

MILESTONES IN THE HISTORY OF MALARIA AND ITS CONTROL

The main chronological landmarks in the advance of our knowledge of malaria and the control or eradication of this disease followed three different and yet related roads.

The human malaria parasites and their transmission

1847	Dempster in India introduced spleen palpation of children as an index of epidemicity of malaria.
1848	Virchow and Frerichs in Germany recognised that the presence of pigment in internal organs may be related to deaths from intermittent fevers.
1877	Manson in China showed that a mosquito (*Culex fatigans*) can act as a vector of human filaria.
1880	Laveran in Algeria discovered and described malaria parasites in human blood.
1886	Golgi in Italy described in detail two species of human malaria parasites (*P. vivax* and *P. malariae*)
1889	Danilewski in Russia described the morphology of avian parasites and indicated their wide distribution.

1889–90	Celli and Marchiafava in Italy described *Plasmodium falciparum*.
1889–93	Smith and Kilborne in the USA demonstrated the role of an arthropod vector (tick) in the transmission of Texas fever (piroplasmosis) of cattle.
1891	Romanowsky developed his polychrome staining method for demonstrating plasmodia in blood smears.
1894–96	Bruce, in Zululand, working on nagana, a disease of horses and cattle, showed that an infection caused by a protozoan parasite can be transmitted by a true insect (tsetse fly).
1894	Manson put forward the theory that malaria is transmitted from man to man by mosquitos.
1897	Ross discovered pigmented cysts (oöcysts) on the stomach wall of an Anopheles mosquito (probably *A. stephensi*) in Secunderabad, India.
1897	MacCallum in the USA described the sexual phase of *Haemoproteus* in the blood of a crow and observed exflagellation of a male gametocyte in *P. falciparum* and the penetration of a female gametocyte by a 'flagellum'.
1898	Ross worked out the complete cycle of bird malaria in naturally infected sparrows in Calcutta.
1898	Grassi, Bignami and Bastianelli in Italy described the cycle of human malaria parasites in Anopheles mosquitos.
1900	Manson, by experiments with human volunteers in the Roman Campagna and in London, confirmed the mosquito-malaria transmission theory.
1901	Grassi forecast the existence of a third phase in the life cycle of the malaria parasite.
1902	Schaudinn announced, incorrectly, the penetration of a red blood cell by a sporozoite, thus apparently refuting Grassi's theory and retarding this line of research for many years.
1922	Stephens identified and described *Plasmodium ovale*.
1931	James revived Grassi's theory, and suggested that the sporozoite, soon after entering the body, invades reticulo-endothelial cells or cells lining the capillary blood-vessels.
1934	Raffaele, in Italy, described tissue forms in *P. elongatum* and concluded that in avian malaria there is a schizogonic cycle of development in the reticulo-endothelial system as well as in the red blood cells.
1937	James and Tate described schizogonic development of *P. gallinaceum* in fixed tissue cells of the fowl, and showed that the brain is an important place for the localisation of the endothelial stages.
1947	Garnham described exo-erythrocytic forms of *P. kochi*

Historical Outline

	(now classed as *Hepatocystis*) in parenchyma cells of the liver of lower monkeys in East Africa.
1948	Shortt, Garnham and Malamos, in England, described pre-erythrocytic forms of *P. cynomolgi* in parenchyma cells of the liver of *Macaca mulatta* (rhesus) monkeys. Shortt and Garnham also described persistent exo-erythrocytic forms of *P. cynomolgi* in a monkey's liver.
1948	Vincke and Lips in the former Belgian Congo (Zaïre) discovered *P. berghei,* the first plasmodium of rodents.
1948	Shortt, Garnham, Covell and Shute described pre-erythrocytic forms of *P. vivax* in the human liver.
1948	Rodhain showed that the chimpanzee is a host of *P. malariae* in Central Africa.
1949	Shortt, Fairley, Covell, Shute and Garnham described pre-erythrocytic forms of *P. falciparum* in the human liver.
1950	Garnham described pre-erythrocytic forms of *P. inui*, a quartan-like parasite, in a simian liver.
1953	Garnham described pre-erythrocytic forms of *P. ovale* in the human liver.
1966	Discovery by Young of the experimental transmissibility of human plasmodia to the Colombian owl monkey (*Aotus trivirgatus*).
1965–76	Extensive scientific studies on the development of a malaria vaccine culminated by Trager's success in producing a continuous in vitro culture of *P. falciparum*

Treatment of malaria

1600	Juan Lopez, a Jesuit missionary, recorded the use of the 'fever tree bark' by Peruvian Indians.
1643	Cardinal Juan de Lugo carried out trials of the Peruvian bark at the Santo Spirito Hospital in Rome.
1649	Cardinal de Lugo supported a wide use of the bark which became known as 'Jesuit's powder'.
1655	Powdered bark first used in England.
1637–98	Morton and Sydenham in England noted the specific action of the bark in curing certain fevers (agues).
1712	Torti in Italy clearly described the specific action of the bark on intermittent (but no other) fevers.
1735	Condamine leading the French expedition to Peru identified the 'Quina-quina' tree.
1742	Linnaeus in Sweden described the tree and gave it the name of Cinchona.
1820	Pelletier and Caventou in France isolated the alkaloids quinine and cinchonine from the bark of Cinchona.

1854	Hasskarl, a Dutch botanist, brought the seeds of Cinchona to Java and began large-scale cultivation in Indonesia.
1872	Markham, an English geographer, started Cinchona plantations in the Nilgiri Hills in India.
1914–18	Events during the First World War indicated the shortage of quinine especially in countries without direct access to Cinchona plantations.
1924	Development of pamaquine (Plasmoquine) in Germany by Schulemann and his colleagues.
1930	Development of mepacrine (Atebrin) in Germany by Mietzsch and Kikuth.
1934	Development of chloroquine (Resochin) in Germany.
1944	Development of proguanil (Paludrine) by Curd, Davey and Rose in England.
1952	Development of pyrimethamine (Daraprim) by Hitchings in the USA and his co-workers in England.
1952	Development of primaquine by Elderfield in the USA.
1961–65	Reports from Colombia and Brazil on strains of *P. falciparum* resistant to chloroquine. Similar reports from south-east Asia.
1960–66	Re-discovery of the value of sulphones and sulphonamides as antimalarial compounds.
1967–74	Development by the US Army Medical Research and Development Command of a number of new synthetic antimalarials (including mefloquine).

Epidemiology and control of malaria

1899	Ross initiated antilarval measures in Sierra Leone.
1899	Large scale demonstration of successful mosquito control by Gorgas and Le Prince in Cuba.
1901–03	Malaria control by anti-larval measures in Malaya initiated by Malcolm Watson. Anti-mosquito campaign organised by Ross in Ismailia, Egypt.
1904–14	Malaria control campaign carried out by Gorgas and Le Prince in the Panama Canal zone.
1908	Ross carried out a survey of malaria in Mauritius and originated the mathematical approach to the transmission of the infection
1924–26	Roubaud in France, Swellengrebel and Van Thiel in the Netherlands, Falleroni in Italy differentiated the cryptic species of *A. maculipennis* complex and elucidated the importance of mosquito behaviour in the transmission of malaria.
1927	First instance of eradication of an invading vector species (*A. albimanus*) in Barbados.

Historical Outline

1935–39	First large scale control of rural malaria by imagocidal measures (using pyrethrum spraying) in South Africa, Netherlands and India.
1936–39	Discovery of insecticidal action of DDT (synthesised by Zeidler in Germany in 1874) by Muller and Weisman in Switzerland.
1939–40	Eradication of an invading African mosquito (*A. gambiae*) from Brazil.
1942–45	Eradication from northern Egypt of *A. gambiae*.
1942–46	Development of new synthetic insecticides (HCH, dieldrin, chlordane etc.) with residual action.
1946–51	Anti-malaria campaign in Cyprus, Sardinia, Guiana, Venezuela and Greece followed by interruption of transmission.
1950–57	Macdonald in the UK and Moshkowski in the USSR expanded Ronald Ross's mathematical approach to the understanding of epidemiology of malaria.
1955	Adoption of the principle of malaria eradication by the Fourteenth World Health Assembly.
1957	Definition of the practice of malaria eradication by the World Health Organization and the establishment of the Malaria Eradication Special Account.
1957–69	Worldwide malaria eradication programme, stimulated, coordinated and assisted by the World Health Organization.
1969	Revision of the global strategy of malaria eradication.
1976	At the end of 1976 the World Health Organization estimated that out of 2048 million people inhabiting actual or potential malarious areas 1696 million were completely or partly protected from infection but 352 million (17%) lived in areas without any specific anti-malaria measures.
1973–78	Marked resurgence of malaria in endemic tropical countries and especially in southern Asia. Sharp increase of malaria imported into temperate areas of Europe and North America.
1975–77	Setting up of the WHO Special Programme for Research and Training in Tropical Diseases, now known as the UNDP/World Bank/WHO Special Programme.
1978	Reorientation of the malaria control strategy by the 31st World Health Assembly

Chapter 2

The Malaria Parasites

The microorganisms causing malaria are commonly referred to as malaria parasites; this term is usually restricted to the family Plasmodiidae within the order Coccidiida, sub-order Haemosporidiidea, which comprises various parasites found in the blood of reptiles, birds and mammals. The zoological family of Plasmodiidae includes the parasites which undergo two types of multiplication by asexual division (*schizogony*) in the vertebrate host and a single sexual multiplication (*sporogony*) in the mosquito host. The genus Plasmodium has been defined on the basis of one type of the asexual multiplication by division occurring in the parenchymal cells of the liver of the vertebrate host (exo-erythrocytic schizogony); the other characteristic of this genus is that the mosquito host is a species of Anopheles.

There are nearly 100 species of Plasmodia, including some 50 of birds or reptiles and at least 22 different species of Plasmodia of lower monkeys and higher apes. Some of the latter parasites are very close to human plasmodia and one of them (*P. rodhaini*) is now recognised as identical with *P. malariae*.

The discovery of *P. berghei*, a malaria parasite of rodents, by Vincke in 1948, opened a new way for studies in parasitology, immunology and chemotherapy of malaria. Several new species of Plasmodia of various rodents have now been discovered.

The zoological classification of plasmodia is complex and even today there is some difference of opinion with regard to taxonomic position of the parasite causing falciparum malaria. In this malaria parasite the exo-erythrocytic schizogony occurs for one generation only in the parenchymal tissue of the liver while in some other parasites of human malaria the exo-erythrocytic (or tissue) schizonts occur in multiple generations. This is one of the reasons why some authors suggested that the parasite of falciparum malaria should be recognised as belonging to a separate genus Laverania, as *Laverania falcipara*. While this argument may be valid in a zoological context the rejection of the familiar name *Plasmodium falciparum* might be disturbing and since the use of this well-known name is still taxonomically permissible it is proposed to retain it in the present text.

There are four generally recognised species of malaria parasites of man:

P. malariae (Laveran, 1881)[1]
P. vivax (Grassi and Feletti, 1890)
P. falciparum Welch, 1897
P. ovale Stephens, 1922

Infections caused by the various human species of plasmodia have been given a number of colloquial names:

P. vivax	Benign tertian, Simple tertian, Tertian
P. malariae	Quartan
P. falciparum	Malignant tertian (M.T.), Subtertian, Aestivo-autumnal, Tropical, Pernicious,
P. ovale	Ovale tertian

These colloquial names have now become obsolete. Their replacement by the unitalicised specific names of the relevant plasmodia is recommended. Thus one refers to vivax malaria, ovale malaria, falciparum infection etc. An exception may be made with regard to 'malariae' as this could be confusing; a term such as 'quartan malaria' is acceptable.

Some authors refer to the mosquito as the definitive host while man and animals are regarded as intermediate hosts of the malaria parasite. This nomenclature may be zoologically correct since the sexual development of plasmodia is the more important function in the perpetuation of the species. However this terminology gives rise to some confusion and it may be preferable to speak of invertebrate and vertebrate hosts.

The term 'malaria' is common in several languages and is generally used in scientific texts. It originated in Italy and refers to the connection between the disease and 'spoiled air' (mal aria) that was believed to cause it. In French the disease is known as 'paludisme', a term indicating the relationship of the disease with marshes (palus – in Latin). In other languages the common names, nowadays rarely used, link the disease with the periodic attacks of fever or with the season of the year.

It is not uncommon to observe that some morphological or other characteristics of one well defined species of malaria parasite may vary somewhat from one geographical area to another. The best known differences are biological variations which may be so distinctive that they provide an acceptable basis for referring to these parasite populations as 'strains'. A parasite strain has been defined as 'a

---

[1] In formal zoological nomenclature the binominal designation of species is completed by adding the name of the author of the original description and the relevant date. If the generic placing is not that of the original author then the name of the author and the date of description are given in parentheses.

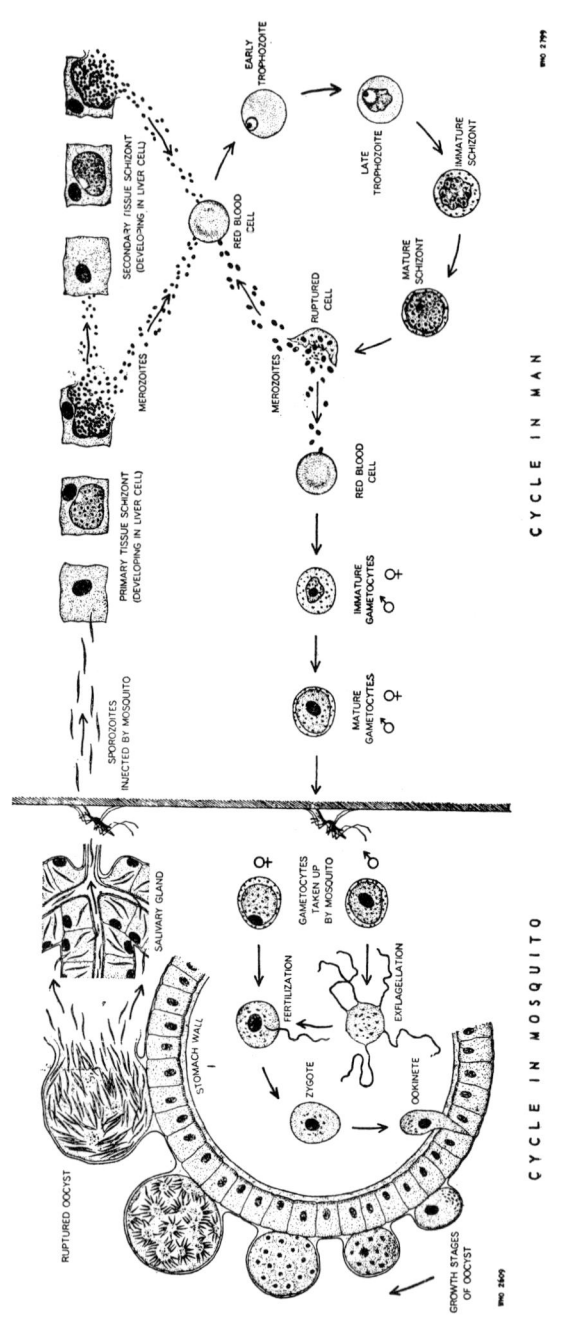

Fig 1 The life-cycle of malaria parasite in the mosquito and in the human hosts. (WHO, 1963)

population of common stock descending from a single ancestor or derived from a single source and maintained without intermixture from other sources through a number of generations'. This definition is not easily applicable to designation of a group of parasites in field condition. At the present time the term 'isolate' is favoured when we refer to a sample of parasites, not necessarily genetically homogeneous, collected on a single occasion from an infected host and preserved in the laboratory either by passaging to other hosts or maintained in a deep frozen state.

The differentiation of strains of malaria parasites, based in the past on morphological characteristics, relapse pattern, drug response, infectivity to various vectors and immunological differences has been given recently more attention thanks to a new biochemical and genetic approach.

The composition of a 'strain' depends on knowledge of the basic genetic organisation of the parasite and on the way in which the genetic factors are inherited and distributed within the parasite population. The biochemical techniques used for detection of genetic differences between isolates of human and animal plasmodia are twofold. Enzyme electrophoresis reveals subtle differences related to products of separate gene loci. Biochemical characteristics of DNA reveal differences in the total genetic information of the parasite. While most of these studies have been carried out on rodent and simian plasmodia, there is enough evidence that these methods may be of value for differentiation of strains of malaria parasites of man.

LIFE CYCLE AND MORPHOLOGY OF HUMAN MALARIA PARASITES

The life cycle of all species of human malaria parasites is essentially the same. It comprises an exogenous sexual phase (sporogony) with multiplication in certain Anopheles mosquitos and an endogenous asexual phase (schizogony) with multiplication in the vertebrate host. The latter phase includes the development cycle in the red corpuscles in the blood (erythrocytic schizogony) and the cycle taking place in the parenchyma cells of the liver (exo-erythrocytic schizogony). In the latter, often referred to as the *tissue stage*, one should distinguish between the primary or *pre-erythrocytic schizogony* which follows the development of the sporozoite and the secondary *exo-erythrocytic schizogony* which takes place in the liver (Fig.1).

The parasite in the mosquito host

When a female Anopheles mosquito ingests the blood of a human host, with malaria parasites in the circulation, the infected erythrocytes set the parasites free in the mosquito stomach. The asexual parasites are digested together with the red blood cells while the mature sexual cells (*gametocytes*) undergo further development. In the male gametocytes the nucleus divides into 4 to 8 nuclei each of which then forms a long thread-like structure 20 to 25 μ in length (*flagellum*); they shoot out from the original cell, lash about for a while and then break free. This process (*exflagellation*) takes only a few minutes at the appropriate temperature and can be seen in a fresh blood drop under the microscope.

The female gametocyte undergoes a maturation process and forms a *female gamete* or *macrogamete;* the flagellum or *male gamete* is called a *microgamete.*

In the stomach of the mosquito a microgamete is attracted by a macrogamete; the latter forms a small projection through which the microgamete enters and thus completes the fertilisation. The product of fusion of male and female gamete is called a *zygote*. This is at first a motionless globular body but within 18 to 24 hours of its formation it elongates and becomes mobile; this worm-like stage measuring 18 to 24 μ in length is known as *oökinete* (Fig.2).

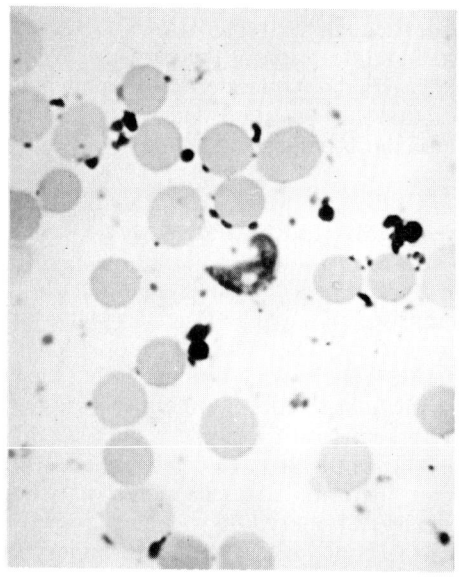

Fig 2 An oökinete in the stomach of an Anopheles mosquito; this stage of the malaria parasite proceeds to the outer epithelium of the midgut of the mosquito to form an oöcyst. (Wellcome Museum of Medical Science)

The Malaria Parasites

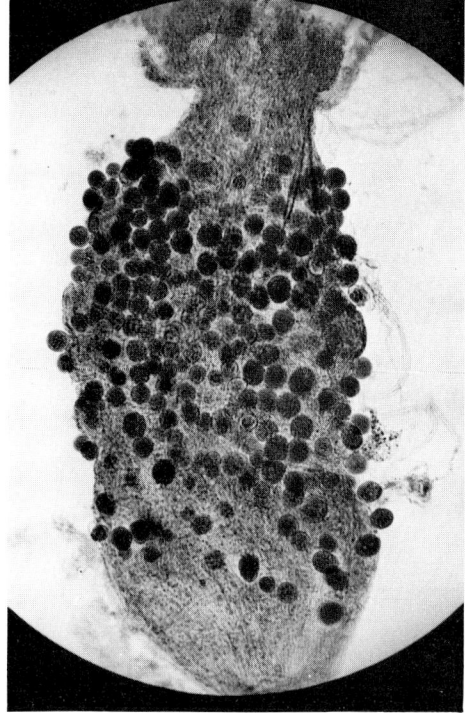

Fig 3 Midgut of an Anopheles mosquito heavily infected with oöcysts of *Plasmodium vivax*. Magnification × ca 40 (Wellcome Museum of Medical Science)

The oökinete soon forces its way to the stomach wall, passes between the epithelial cells to the outer surface of the stomach and settles down. It becomes rounded up into a small sphere with an elastic membrane and is now called an *oöcyst*. The number of oöcysts on the stomach of an Anopheles may vary between a few and several hundreds (Fig. 3).

The oöcyst gradually increases in size and appears in the stomach as a semi-transparent globular body, some 40 to 80 µ in size containing grains of pigment. The distribution and size of pigment grains, and their colour are characteristic for the given species of plasmodium. As the oöcyst enlarges and the nucleus divides repeatedly the pigment is obscured. The divided nuclei form finger-like processes at the periphery of which appear great numbers of spindle-shaped bodies, 10 to 15 µ in length with pointed ends and a central nucleus (*sporozoites*) (Fig. 3). Later the oöcyst bursts and liberates thousands of mobile sporozoites into the body cavity of the mosquito from where many sporozoites reach the salivary glands and the female mosquito now becomes infective. When she feeds on blood after piercing the human skin the sporozoites are injected into the wound and pass into the bloodstream of the vertebrate host (Figs 4 and 5).

While the conventional light microscopy revealed the main differences between various species of human and animal plasmodia newer techniques of electron microscopy have been increasingly used during the past two decades and showed the presence of many details of fine structure of several organelles of these parasites. The erythrocytic, exo-erythrocytic and sporogonic (viz. mosquito stages) forms of plasmodia were compared and showed a number of differences. The major differences are in the surface structure of motile asexual stages in the blood, in the structure of the mitochondria and the ingestion and digestion of nutrients. The characteristic alterations on the infected

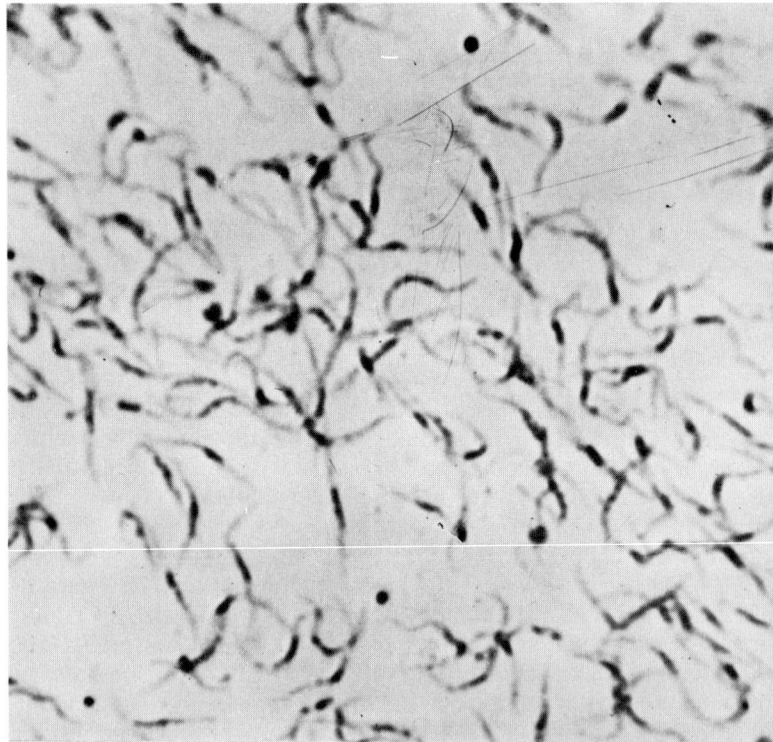

Fig 4 Sporozoites of *P. falciparum* released from a ruptured mature oöcyst. Magnification × 2000. (Wellcome Museum of Medical Science)

The Malaria Parasites

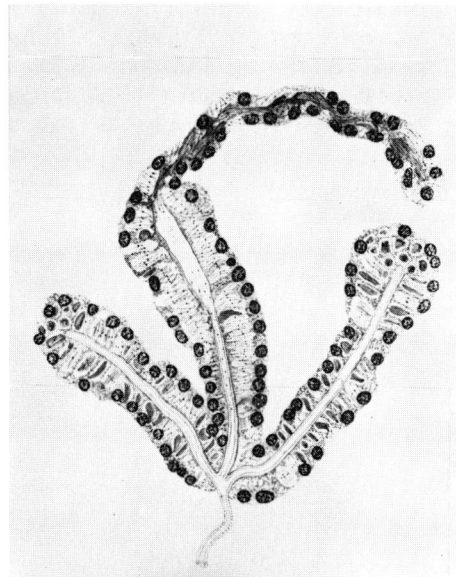

Fig 5 Salivary gland of an Anopheles mosquito infected with a large number of sporozoites of *P. falciparum*. Magnification × ca 250. (Wellcome Museum of Medical Science)

erythrocytes examined by electron microscopy are now better understood although the significance of these changes is still unclear.

The parasite in the vertebrate host

Tissue phase. Following the inoculation of sporozoites by the mosquito bite, there is a brief period of about half an hour when the blood is infective. Later the sporozoites disappear from the blood. Many are destroyed by phagocytes, but some enter the parenchymal cells of the liver where they undergo a process of development and multiplication known as *pre-erythrocytic schizogony*. The nucleus of the parasite undergoes repeated division and the *tissue schizont* increases in size until it reaches between 45 μ and 60 μ in diameter. The division of nuclei is accompanied by the collection of the cytoplasm around each nucleus resulting in a formation of many thousands of uninucleate *merozoites*, each of them measuring 1.0 to 1.8 μ. The nucleus of the liver cell is displaced towards the periphery but there is no other reaction on the part of the surrounding liver tissue (Fig. 6).

The duration of this phase, the size of the fully grown schizont and the number of merozoites it contains, depend on the species of the malaria parasite as shown below:

Species	Duration of pre-erythrocytic phase	Size of schizont	Number of merozoites
P. vivax	6–8 days	45 μ	about 10 000
P. malariae	12–16 days	45 μ	about 2000
P. ovale	9 days	70 μ	15 000
P. falciparum	5½ days–7 days	60 μ	40 000

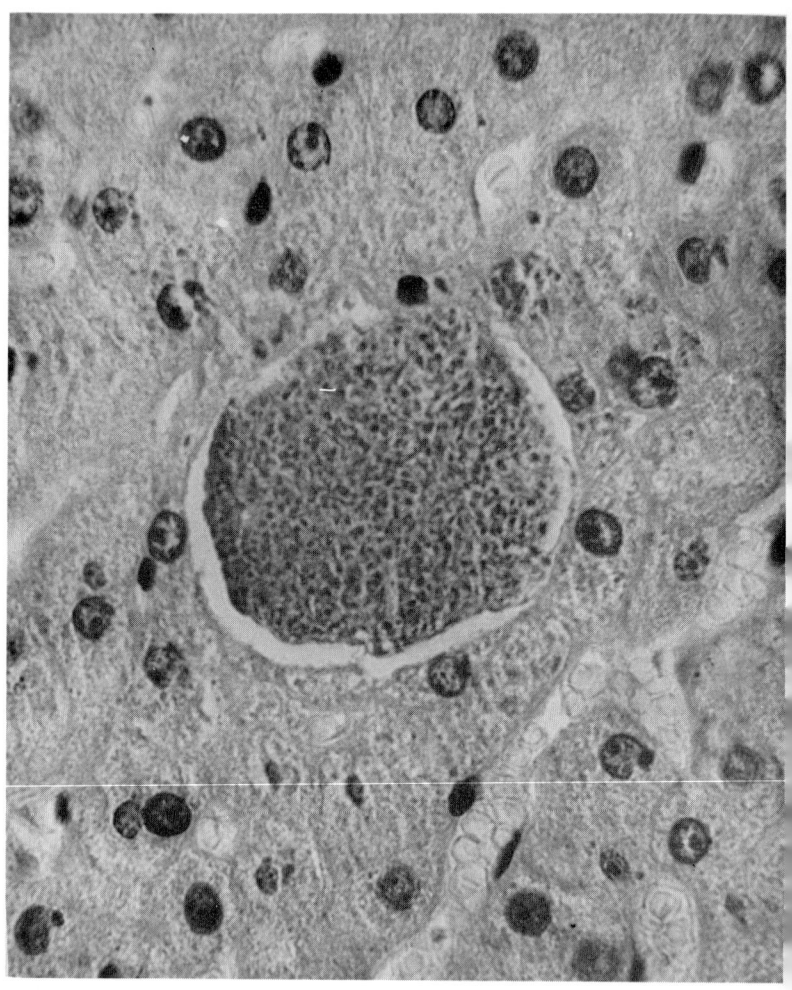

Fig 6 Pre-erythrocytic schizont of *P. falciparum* in the liver. Magnification × 1000 (Wellcome Museum of Medical Science)

At the end of the pre-erythrocytic phase, after about 6 to 16 days from the time of infection the envelope of the cell containing the schizont ruptures and the merozoites are set free into the surrounding tissue and thence into the blood circulation. Most of them invade the red blood cells present in the sinusoids of the liver, but some are phagocytosed.

The completion of the pre-erythrocytic or *primary exo-erythrocytic schizogony* may be followed by the *secondary exo-erythrocytic schizogony* during which merozoites of *P. vivax*, *P. ovale* and perhaps *P. malariae* re-enter fresh liver cells and repeat the process of schizogony. This was thought to be the cause of relapses that occur in some of these infections at a later date.

It is still not certain if the late liver schizonts are the results of a continuous process of secondary exo-erythrocytic division as originally postulated by Garnham or due to a condition of 'dormancy' of the primary exo-erythrocytic tissue phase. It now appears that the latter explanation is more probable. Moreover, it now seems that the prevalent idea of relapses being caused by revival of exo-erythrocytic schizogony may not be quite true for all species. It is not unlikely that at least some strains of *P. malariae* are capable of survival for many years in erythrocytic forms in the internal organs and relapses in these infections are not related to the persistence of exo-erythrocytic schizonts. The question is still somewhat controversial and may be answered only by future studies.

An important point that distinguishes the tissue schizonts from the schizonts in the erythrocytes is that the former show no pigment while the latter are pigmented.

Erythrocytic phase. The interval between the date of the infection and the time when the malaria parasites are detectable in the peripheral blood is known as the *pre-patent period.* This should be distinguished from the *incubation period* which is related to the first appearance of clinical symptoms of the disease.

The merozoites released from the tissue schizont invade the erythrocytes. The youngest stages in the blood are small, more or less rounded forms, some of which contain a vacuole which displaces the cytoplasm to the periphery, while the nucleus is situated at the pole (Fig. 7). In optical section the cytoplasm has an annular appearance and the young parasites are known as *ring forms*. As these grow in size they become more irregular in shape. All these early stages of the parasite are termed *trophozoites*. In the course of their development they absorb the haemoglobin of the red blood cell leaving as the product of digestion a pigment (*haematin*) or *haemozoin*, a combination of haematin with protein. This iron-containing pigment is seen in the body of the parasite in the form of dark granules, which are more obvious in the later stages of development.

After a period of growth the parasite multiplies by an asexual dividing process of *schizogony*. The nucleus of the parasite divides into a variable number of small nuclei. This is soon followed by the division of cytoplasm forming a *schizont*. Mature *schizonts* are fully developed forms in which, as a result of the segmentation of the nucleus and the cytoplasm, a number of small rounded forms (*merozoites*) are produced. When the process of schizogony is completed the red blood cell bursts and the merozoites are released into the blood stream. The merozoites then invade fresh erythrocytes in which another generation of parasites is produced by the same process. This *erythrocytic cycle of schizogony* is repeated over and over again in the course of infection leading to a progressive increase of parasitaemia until the process is slowed down by the immune response of the host.

The development of parasites in the red blood cell brings about certain changes of it: among these abnormal appearances the most important are *enlargement, decolorisation* and certain forms of *stippling*. These changes are characteristic for the particular species of plasmodium involved.

The length of the erythrocytic phase is known as *schizogonic periodicity*. It differs according to the species of the parasite, being 48 hours in the vivax, ovale and falciparum malaria and 72 in the quartan. In the early stage of infection there may be groups ('broods') of parasites developing at different times so that the febrile symptoms show no characteristic periodicity. Later the schizogonic periodicity is better synchronised and the febrile paroxysms assume a more definite three- or four-day pattern.

After several generations of merozoites have been produced, some of these give rise to sexually differentiated forms (*gametocytes*). After invading fresh erythrocytes these sexual forms grow, but the nucleus remains undivided. The mature gametocytes have different forms in different species of plasmodia: in *P. falciparum* they are usually crescent-shaped when mature, while in other species they are round. In all species of plasmodia the female (*macrogametocyte*) has a deeply staining cytoplasm and a small compact nucleus while the male (*microgametocyte*) stains pale blue or pink and has a larger, diffuse nucleus. Both contain numerous granules.

Ultrastructure. The study of the inner structure of all stages of development of malaria parasites has been revolutionised by the new techniques of electron microscopy. The ultrastructure of different human plasmodia is generally similar, with a few exceptions of the blood stages, in which the parasites depend essentially upon the uptake and digestion of nutrients from the host cells.

The gametocytes show a three-layered pellicle and a dense nucleolus within the nucleus. In the process of exflagellation of micro-

The Malaria Parasites

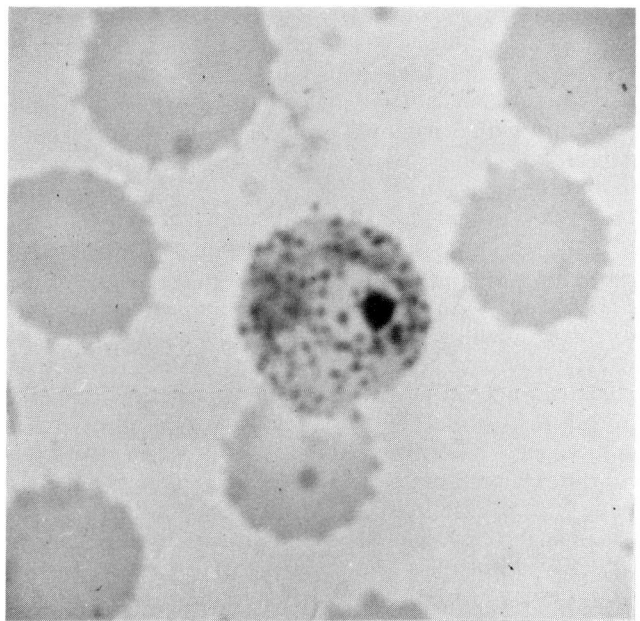

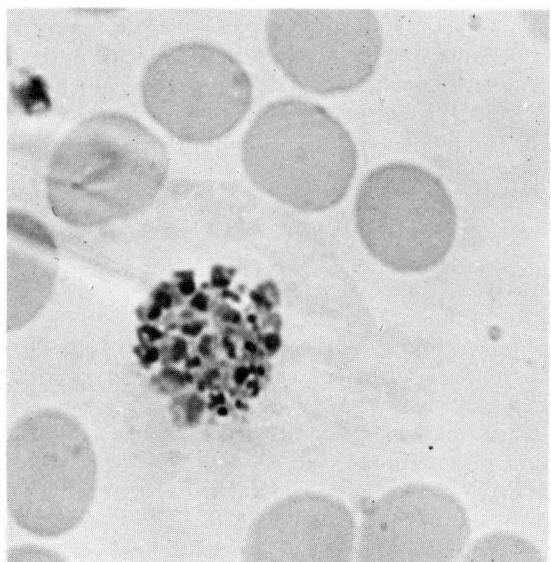

Fig 7 *Plasmodium vivax.* Trophozoite (top) with pronounced Schüffner's stippling in an enlarged erythrocyte. Fully developed schizont (bottom) with about 20 merozoites ready to burst and to invade new red blood cells. Magnification × 1300 top, × 800 bottom. (Wellcome Museum of Medical Science)

gametocytes the nucleus divides three times; a centriole migrates to the nucleus and becomes a basal body from which fibrils grow out to become part of the microgametes.

The oökinete has a number of unusual features and especially a polar structure with a narrow retractile protuberance. There is also a crystalloid body in the early stage of the oökinete, probably of a protein nature.

Oöcysts have a number of interesting features and especially centriole-like structures surrounded by peripheral tubules. A meiotic division of the nucleus has been observed in oöcysts.

All plasmodial sporozoites seem to have the same structure, namely a thick external membrane modified at the anterior end into an apical cap, with a polar ring and a conoid body. To this end are attached sub-pellicular microtubules; there are also paired organelles, convoluted rods (*toxonemes*) and a pit (*cytostome*). The sporozoites also contain a nucleus, mitochondria and an endoplasm with ribosomes.

The erythrocytic asexual stages have relatively simple internal structure. Food is ingested through a cytostome, with the production of a large vacuole. During schizogony merozoites bud off the residual body. The new techniques of electron microscopy have now shown how the erythrocytic merozoite penetrates into the red blood cell. In this process (*endocytosis*) special organelles of the merozoite (rhoptries and micronemes) seem to open a hole in the erythrocyte, probably by secreting a substance that invaginates the membrane of the cell. As the merozoite enters, its surface coat appears to be pinched off. At the point of entry of the merozoite a vacuole is formed but it rapidly vanishes. The whole process takes about 30 seconds.

HUMAN PLASMODIA

Plasmodium vivax

This species of malaria parasite of man occurs throughout most of the temperate zone and also in large areas of the tropics. It is much less common in tropical Africa, especially so in West Africa. It causes so-called 'benign tertian' malaria with frequent relapses, the pattern of which varies, in relation to various strains of *P. vivax*. The development of this plasmodium includes the *pre-erythrocytic* and *exo-erythrocytic* cycle in the liver. The existence of the pre-erythrocytic cycle was proved experimentally in 1948 by Shortt, Garnham, Covell and Shute, thus confirming the early hypothesis of Grassi and refuting the notoriously erroneous description by Schaudinn (1903) of the penetration of an erythrocyte by a sporozoite.

The duration of the pre-erythrocytic phase is eight days after the sporozoite infection; the secondary exo-erythrocytic forms are

Table 1

Some characteristics of infection with four species of human plasmodia

Species	Plasmodium vivax	Plasmodium ovale	Plasmodium malariae	Plasmodium falciparum
Pre-erythrocytic cycle (days)	8	9	13	5½–6
Pre-patent period (days)	11–13	10–14	15–16	9–10
Incubation period (days)	13 (12–17) or up to 6–12 months[1]	17 (16–18) or longer	28 (18–40) or longer	12 (9–14)
Exo-erythrocytic cycle (secondary)	Present	Present	Present in some strains?	Absent
Approximate number of merozoites per tissue schizont	Over 10 000	15 000	2000	40 000
Erythrocytic cycle (hours)	48	49–50	72	48
Parasitaemia per μl (mm³)				
Average	20 000	9000	6000	20 000–500 000[2]
Maximum	50 000	30 000	20 000	2 000 000
Primary attack severity	Mild to severe	Mild	Mild	Severe in non-immunes[2]
Febrile paroxysm (hours)	8–12	8–12	8–10	16–36 or longer
Relapses	++	++	+++	—
Period of recurrence	Long[1]	Long	Very long	Short
Duration of infection (years)	1½–3	Probably the same as *P. vivax*	3–50	1–2

Notes: [1] Patterns of infection and of relapses vary greatly in different strains.
[2] The severity of infection and the degree of parasitaemia are greatly influenced by the immune responses.

believed to be responsible for relapses. The number of merozoites in a mature tissue schizont on the eighth day is between 8000 and 20 000. In the blood most stages of *P. vivax* are larger than the other species of human plasmodia. The young trophozoite or ring grows rapidly and soon exhibits the characteristic malaria pigment. The parasite when alive has a pronounced amoeboid activity and the presence of cytoplasmic 'pseudopodia' seen in a stained blood film is typical for this parasite. A large vacuole forms a 'hole' in the ring until the division of the nucleus begins. After the nuclei have ceased to divide the mature schizont, which has on the average 12 to 18 merozoites, fills the entire host cell. Segmentation is followed by the rupture of the infected erythrocyte and release into the blood of merozoites and pigment. The merozoites, each measuring about 1.5 µ, invade fresh erythrocytes and the entire asexual erythrocytic cycle is repeated approximately every 48 hours. The degree of infection in vivax malaria rarely exceeds 50 000 per mm^3 of blood. Infections of one erythrocyte by two or more parasites may be seen but are not very common.

P. vivax has a striking effect on the invaded red blood cell, which gradually enlarges and becomes decolorised. A characteristic *stippling* in the form of small reddish points appears in the infected erythrocyte and is known as *Schüffner's dots*.

Gametocytes may appear in the blood within three days after the first appearance of asexual parasites. Both male and female gametocytes are large, round or oval, filling nearly the whole enlarged and 'stippled' host cell. The *macrogametocyte* has a dense cytoplasm staining dark blue and a small compact nucleus; the *microgametocyte* has a greyish-blue cytoplasm and a large diffuse nucleus. Both contain numerous pigment granules.

The periodicity of the asexual cycle of *P. vivax* is typically tertian with gametocytes developing in the peripheral blood. The course of development of the parasite is well synchronised.

The gametocytes develop into gametes in the midgut of the Anopheles. After the exflagellation of the male and fertilisation of the female gamete the sexual cycle takes 16 days at 20°C, and 8–10 days at 28°C. Below 15°C the completion of the sporogonic cycle is unlikely.

The young oöcyst has a light brown pigment distributed in the form of fine granules without any distinctive pattern. In an older oöcyst the granules are often arranged in a single or triple line.

Plasmodium falciparum
Of all the species of human plasmodia, *P. falciparum* is the most highly pathogenic, as is indicated by the name *malignant* often applied to the type of malaria associated with it. This, in a non-immune subject, usually runs an acute course, and unless promptly treated with specific drugs, frequently terminates fatally. It is the chief infection in

areas of endemic malaria in Africa, and is also responsible for the great regional epidemics which were a feature of malaria in north-west India and Ceylon. It is generally confined to tropical or subtropical regions, because development in the mosquito is greatly retarded when the temperature falls below 20°C. Even at this temperature, about three weeks are required for maturation of the sporozoites.

The asexual development of *P. falciparum* in the liver involves a pre-erythrocytic phase only; there is no exo-erythrocytic phase giving rise to long term relapses, such as occur in vivax and ovale infections. The earliest forms hitherto seen in the liver are schizonts measuring about 30 μ in diameter on the fourth day after infection. The number of merozoites in a mature schizont averages about 40 000.

The young ring forms of *P. falciparum*, as usually seen in the peripheral blood, are very small, measuring about one-sixth of the diameter of a red blood cell. In many of the ring forms there may be two chromatin granules, and marginal (*accolé*) forms are fairly common. There are frequently several ring forms to be seen in a single host cell.

Although marginal forms, rings with double chromatin dots and multiple infections of red cells occur in other human plasmodia, they are much more common in *P. falciparum* and their presence is an important aid to diagnosis.

Later in the attack the ring forms of *P. falciparum* may be considerably larger, measuring one quarter and sometimes nearly one half the diameter of a red cell, and may be mistaken for parasites of *P. malariae*. They may have one or two grains of pigment in their cytoplasm.

In acute infections with numerous parasites, atypical forms are sometimes seen and these have erroneously been described under different specific names. These amoeboid forms have been designated under the name of *P. tenue*, but this is not regarded as a valid species.

The succeeding developmental stages of the asexual erythrocytic cycle do not generally occur in the blood, except in severe 'pernicious' cases. The presence of maturing or mature schizonts of *P. falciparum* in a blood film is therefore often an indication for prompt and vigorous treatment. Segmenting forms of *P. falciparum* are easily recognised by having one or at most two solid blocks of pigment. In other species of human malaria parasites beyond the half grown stage there may be 20 or more pigment granules.

The ring forms and older trophozoites usually disappear from the peripheral circulation after 24 hours and are held up (*sequestered*) in the capillaries of the internal organs, such as the brain, heart, placenta, intestine or bone marrow, where their further development takes place. In the course of the next 24 hours the parasites in the capillaries multiply by schizogony. When the schizont is fully grown it occupies about two-thirds of the red cell. Finally it undergoes segmentation giving rise to from 8 to 24 merozoites, the average number being 16. The mature schizont of *P. falciparum* is smaller than that of any of the other malaria parasites. The degree of infection in this type of malaria is considerably higher than in the other forms, the density of parasites sometimes exceeding 500 000 per µl (mm^3) of blood.

The distribution of the parasites in organs and tissues of the human body varies in different cases, thus accounting for the diversity of clinical manifestations observed in falciparum malaria. Most of the severe and fatal cases are due to blocking (occlusion) of the capillaries by clumps of red blood cells harbouring developing parasites, enormous numbers of which can be seen in smears and sections of post mortem material.

In falciparum malaria the infected red cells retain their normal size throughout all stages of development of the parasite. Cells harbouring the older trophozoites and schizonts are frequently stippled with a few coarse reddish dots (Maurer's dots), scattered over about two-thirds of the erythrocyte.

The development of the gametocytes takes place in the inner organs, but sometimes young forms are seen in the blood. The young gametocytes tend to be elongated, becoming spindle-shaped or elliptic as they grow. Finally, they assume the characteristic curved shape of the mature gametocytes. These first appear in the peripheral blood after several generations have undergone schizogony, usually about 10 days after the initial invasion of the blood. The body of the mature gametocytes may be sausage-shaped, banana-shaped or crescentic; they are usually referred to as *crescents*. The female form or macrogametocyte is usually more slender and somewhat longer than the male, and the cytoplasm takes up a deeper blue colour with Romanowsky stains. The nucleus is small and compact, staining dark red, while the pigment granules are closely aggregated round it. The male form or microgametocyte is broader than the female and is more inclined to be sausage-shaped. The cytoplasm is either pale blue or tinted with pink and the nucleus, which stains dark pink, is large and less compact than in the female, while the pigment granules are scattered in the cytoplasm around it. The number of gametocytes present in falciparum infections is variable, occasionally amounting to 50 000 to 150 000 per µl of blood, a figure never attained by the other species of human plasmodia.

Though erythrocytic schizogony in *P. falciparum* is completed in 48 hours and the periodicity of development is therefore of typically tertian type, there frequently occur in this species two or more broods of parasites, the segmentation of which is not synchronised, so that the periodicity of symptoms in the patient tends to be irregular, especially in the early stages of the attack.

The sexual cycle of *P. falciparum* in the mosquito conforms with that described for mammalian plasmodia in general. Its duration at 20°C is 22 days; at 23°C – 15 to 17 days, and at 25° to 28°C – 10 to 11 days. The pigment in the oöcyst is almost black and the granules are relatively large. It forms a pattern over the cyst, usually a double circle around the periphery, but it may be arranged as a small circle in the centre, or even as a double straight chain. By the eighth day much of the pigment becomes obscured but a few grains can usually still be seen.

Plasmodium malariae

P. malariae is the causal organism of quartan malaria, so named because the paroxysms recur on the fourth day, after two days' interval. The parasite differs from the other species affecting man, by its morphological characters and also by its slow development in both the human and the insect host. The course of the disease is not unduly severe but its long persistence is notorious. The geographical range of quartan malaria extends over both tropical and sub-tropical areas but its presence in various zones tends to be patchy.

No direct evidence is available of pre-erythrocytic stages of *P. malariae* after the inoculation of sporozoites into the human host but the evidence of such a stage has been obtained indirectly, by infecting Anopheles mosquitos on human *P. malariae* and inoculating sporozoites into a chimpanzee in whose liver exo-erythrocytic schizonts were demonstrated. *P. malariae* occurs naturally in chimpanzees and these animals may be potential reservoirs of quartan malaria. The old name of *P. rodhaini*, a parasite naturally found in chimpanzees is synonymous with *P. malariae*. The pre-erythrocytic schizonts in the liver do not reach maturity until the 13th day after inoculation of sporozoites. When the mature schizont discharges the merozoites into the blood circulation, the asexual erythrocytic cycle begins and shows a 72 hours periodicity. The existence of the late erythrocytic phase, responsible for long term relapses, is probable though it has not been demonstrated and now several authors doubt if it exists.

The young trophozoites in the blood are not very different from those of *P. vivax*, though their cytoplasm is thicker and they stain more deeply.

Older trophozoites when rounded are about half the size of the host cell. In thin films the trophozoites may stretch across the entire width of the cell; such *band forms* are a characteristic feature of *P. malariae*. The pigment granules are numerous, large and dark.

The entire development of the trophozoite takes about 54 hours and during the succeeding 18 hours the parasite undergoes the schizogonic development. Young schizonts divide repeatedly and finally the mature schizont has an average of eight merozoites. The merozoites occupy almost the entire erythrocyte and form either an irregular cluster or are arranged symmetrically around the centre, in the form of a daisy. The term *rosette* is often applied to such schizonts.

P. malariae produces no evident changes in the host cells although they may often appear somewhat smaller than uninfected erythrocytes. A special staining may show the presence of discrete stippling, often called Ziemann's stippling.

The degree of parasitaemia in quartan malaria is lower than in any other plasmodial infections and the parasite count rarely exceeds 10 000 per µl of blood.

The gametocytes develop probably in the internal organs and appear in the peripheral blood when fully grown. The female gametocyte has a deep blue cytoplasm and a small, dense nucleus; the male stains pale blue and has a diffuse larger nucleus.

The 72 hours periodicity of the asexual cycle of development is usually well synchronised with the forms of parasite seen in the blood.

The sporogonic cycle in the Anopheles takes 30–35 days at 20°C; at 23–28°C it may be as short as 16 days though the average period is 26–28 days.

The pigment in the oöcysts is in the form of large dark-brown granules and has a characteristic peripheral distribution. The clumping of the pigment in a small area of the oöcyst is of value in identifying the infection in the mosquito.

Plasmodium ovale

P. ovale infection produces a tertian type of fever similar to that of vivax malaria, but often with prolonged latency, lesser trend to relapse, and generally milder clinical symptoms. It was described only in 1922 by Stephens who saw it in the blood of a soldier who had returned from East Africa. *P. ovale* has been recorded chiefly from tropical Africa in the west of which it is quite common. It has been reported sporadically from the West Pacific region and from other parts of the world. Some of these identifications are not absolutely certain.

The asexual erythrocytic cycle of development of *P. ovale* is similar to that of *P. vivax* and extends over 48 hours. The pre-erythrocytic stage has a pre-patent period of nine days and the mature liver schizonts, some 70 µ in diameter, contain some 15 000 merozoites. *P. ovale* resembles *P. malariae* but its effect on the infected erythrocytes is similar to that produced by *P. vivax*. The young trophozoites measure about one-third the diameter of the red blood cell. Schüffner's stippling appears quite early and is more pronounced than in the case of *P. vivax*. As the trophozoites grow they show some resemblance to *P. malariae* though the band forms are seldom seen. Most of them are round and compact with granules of pigment coarser than in *P. vivax* but not as coarse as in *P. malariae*. At this stage many erythrocytes are slightly enlarged and in thin films many of them assume an

The Malaria Parasites

oval shape with ragged or fimbriated margins and heavy stippling. The schizonts resemble those of *P. malariae*. They are rounded, compact and when mature contain 8–10 nuclei which are arranged peripherally around the central clump of pigment granules. Occasionally the number of merozoites may be as high as 16.

The gametocytes of *P. ovale* resemble those of *P. malariae*, but the erythrocyte that contains them rarely assumes the oval shape. The female gametocyte has a small, compact, bluish nucleus, the male's diffuse nucleus stains pale blue with a reddish tinge.

The pigment in the oöcyst is dark brown and the granules resemble those seen in *P. malariae* but have a tendency to form chains which cross each other in the centre of the cyst. The completion of the sporogonic cycle in the mosquito takes 16 days at 25°C.

Mixed infections

Infections due to two or more species of malaria parasites are not uncommon, but they are often overlooked. In endemic malarious areas mixed infections are particularly frequent; there is a tendency for one species of the parasite to predominate over the other. The most common types of mixed infections are *P. falciparum* and *P. vivax* in sub-tropical areas while in tropical Africa *P. falciparum* and *P. malariae* are prevalent, though *P. falciparum* and *P. ovale* are also frequent. On rare occasions all three species can be found in one blood film.

The best way of diagnosing a mixed infection with more than one species of plasmodia is by a careful and longer than usual microscopical examination of the blood film.

Physiology of human plasmodia

The metabolic requirements of plasmodia are derived from the haemoglobin of the host erythrocytes and from the nutrients available in the plasma. The main biochemical reactions are fourfold. The energy required for the intracellular growth of the asexual parasites is obtained by the phosphorylation of glucose involving the Embden-Meyerhoff and subsequently probably the Krebs cycle. The oxydative processes are maintained by the oxy-haemoglobin of the infected erythrocyte. The globin portion of the haemoglobin is broken down into large quantities of free amino acids including cystine and methionine which are then built up into parasite protein. Lipids are synthesised from the components available in the plasma of the host. This is accomplished partly by osmosis and partly by formation of food vacuoles within the body of the parasite. Obviously, the state of nutrition of the host has an important bearing on the multiplication of plasmodia. It has been found that para-amino-benzoic acid (PABA) must be present in the diet of the host or in the culture medium. PABA present in milk is one of the essential building stones of the molecule of the folic acid needed for the growth of mammalian plasmodia. The importance of this and other biochemical studies is considerable for the understanding of the action of antimalarial compound and for rational development of new drugs.

The differences in the physiology of the four species of human plasmodia are reflected in their apparent predilection for certain types of erythrocytes. Thus *P. vivax* and *P. ovale* invade preferably the younger red blood cells (reticulocytes); *P. malariae* prefer mature red blood cells while *P. falciparum* seems to be indifferent to the age of its host cell.

ANIMAL PLASMODIA

Avian plasmodia

Malaria parasites of birds are found in nearly every country in the world. This is largely due to the migratory flights of birds and the ample facilities for transmission of the infection by many genera and species of mosquitos. It was Danilewsky in Russia who first observed in 1884 malaria parasites in the blood of birds. His major work published in 1894 indicated the wide distribution of these parasites. Ross in 1897 demonstrated the development of *P. relictum* in culicine mosquitos fed on infected sparrows. Grassi and other Italian workers described in 1899–1900 a number of avian malaria parasites and their transmission by mosquitos.

The main characteristics that distinguish avian malaria parasites from those of primates are: (1) Avian parasites are found in nucleated erythrocytes. (2) They are transmitted mainly by mosquitos of the genera *Aedes* and *Culex* and very rarely – *Anopheles*. (3) The exo-erythrocytic stages of avian parasites are found in mesodermal tissue, the primary cycle occupies two generations and can arise from blood stages.

Over 450 species of birds have been found infected with malaria parasites. Avian malaria parasites are classified into the subgenera: *Haemamoeba, Giovannolaia, Novyella* and *Huffia*. The identification of species is not easy and must be based on observation of various stages of the life cycle and certain biological features.

After the discoveries of Ross and Grassi it seemed that the knowledge of the life cycle of the malaria parasites was complete, but it soon became obvious that there must be an unknown phase between the introduction of the sporozoite and the appearance of parasites in the blood. Grassi formulated this idea in 1906, but there was no definite proof of the presence of these forms in the body of the host. It was not until 1934–36 that Raffaele described the exo-erythrocytic forms of *P. elongatum* and *P. relictum* in the bone-marrow and brain of birds.

The Malaria Parasites

These findings were soon confirmed in *P. gallinaceum* by James and Tate and were a precursor to the discovery of exo-erythrocytic schizogony in malaria parasites of primates.

In 1926 Roehl in Germany introduced the method of quantitative assessment of antimalarial action of new compounds. The Roehl's test was based on infecting canaries with *P. relictum*; untreated birds showed parasites in the blood after 4–5 days, while birds given quinine by a stomach tube showed no parasitaemia. This method was used as a primary screening test of a number of antimalarial drugs developed by the Germans during the 1930s.

Experimental chemotherapy of malaria benefited greatly from the discovery of avian plasmodia. They were widely used in the USA for studies on synthetic antimalarial drugs in 1940–45 and are still of value at the present time, even though rodent and simian plasmodia are increasingly employed for this purpose.

Rodent plasmodia

Plasmodium berghei. The discovery of a new species of malaria parasite in a rodent was made in 1948 by Vincke and Lips in the former Belgian Congo (today's Zaïre). It was not a chance discovery but a purposeful search for an animal host which might have infected an Anopheles mosquito (*A. dureni*) commonly found in a forest gallery in the Katanga province. This animal host was eventually discovered and proved to be a tree rat *Thamnomys surdaster*. It was soon found that the new parasite named *Plasmodium berghei* could be easily transmitted by injection of blood to laboratory mice and rats.

However, experimental, cyclical, transmission of *P. berghei* through its original vector or through other Anopheles was not successful until 1964 when Yoeli demonstrated that three conditions must be fulfilled: (1) A newly isolated strain of the parasite is needed, (2) The mosquitos must be fed on the animal during the early stage of parasitaemia, (3) The mosquitos must be maintained at a comparatively low temperature of 19–20°C. The latter factor corresponds to the environment of the forest gallery in Katanga.

Exo-erythrocytic stages of *P. berghei* become mature about 50 hours after sporozoite inoculation. They are present (as in primate malaria) in parenchymatous cells of the liver.

The asexual cycle in the blood, from trophozoites to schizonts, averages 24 hours; multiple infections of the red blood cells are common and occur particularly in young erythrocytes. The number of merozoites in fully developed schizonts varies between six and twenty. Gametocytes have a typical appearance but their numbers decline markedly after a series of blood passages.

P. berghei is lethal to white mice and to young rats. At least 50 different species of rodents are susceptible to the infection with this parasite. There are about 200 different strains of *P. berghei* isolated from various rodents or from the natural vector. A closely related parasite, *P. berghei yoelii*, was isolated in the Central African Republic and may represent a new species.

P. berghei has been widely used for experimental work on parasitology, immunology, and chemotherapy of malaria. Over 2000 papers on these various subjects have been published, pointing out the importance of rodent malaria in scientific research, and most of the primary screening of some 300 000 compounds developed during the past ten years in the USA was done using this rodent plasmodium.

Several new species and subspecies of rodent plasmodia have been discovered and described during the past decade. They are increasingly used for parasitological and chemotherapeutic studies. For the latter use rodent plasmodia have some limitations since the biochemical characteristics of these parasites are somewhat different from those of human plasmodia.

Simian plasmodia

The presence of malaria parasites in the blood of monkeys was observed already in 1893 and one of these parasites found in an East African monkey received the name of *Plasmodium kochi* (later renamed *Hepatocystes kochi* by Garnham). In 1907 the discovery of *P. cynomolgi* in *Macaca irus* from Java was of particular interest because of its resemblance to the *P. vivax* of man and during the first quarter of the present century a series of other simian plasmodia were found in monkeys in the field or in the zoos in various parts of the world. Much of the early work on simian malaria was done in India where *P. knowlesi* was isolated in 1932 from *Macaca irus* and subsequently transmitted to man. The study of plasmodia of higher apes (chimpanzees and gorillas) was given great impetus by Rodhain who showed in 1940 the identity of *P. malariae* of man with that of *P. rodhaini* of chimpanzees.

In 1947 Garnham demonstrated the true nature of *Hepatocystes kochi* in the East African monkey *Cercopithecus aethiops*. He showed that the blood forms of this parasite are composed of gametocytes only and discovered the presence, in the liver of infected monkeys, of the exo-erythrocytic stages of the parasite. The final stage of development in the tissue is a merocyst with a large vacuole; the numerous merozoites present in a simple merocyst invade the blood stream.

This finding was the first step to the subsequent discovery of exo-erythrocytic stages of the true malaria parasites. The vector of *H. kochi* is a *Culicoides* as found by Garnham in 1951.

The importance of studies on simian malaria was brilliantly demonstrated by Shortt and Garnham in 1948. The discovery of exoerythrocytic stages in the liver of monkeys infected with *P.*

cynomolgi pointed the way to finding the tissue stages of *P. vivax* in man.

Although the relationship between the plasmodia of monkeys and those of man became obvious already in the 1930s, when *P. knowlesi* was used in Romania for malaria therapy by blood infection, the question of simian malaria as a zoonosis became important in the 1960s. In that year American workers described the case of an accidental laboratory infection by *P. cynomolgi bastianellii* transmitted from *Macaca irus* through mosquitos. The tertian periodicity of the febrile illness and the presence of vivax-like parasites in the blood of the accidentally infected individual drew attention to the possibility of natural transmission of the disease from monkeys to man.

P. cynomolgi infections in the rhesus monkey have occupied an important place in the search for new antimalarials between 1950 and 1960. This model offered a precise biological and chemotherapeutic counterpart of *P. vivax* infection of man. It was thanks to this model that identification of primaquine as an answer to radical cure of relapsing malaria became possible.

Further work especially in Malaysia and Brazil was responsible for a surge of new knowledge of simian malaria. Within five years the number of species of plasmodia of lower monkeys increased to about a dozen.

It was soon found that in addition to the confirmed possibility of transmission to man of *P. cynomolgi* through mosquitos, other plasmodia of lower monkeys such as *P. brasilianum* and *P. inui* could also be transmitted in the same way.

Although the possibility of the two-way transmission (monkey – vector – man) of simian malaria in natural conditions was experimentally established, the proof that it can happen in nature was provided in one case of human infection with *P. knowlesi* in Malaya and in another case of a similar infection with *P. simium* in Brazil. These exceptional occurrences, while stressing the close relationship between human and some simian plasmodia, do not invalidate the fact that in nature the only true reservoir of human malaria parasites is the infected human being.

During the past ten years, an increasing amount of research has shown not only that some plasmodia of monkeys or apes can be transmitted to man, but also that human malaria parasites can be successfully transmitted to some lower primates and especially to several species of neotropical monkeys.

The latter finding by Young and his colleagues in Panama in 1960 was of special significance since it opened an entirely new field for experimental chemotherapy of malaria.

Thus *P. vivax, P. falciparum* and *P. malariae* can now be transmitted by *Anopheles* to the Colombian night monkey *Aotus trivirgatus*. Other

South American monkeys (*Ateles, Saimiri, Saguinus*) are also susceptible to infection with human plasmodia but the *Aotus* is by far the most useful experimental animal in this respect.

The value of this species is so great that its wide use in various research centres has now led to a great shortage of *Aotus* and to an embargo imposed by some South American governments on trapping and exportation of these animals.

Plasmodia of other animals

In addition to a number of plasmodia of rats and mice newly described during the past few years, malaria parasites were found in an Indian buffalo, in some African and Asian deer, in Malagasy lemurs and in an African fruit-bat.

A large number of species of malaria parasites have been described in various lizards or lizard-like animals mainly living in the tropics and ranging from skunks to iguanas and chameleons. None of these plasmodia can infect man.

Chapter 3

Clinical Course of Malaria

The clinical course of malaria consists of bouts of fever accompanied by other symptoms and alternating with periods of freedom from any feeling of illness. Prominent feature of the febrile response is its tendency to periodicity (Fig. 8).

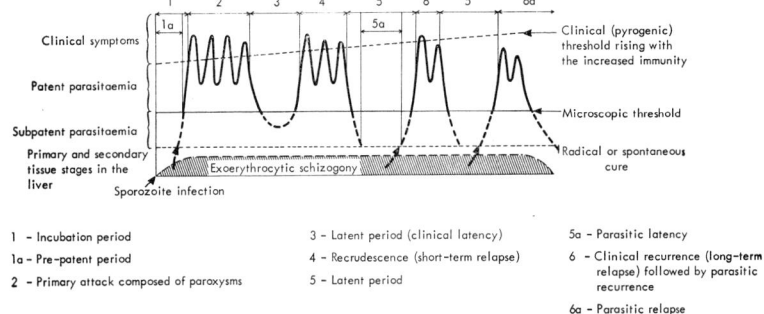

Fig 8 Diagram of the course of a malaria infection showing the primary attack and relapses of the recrudescent and recurrent types. (WHO, 1963)

The incubation period in malaria covers the time between the infection and the first appearance of clinical signs, of which fever is the most common. The length of the incubation period is usually between 9 and 30 days and varies with the species of the parasite (shortest for *P. falciparum*, longest for *P. malariae*), with the intensity of the infection and with the previous treatment or the degree of resistance of the host. It also depends on the circumstances of the infection, whether natural by mosquito bite or artificial, e.g. by injection of infected blood.

The *pre-patent period* extends from the time of infection to the first finding of malaria parasites in the blood.

Average incubation periods for mosquito transmitted malaria are 12 days for falciparum malaria, 13–17 days for vivax and ovale and 28–30 days for quartan malaria. However, some strains of *P. vivax* show much longer incubation periods, up to 9 months. These strains were particularly common in northern Europe and Russian authors (Nikolaev) proposed that they should receive a sub-specific status as *P. vivax hibernans*. The mechanism of such long incubation periods is not clear; while some investigators believe that it is due to a small number of sporozoites injected by the Anopheles, other studies suggest that we are dealing here with a genetic polymorphism of sporozoites of *P. vivax* so that some of them produce a short incubation period of the disease while others remain in the liver for a long period before maturation and formation of tissue forms. This being so, a small inoculum of sporozoites is likely to contain only those with a long incubation period, predominant in temperate countries. However, large inocula of sporozoites contain those with a short incubation period which dominate the clinical picture, especially in tropical countries.

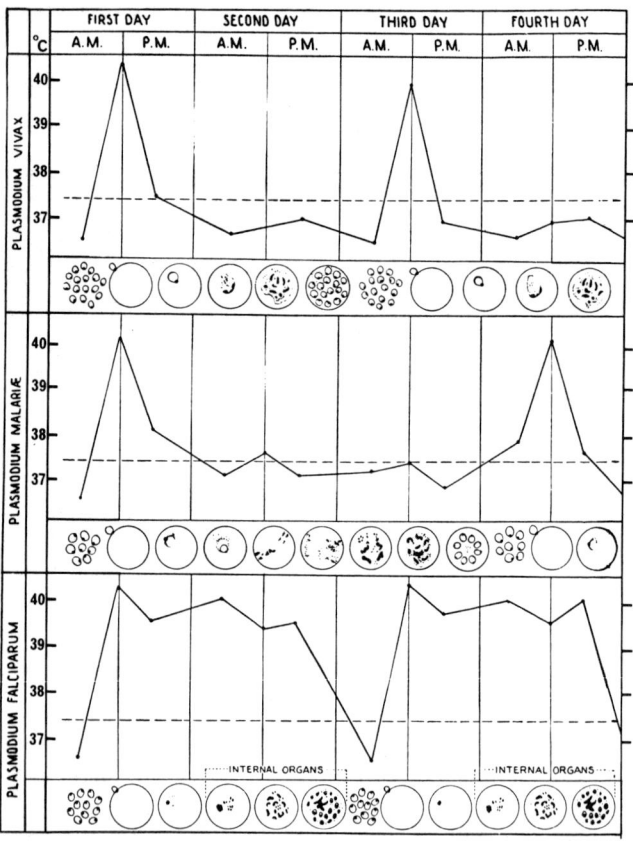

Fig 9 Temperature curves in malaria showing relation to growth and schizogony of malaria parasites of three species of Plasmodia.

In all types of infection the periodic febrile response is related to the time of the rupture of a sufficient number of mature schizonts and consequent discharge of merozoites into the blood stream. In vivax and ovale (tertian) malaria the schizonts of each brood of parasites mature every 48 hours so that the periodicity of fever is tertian; in quartan malaria, due to *P. malariae*, this occurs at intervals of 72 hours (Fig. 9).

The onset of a *primary attack* marks the end of the incubation period. The attack is composed of a number of *paroxysms* and is usually succeeded (except when parasites have been eliminated by adequate treatment) by a more or less prolonged period in which the trend of the infection depends on the process of multiplication of parasites and on the counteraction of immune response of the host.

A reappearance of symptoms of infection following the primary attack is generally known as a *relapse*. However, the term *recrudescence* (or short term relapse) is often used for a return of symptoms and parasitaemia within eight weeks from the termination of the primary attack; the term *recurrence* (or long term relapse) often refers to the return of fever and parasitaemia 24 weeks or more after the primary attack.

The malaria paroxysm is usually preceded by a premonitory stage with lassitude, headache, anorexia, occasional nausea and vomiting. A typical paroxysm comprises three successive stages: *The cold stage* starts with shivering (rigor) and a feeling of intense cold. The teeth chatter and the patient covers himself with any available clothing and blankets. His pulse is rapid but weak, his lips and fingers are cyanotic, his skin is dry and pale with a goose-flesh appearance. Vomiting may occur and children often have convulsive seizures. This stage lasts between 15 minutes and one hour. *The hot stage* follows when the feeling of intense cold gives way to one of distressing heat. The face is flushed, the skin dry and burning, headache becomes intense, nausea and vomiting are common, the pulse is full and bounding. There is often intense thirst while the temperature may rise to 41°C (106°F) or more. This stage lasts from two to six hours.

In *the sweating stage* the patient breaks out in profuse sweat, so that his bedding becomes drenched. The temperature falls rapidly, often below the normal level. He usually falls into a deep sleep and on waking feels weak but otherwise normal. This stage lasts from two to four hours.

The total duration of the typical attack which often begins in the early afternoon is from eight to twelve hours. However, the clinical symptoms vary considerably in relation to the species of the infecting parasite and the age of the patient.

Falciparum malaria

The incubation period of falciparum malaria varies between nine and fourteen days. The disease starts with headache, pains in the back and limbs, prostration, a feeling of chill, nausea, vomiting or mild diarrhoea. Scanty parasites may be present in the blood before the onset of acute symptoms in persons who have taken small doses of suppressive drugs. Fever may be low or absent and the patient may not appear to be very ill; the diagnosis at this stage depends on the knowledge of the recent exposure to the infection in a tropical, possibly malarious area.

As the disease develops, headache, pains in the back and limbs and general malaise increase in intensity. Anxiety, mental confusion are common at this stage. Fever is irregular and shows no distinct periodicity. (Fig. 9)

Sweating may be present even when the fever is low. The pulse and respiration rates are rapid. Nausea, vomiting and diarrhoea increase in severity and there is often some pulmonary involvement producing cough. The spleen shows a degree of enlargement and is tender on palpation. The liver may become enlarged and there may be slight jaundice. There is often albumin in the urine and hyaline or granular casts. There may be a degree of anaemia and there is usually some leucopenia with monocytosis.

If the early stage of the disease is diagnosed and adequately treated the infection may quickly subside.

However, if treatment is neglected, symptoms of 'pernicious malaria' may appear with great suddenness. This term is given to severe complications which may develop without warning at any stage of falciparum infections. They may supervene when the blood infection is apparently light, but are much more likely when more that 5% of erythrocytes are infected. Three main groups of symptoms may be distinguished.

Cerebral malaria may begin slowly or suddenly after the initial symptoms. Headache and drowsiness are succeeded by a comatose state with contracted pupils and abolished or exaggerated deep reflexes. There are many neurological symptoms which can simulate meningitis, epilepsy, acute delirium, intoxication, heat stroke etc. These symptoms are due to the blocking of capillaries in the central nervous system by parasitised erythrocytes (Fig. 10). However, recent studies suggest that cerebral malaria is a form of disseminated vasculomyelopathy, a hyperergic response of a central nervous system to the antigenic challenge of *P. falciparum*. The initial event seems to be an alteration of the endothelial permeability of the capillaries of the brain followed by perivascular infiltrates and demyelination.

Algid malaria. In this condition, which resembles surgical shock, the skin is pale, cold and clammy. The breathing is shallow, the pulse weak

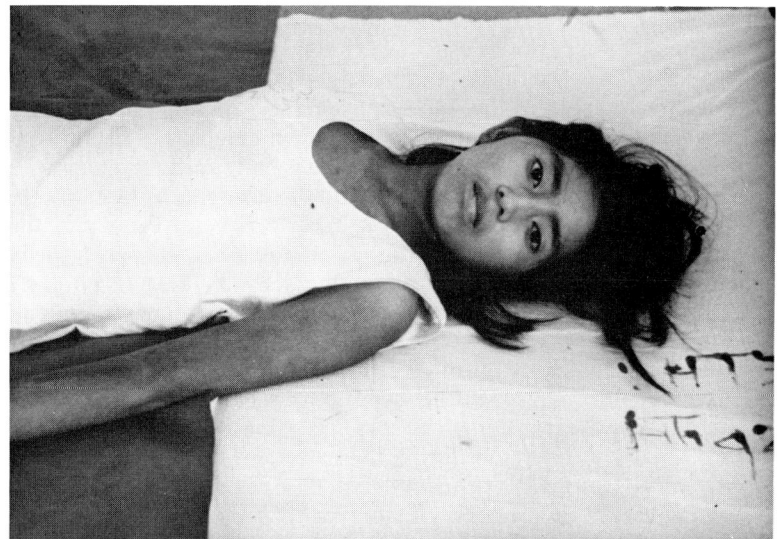

Fig 10 A case of severe *P. falciparum* malaria in an Amerindian girl in Guiana. (Photograph by Dr M Giglioli)

and rapid; the face is drawn and pinched, and the eyes are sunken. The blood pressure is low. Vomiting and diarrhoea may occur. It is thought that this usually fatal condition is due to adrenal insufficiency.

Gastro-intestinal symptoms may imitate dysentery or cholera. Frequent stools containing blood, mucus and pus together with abdominal pain and irregular fever suggest the former. Profuse watery diarrhoea, muscular cramps and dehydration are reminiscent of cholera. The old term 'bilious remittent fever' refers to persistent hiccup and profuse vomiting containing bile or semi-digested dark blood; there are watery stools containing blood, enlargement of the liver and jaundice. Renal failure with anuria may supervene and death occurs from uraemia, vascular collapse or pulmonary oedema.

Other systemic manifestations of falciparum malaria include nephritis, pulmonary involvement resembling pneumonia, neuritis etc. Massive intravascular haemolysis may then occur, leading to the striking clinical picture of 'blackwater fever'. This syndrome is fully described in a separate section. Acute pulmonary oedema may develop spontaneously, though at times it is due to excessive fluid administration.

Malaria may be a serious complication of pregnancy causing intra-uterine death of the fetus and simulating toxaemia of pregnancy in the mother.

Vivax malaria

The incubation period is usually between 12 and 17 days, but it may be prolonged to 6–9 months or even longer. The primary attack begins with headache, pain in the back, nausea and general malaise; these prodromal symptoms are mild or absent in relapses. The fever is irregular for 2–4 days, but soon becomes 'intermittent', viz. with marked swings between the morning and the evening. At first there is no regularity in the pattern of fever because several broods of the parasite are not synchronised, but soon the 48 hours periodicity becomes established. Paroxysms occur chiefly in the afternoon or evening and the classical cold, hot and sweating stages become evident. The temperature may rise to 40.6°C (105°F) or higher. Nausea and vomiting may be distressing and herpes of the lips is common. (Fig. 9)

Dizziness, drowsiness or other symptoms of cerebral irritation may occur, but they are transient. The spleen is palpable during the second week. Polyuria is common during the early part of the paroxysm.

Anaemia develops as a result of destruction of erythrocytes and may become severe in children. Fulminant types of vivax malaria have been described in the past in children in the USSR, but this complication is related to malnutrition or other intercurrent diseases. Vivax malaria is important not because of its fatality rate but mainly on account of debility that it produces as a result of relapses.

Rupture of the enlarged and soft spleen, following a minor accident may occur, though this is a rare complication.

During the early phase of the primary attack parasites are scanty in the peripheral blood, but they are common when the tertian rhythm of fever is well set. Gametocytes appear in the blood about one week after the onset of the primary attack.

Relapses. A single untreated attack may last for several weeks, with repeated paroxysms. In about 60% of untreated or inadequately treated cases clinical symptoms recur after a period of quiescence, the length of which depends largely on the particular strain of the parasite.

Renewed clinical activity is seen either during the first 8–10 weeks after the primary attack, when it is referred to as *recrudescence* or *short-term relapse*, or around the 30th to 40th week after the primary attack, when it is known as *recurrence* or *long-term relapse*.

Vivax infections acquired in different parts of the world show striking differences in the duration of the incubation period and the occurrence of long periods of latency. These differences have been broadly correlated with climatic zones. Prolonged latency has been observed chiefly in temperate regions.

When malaria infection is symptomless between the primary attack and the relapse it is said to be *clinically latent* even though there may be a degree of parasitaemia and such other signs as large spleen; *parasitic latency* occurs when plasmodia are undetectable in the peripheral blood though the exo-erythrocytic forms survive in the tissues.

Three characteristic relapse patterns are recognised in vivax infections, when the initial attack has been terminated by schizontocidal drugs which have no effect on relapses.

Type I   Incubation period short (12–20 days).
         Relapses frequent; no prolonged latency.
Type II Incubation period short (12–20 days).
         Prolonged (7–13 months) latency followed by one or several relapses at short intervals.
Type III Incubation period long (6 months or longer).
         Delayed primary attack succeeded by a series of relapses at short intervals and by a second long latency followed by relapses.

In the USSR the geographical areas of distribution of Types II and III are separated by the latitude 52°N. To the north of this line long incubation period of the infection was reported in 60% of cases. The Russian authors believe that the relevant strain of *P. vivax* should be recognised as sub-species *hibernans*.

Strains of *P. vivax* show some differences in their response to antimalarial drugs. The mean duration of the untreated infection with *P. vivax* is three years, though in some cases the infection may last longer.

Ovale malaria

The clinical picture of malaria due to *P. ovale* resembles closely that of vivax malaria. The paroxysms may be equally severe but spontaneous recovery is more common and there are fewer relapses. It should be stressed that the parasite often remains latent and is easily suppressed by other more virulent species of plasmodia. It may appear in the blood when these have declined. Mixed infections in which *P. ovale* is found are common in persons exposed to malaria in tropical Africa.

Quartan malaria

The incubation period in infections with *P. malariae* is never less than 18 days and may be considerably longer (30–40 days). The clinical picture of the primary attack resembles that of vivax malaria, but the rigors may be more severe. The paroxysms are more regularly spaced and occur often in the late afternoon. Anaemia is usually less pronounced than in vivax malaria and other complications are less common. Splenomegaly is frequent and may attain considerable size. The untreated infection may persist for very long periods and relapses have been recorded 30–50 years after the infection.

Asymptomatic parasitaemia is not uncommon and presents a problem in donors of blood for transfusion. Quartan malaria nephrosis frequently found in African children is very rare in non-immunes infected with *P. malariae*.

All stages of asexual parasites are usually present in the peripheral blood at the same time, but parasitaemia is never very high and seldom exceeds 1% of the red blood cells. The mechanism of relapses in quartan malaria still remains something of a mystery. The view that long term relapses originate from a secondary exo-erythrocytic cycle within the liver cells was widely held after the discovery of the existence of pre-erythrocytic forms of *P. vivax* and other species of plasmodia. There is now some doubt if the relapses of *P. malariae* infections are always related to the tissue forms. It is likely that in some strains of this species asexual erythrocytic parasites can survive in the body, in some way, where they are protected from the cellular and humoral immune defences of the host. They may depend for their survival on continued repeated antigenic variation, and cause subsequent relapses.

MALARIA IN CHILDREN AND IN PREGNANCY

In children the classical features of the malarial paroxysm as seen typically in non-immune adults are not common. Indeed the clinical picture varies greatly according to the play of various factors. Firstly, even when primary attacks occur among non-immune children, many of the classical features may be masked; secondly, in children who have some tolerance of malaria, and are born in an endemic area, the disease often smoulders on almost unsuspected, although occasionally it may flare up into a severe complication.

In non-immune infants and children who contract an acute primary attack, some variability often occurs. The child at first appears restless or drowsy, refuses food and may complain of headache and nausea. Some pallor of the skin may be noted in those having little natural skin pigment. Severe cases may show pallor of the nails and of the mucous membranes; slight cyanosis may be noted. As the temperature rises thirst may be marked; in breast-fed infants this displays itself as frequent attempts to suck the breast, but soon this is abandoned, possibly due to nausea. A clear-cut cold stage and a definite rigor are uncommon in infants and children. Vomiting is often marked, and the vomitus is tinged with bile; although it may render oral therapy difficult, it is seldom sufficiently frequent or copious to cause severe dehydration or loss of electrolytes. Likewise the stools are often loose and dark green, mucus may be seen, but blood or leucocytes are rare. Infants may appear in abdominal distress. Older children may refer pain to the liver or spleen and they may be constipated.

The temperature is very variable; in some it is only moderate, but in the majority it is high (40°C), often continuous and irregular, the child is flushed and perspires freely. Even when the temperature is moderately high, convulsions often occur. They usually last only a few minutes and reflect some cerebral irritation. Unless consciousness quickly returns they must arouse fears of more serious brain damage due to cerebral malaria. The liver often enlarges and may be slightly tender, likewise the spleen; many days however may pass before splenic enlargement can be detected clinically, especially in the primary attack of non-immune children. Splenomegaly develops earlier in vivax malaria, less rapidly in falciparum malaria and very slowly in quartan malaria. In most cases the urine shows no abnormalities save those occurring in any fever; some cases show slight albuminuria, even scanty casts and possibly a few leucocytes and red cells – indicating some renal damage.

The manifestations of malaria in infants and children inhabiting highly endemic areas are even more variable. In tropical Africa, a small proportion of infants may show, after an acquired primary infection, a low grade parasitaemia with few clinical symptoms or even none. There might be slight restlessness, lack of appetite, sweating, anaemia and occasional rises of temperature. After some time, which varies from one infant to another, inherited immunity declines and the clinical attacks often become more severe. Generally speaking children living in highly endemic malarious areas without any protection from malaria and continuously exposed to the infection are, until the age of about five years, at a particularly critical stage of their host–parasite relationship and many of them die either of cerebral malaria or of an acute general infection. Some, after several successive attacks, achieve a relative tolerance to the infection and these the clinical picture of malaria may be mild: fever, fretfulness, tiredness, cough, diarrhoea etc. Many indigenous children particularly in tropical Africa may have enlarged spleens and livers and malaria parasites in their blood without any other signs of the disease other than a degree of anaemia, which may in part be due to other factors such as malnutrition, schistosomiasis, intestinal parasites etc.

Nevertheless, it would be wrong to disregard the importance of malaria in partially immune children. The high mortality rate among them might be due to a number of diseases rather than to a single entity. If the diet is excellent the effects of malaria are not marked, but in children on marginal diets loss of weight, anaemia, oedema or even frank kwashiorkor may occur and are not easily or completely cured until the malaria itself is treated. At any time one of these thin and anaemic children may succumb easily to a respiratory or intestinal infection and it may be impossible either in life or at autopsy to say how far malaria, malnutrition, bacterial infection or other factors were responsible.

The high invasive power of *P. falciparum* leads to the rapid destruction of erythrocytes and the resulting anaemia can be very severe. Infections in which 5–10% of red blood cells contain parasites are not uncommon. The progressive blood-loss leads to local anoxia of various organs and the resulting changes in the brain, liver, kidneys, bone marrow etc. are responsible for complications of falciparum malaria which can be very serious, especially in those who have little immunity to the disease. These effects occur in endemic regions most commonly between the ages of 6 months and 3 years and are responsible for almost all the deaths directly due to malaria in these areas.

The term 'chronic malaria' is sometimes applied to the condition seen in children who in highly endemic areas suffer from many attacks, often untreated, of malaria. This is seen more often in vivax and quartan infections and results in 'malarial cachexia' characterised by stunting of growth, wasting, anaemia and much enlargement of the liver and spleen. The temperature is often normal, at other times low fever occurs; parasitaemia is variable, and the thick blood film may be often negative; only prolonged observation can establish the diagnosis, which is not finally clinched until improvement occurs under the appropriate therapy.

Complications of an acute attack of vivax or quartan malaria are relatively uncommon but the infection may undermine the general defences of the growing organism and aggravate other intercurrent diseases. High temperatures seldom persist for more than brief periods. Cerebral and intestinal symptoms are rare, but the nephrotic syndrome is a complication often seen in quartan malaria.

Malaria in pregnancy

There is evidence of general maternal immunosuppression during the second half of pregnancy. This results possibly from the presence in the blood of high adrenal steroid levels, as well as placental chorionic gonadotrophin and alpha-fetoprotein: there may also be depression of the lymphocyte activity. It is likely that recrudescences or relapses of previous malaria infection seen in pregnant women are due to this multifactorial transient immunosuppression.

The importance of childbirth in waking up a latent malaria infection in the mother must not be forgotten and adequate treatment of this disease should not be withheld from a pregnant woman for fear of any adverse effect of the drugs on her or the unborn baby.

The syndrome of acute renal insufficiency as a complication of falciparum malaria appears to be not uncommon in pregnancy and can be superimposed on other diseases such as toxaemia of pregnancy. Proper treatment of the malaria infection should be associated with other measures. Diuresis often returns to normal after delivery. Malaria is usually an aggravating factor in anaemias of pregnancy, so common in tropical areas.

There is no doubt that intra-uterine transmission of malaria from the mother to her child can occur, although the mechanism of the transplacental passage of the parasite is obscure. The efficacy of the placenta as a barrier to the malaria parasite seems to depend on the degree of immunity of the mother. The frequency of transplacental infections of new-born babies is far greater in non-immunes than in immunes. Among the indigenous inhabitants of malarious regions, with a high tolerance of malaria, although massive infections of the placenta are frequent, the incidence of congenital malaria is very low.

It has been suggested that in non-immunes the placental barrier may be broken down as the result of pathological changes. This is probably correct, but congenital malaria can also occur in the absence of demonstrable damage to the placenta and even without any evidence of clinical malaria in the mother during pregnancy. Congenital malaria can occur in association with any species of malaria parasite. The pre-natal transfer of protective substances from the immune mother to the fetus through the placenta has now been confirmed; its importance to the newborn is very great even though the duration of such passively transmitted immunity does not exceed a few months. On the other hand the amount of antibody transmitted through maternal milk is very small, if any.

Epidemic malaria is an important cause of abortions, miscarriages, stillbirths and neonatal deaths. The effects of endemic malaria on the 'reproductive wastage' in indigenous populations in highly malarious regions vary inversely with the degree of tolerance of the disease possessed by the community. There is much evidence that low birth weights are commoner in deliveries in which the placenta is infected with malaria parasites. Consequently in all endemic areas, expectant mothers should be kept on a prophylactic treatment for at least 3 months before the expected date of delivery.

IMPORTED MALARIA

The problem of malaria imported into Europe, North America and other temperate parts of the world has assumed, during the past decade, increasing public health importance and created much concern among the clinicians. The annual number of notified cases of malaria brought into Europe from tropical countries by the rising tide of air travel, tourism and immigration went up from about 800 in 1967 to nearly 4000 in 1979. The latter figure is certainly an understatement because notification of malaria is obligatory only in a few countries and even there many cases remain unrecorded.

It is obvious that cases of malaria imported into countries where the local Anopheles are abundant and climatic conditions are suitable for transmission, may become sources of new infections for people who never travelled abroad. The high fatality rate of *P. falciparum* malaria in non-immune individuals is disturbing. The list of wrong diagnoses of malaria includes dysentery, dengue, influenza, hepatitis, heat stroke, nephritis and many other diseases. It is not uncommon that a patient, after first seeing his doctor and being given a palliative drug, develops within a few days, and with dramatic suddenness, signs of cerebral involvement, hyperpyrexia or renal failure. An emergency admission to the hospital may lead to a correct diagnosis of cerebral malaria but such severe infections with *P. falciparum* may not always respond to belated treatment.

According to available data the fatality rate of such undiagnosed cases varies between 3% and 11% and in some reports it is as high as 25%. The interval between the infection contracted abroad, usually in Africa or Asia, and the onset of symptoms, may be as long as one month in cases of falciparum malaria. This adds to the probability of overlooking malaria in a febrile patient, especially when gastro-intestinal symptoms, myalgia, arthralgia and jaundice complicate the clinical picture. Attacks of vivax or quartan malaria may be seen in some patients up to seven or nine months after their return from the tropics. One should bear in mind that the usual prophylactic drugs taken by the traveller while in the tropics and for one month after his return may not protect him from true relapsing infections with vivax, ovale or quartan malaria. The suppressive action of antimalarial drugs on the primary attack may not extend to the secondary relapse after the latent period. Moreover, some strains of *P. vivax* have an inherently long incubation period.

The possibility of transfusion malaria in a patient who has never been abroad but has been infected by a symptomless blood donor should also be kept in mind.

Thus malaria must be suspected in any patient with fever of unknown or doubtful origin who has been to a malarious tropical area during the previous one or two years or who has had a blood transfusion up to about 3 months before the start of his febrile illness. Simple questioning of the patient about his recent visits abroad will often lead to the correct diagnosis and treatment.

Information on malaria risk for international travellers is collected and published annually by the World Health Organization. This may be of considerable assistance to the medical practitioner or medical adviser of any organised group or agency in assessing the need for personal protection of prospective travellers and in evaluating the probability of malaria infection on their return.[1] (See Annex III)

TRANSFUSION MALARIA

While natural malaria infection takes place through the bite of an infective Anopheles mosquito, direct transfer of erythrocytes containing plasmodia may also be responsible for the infection. This may occur accidentally by usage of syringes or needles contaminated by blood, as happens among groups of drug addicts. Another more common occurrence is accidental infection of a recipient by blood transfusion from an infected blood donor.

Estimates of the total number of cases of malaria related to blood transfusion are approximate. Only a proportion of such episodes has been reported and the information ranges from a brief mention of malaria as a complication of surgery to a comprehensive analysis of a series of cases, reported singly by different authors.

During the past 60 years not less than 2500 cases of transfusion malaria were recorded. Transfusion malaria is particularly common in countries where blood donation has become a commercial transaction and where the blood donors come from the less affluent social classes. *P. vivax* infections are most commonly incriminated in accidental infections following blood transfusion; however *P. falciparum* infections occur not infrequently and more recently *P. malariae* were reported with increasing frequency, because of the asymptomatic, long-term carrier state of donors infected with this plasmodium.

While the longevity of *P. falciparum* in man seldom exceeds one year and *P. vivax* or *P. ovale* usually die out within 3 years, *P. malariae* which is prone to long term relapses, with or without febrile symptoms, may remain in the infected host for 10, 20, 30 or over 40 years. In fact, one may say that in some cases a quiescent infection with *P. malariae* may be maintained for life and the epidemiological implications of this special position of *P. malariae* with regard to its human host are considerable.

The viability of malaria parasites depends on that of their erythrocyte hosts. A series of studies carried out during the 1940s showed that malaria parasites of all species can remain viable in the blood destined for transfusion for at least one week. Further studies revealed that both *P. falciparum* and *P. malariae* remain viable for well over 10 days

---

[1] The latest information on malaria risk for international travellers was published in the *WHO Weekly Epidemiological Record*, 1978, **53**, No 25–26. A reprint of this document is available on request from the WHO Division of Malaria and other Parasitic Diseases, CH 1211, Geneva, 27, Switzerland.

in blood stored at 4°C, especially when the anticoagulant contains dextrose.

The time of appearance of symptoms of blood-induced infection depends on the number of parasites introduced, on the method of inoculation, and on the susceptibility of the recipient. Much information on this subject has been gathered in the course of malaria therapy.

Generally speaking the main symptoms of accidental infection with *P. falciparum* develop within 10 days after transfusion, *P. vivax* takes 16 days, while *P. malariae* – 40 days or longer. The interval between the onset of symptom and diagnosis depends on the amount of infected blood transfused, the degree of awareness of the possibility of transfusion malaria, but it can vary from 1 week to 1 month or considerably longer: in one case the disease was finally diagnosed 6 months later.

When any patient who has received a blood transfusion up to 3 months previously shows an unexplained fever, the possibility of malaria must be considered, and microscopic examination of the blood and, if necessary, serological tests should be carried out.

The prevention of transfusion malaria depends on the screening of possibly infected blood donors and the elimination of actual or possible plasmodial infection in the donor and in the recipient of the blood. Screening of blood donors is primarily based on their history of malaria or exposure to the infection. Regulations governing the acceptance of donors of whole blood for transfusion vary considerably from one country to another and it would be desirable for some internationally acceptable criteria to be established. In many countries the regulations proscribe the acceptance, as donors of whole blood, of persons who have had malaria less than 3 years or less than 5 years previously. In the United Kingdom the following regulations are in force: (a) the blood of those who have had malaria or who are natives of or who have lived until recently in endemic malarious areas may be used only for preparing plasma; (b) the blood of those who were born in the United Kingdom and who are normally resident there, but who have recently visited or passed through endemic malarious areas, may be used as whole blood, provided that they have left the malarious area for at least 2 months before, have had no feverish illness since returning, and have taken antimalarial drugs for 1 month after their return. If there is any doubt, the blood of such donors should be used only for preparing plasma. In the USA, donors of whole blood are excluded if they lived most of their life in an endemic malarious area or if they had clinical malaria during the previous 3 years. Travellers to endemic malarious areas are excluded if they returned from these parts of the world within 2 years and took prophylactic antimalarial drugs. On the other hand travellers to malarious areas who remained symptom-free without taking drugs can be accepted as whole blood donors after 6 months.

The detection of a malaria infection in a blood donor who is suspected on circumstantial evidence may prove very difficult. Microscopic examination of a blood film is of little value for the detection of asymptomatic parasitaemia, since the parasites are usually very few in number. On the other hand modern serological techniques and particularly the indirect fluorescent antibody (IFA) test are very useful for detection of persons who have had malaria in the past, although the test does not always indicate the actual presence of infection.

Pre-medication of donors suspected of having had malaria is impracticable as a rule though it may be possible in exceptional cases. The general consensus of authoritative opinion is that a dose of 600 mg of chloroquine (base), given to an adult recipient of infected blood 24 hours before transfusion or immediately after it, protects from induced malaria. It seems that this is the best solution where there are unusual risks of accidentally induced infection.

THERAPEUTIC MALARIA

Hippocrates and Galen mentioned that malaria seemed occasionally to have beneficial effects on other diseases. In England John Macculloch (1828) described an attempt to 'acquire an ague for removing a previous chronic disorder'. Deliberate infection with malaria for treatment of general paralysis was proposed by Wagner von Jauregg in Vienna in 1887, though the first trials started only in 1918. The initial method consisted of infecting patients by injection of blood obtained from other persons suffering from malaria. In 1922 Warrington Yorke in Liverpool began inducing malaria by the bites of infected mosquitos since this method had many advantages over blood inoculation. Therapeutic malaria has been widely used in many countries and with generally satisfactory results. The explanation of the beneficial effects of malaria on late neurosyphilis is not clear. In addition to the possible effect of febrile paroxysms it is likely that the plasmodial infection stimulates some specific defence mechanism against *Treponema pallidum*. The benefit depends on the degree of fever and on the number of paroxysms.

Many aspects of transfusion malaria were studied in the course of therapeutic malaria. The main difference between the two is that in the former the infection is accidental and presents an added hazard to the recipient of the blood. In therapeutic malaria the induced infection is deliberate; the species of the parasite is known in advance, the dosage of plasmodia as well as the number of injections are related to the state of health of the patient and the course of the infection can be easily changed by the use of appropriate drugs.

It is obvious that the 'incubation period' of therapeutic malaria induced by blood injection depends on the species of the parasite and on the numbers of plasmodia used; it varies between three days (0.5–1 million plasmodia) and ten days (1000–2000 plasmodia). On the other hand the true incubation period related to the mosquito transmission of the infection depends primarily on the species of the malaria parasite involved.

Therapeutic malaria was widely practised in many countries between 1920 and 1950. In the United Kingdom a special unit for malaria therapy was established in 1925 at Horton Hospital, Epsom, and over the next forty years many thousands of patients have benefited from this treatment. The advent of penicillin for treatment of syphilis has greatly reduced the demand for therapeutic malaria and the procedure is now employed only in exceptional cases or for scientific purposes.

P. vivax has been used in preference to any other species largely because of the relatively benign infection that it causes.[1] However, in some cases *P. malariae*, *P. falciparum* or *P. ovale* have been employed. A simian malaria parasite *P. knowlesi* has been used occasionally: it causes moderate fever and is easily controlled by drugs.

Various species of Anopheles have been preferred by different specialists for transmission of induced malaria by mosquitos. In Europe *A. atroparvus* has been most commonly used, though more recently the Indian *A. stephensi* proved to be an efficient vector. In the USA *A. quadrimaculatus* was generally employed.

Therapeutic malaria offered great opportunities for research in various fields of parasitology, immunology, and chemotherapy.

In the United States much of the advance of chemotherapy of malaria during the past thirty years was due to the existence of 'human malaria research centres' where the infection could be induced in volunteers. In Brazil induced malaria was tentatively given for treatment of non-syphilitic psychiatric disorders.

In the United Kingdom over the past fifty years the scientific contribution of the malaria therapy unit at the Horton Hospital, later known as Malaria Reference Laboratory, Horton Hospital, was immense. The characteristics of various strains of the three species of plasmodia were determined, the development of the parasite in different Anopheles species was elucidated, the pattern of relapses in malaria became clearer, much knowledge of the immune response to the infection in man was gained in the course of long-term observations; the action of various drugs on the course of the disease and its prevention contributed substantially to the development of synthetic

---

[1] It should be remembered that in malaria induced by injection of infected blood there are no relapses due to the absence of exo-erythrocytic forms in the liver, since the infection took place without the involvement of sporozoites. Thus the treatment of induced malaria is relatively simple.

antimalarials. In 1948 the discovery of pre-erythrocytic stages of *P. vivax* was made after the infection of a volunteer with the Madagascar strain of *P. vivax* and subsequent biopsy of his liver.

More recently an international collaborative project studied the parasitological and epidemiological characteristics of *P. vivax* North Korean strain on patients infected with malaria for therapeutic purposes.

With the discovery in the 1960s that human malaria can be transmitted to the owl monkey (*Aotus trivirgatus*) the importance of deliberately induced malaria to human volunteers declined still further. Nevertheless, for the final testing of some new antimalarial drugs or immunological methods, the value of the study of the course of infection in man is beyond any doubt.

Chapter 4

Pathology and Immunology of Human Malaria

The invasion of red blood cells which follows the pre-erythrocytic phase of the life cycle is the basic pathological process in malaria infections.

The degree of parasitaemia produced by the different species of plasmodia varies considerably. *P. vivax* develops most readily in the youngest red blood cells (reticulocytes); the same is probably true for *P. ovale*. *P. malariae* tends to invade the older erythrocytes. *P. falciparum* invades red blood cells of any age.

The factors which determine the reaction of the host to the parasite include: (1) The action of plasmodia on the blood; (2) General changes of blood flow related to pyrexia and altered biochemistry of the body; (3) Local changes due to the damage to the endothelial cells of blood vessels and tissue anoxia.

With each maturing of the schizont there occurs the subsequent rupture of the infected erythrocyte. Large numbers of non-parasitised red blood cells are also affected and both parasitised and non-parasitised cells undergo phagocytosis in the spleen and liver. No satisfactory evidence has as yet been produced to show that the parasite produces a toxic substance but a circulating soluble antigen has been shown to exist in severe infections and it is possible that it is liberated at the time when the erythrocyte distintegrates. This is partly responsible for a degree of anaemia always present in malaria infection.

The pathogenesis of fever in man is still little understood but the recent studies indicate that in response to exogenous stimuli (toxic products or infectious agents) endogenous pyrogen is released from leucocytes and enters the circulation. The interaction of this pyrogen with specialised receptors on thermosensitive centres of the hypothalamus causes a release of prostaglandin, monoamines etc. The information transmitted to the posterior hypothalamus and to the vasomotor centres directs sympathetic nerve fibres to constrict peripheral vessels and decrease heat dissipation: this results in the classical rigor of a malarial paroxysm.

Anaemia usually develops, its degree largely depending on the species of invading plasmodia. It is most pronounced in falciparum infections where the destruction of erythrocytes may be extensive and rapid. The type of anaemia is haemolytic, normochromic and normocytic and in the acute attack there may be a striking fall in the haemoglobin values of the blood. Haematological changes in malaria are particularly evident in falciparum infections. About 20% of patients with acute malaria show a significant degree of anaemia with haematocrit levels below 35%; this may delay the recovery after the infection has been eliminated. Other effects of the infection include thrombocytopenia which leads to coagulation defects evidenced by decrease of prothrombin and increase of fibrin degradation products. Leukopenia, which is common during the acute stage of the infection, usually returns to normal following specific therapy. The peripheral blood film shows many parasitised cells, polychromasia, anisocytosis, poikilocytosis, target cells and in severe cases, nucleated red cells. Malaria pigment (haemozoin) in the form of granules is present in large monocytes.

There are also changes on the surface of the erythrocytes leading to their clumping and this interferes with the circulation of the blood in the capillaries. Such 'sludging' process due to the aggregation of red blood cells and to the pressure of swollen and overladen phagocytes is seen in various organs where it interferes with local circulation and causes through anoxia important lesions in various organs. This is seen mainly in falciparum infections (Fig. 11).

The cause of fever in malaria is obscure and various factors including sensitivity to the products from released merozoites, the sudden release of potassium, haemozoin and cell debris have all been considered in this connection. It is not easy to relate the presence of the malaria parasite within the erythrocyte to the varied pathological processes in the human host leading to general symptoms of rigors, hyperpyrexia, sweating, algid malaria etc. On the other hand various more local disturbances can be traced to the changes in individual organs. Thus the failure of renal circulation results in urinary suppression and uraemia; changes in the liver blood flow lead to centrilobular congestion and degeneration. The effects of such dynamic changes are evident from the description of the pathology of the individual organs.

PATHOLOGICAL PICTURE IN INDIVIDUAL ORGANS

The following descriptions refer mainly to infections with *P. falciparum*. However, *P. malariae* which may cause the nephrotic syndrome shows a more specific picture in the affected organ.

The central nervous system presents severe lesions in 'cerebral malaria' due to *P. falciparum* infection. Three main types of changes can be seen on autopsy: (1) Gross congestion of meninges and the brain itself with the small vessels of the grey matter packed with erythrocytes containing pigmented parasites in all stages of development; (2) Occlusion of the capillaries and pre-capillaries of the cortex,

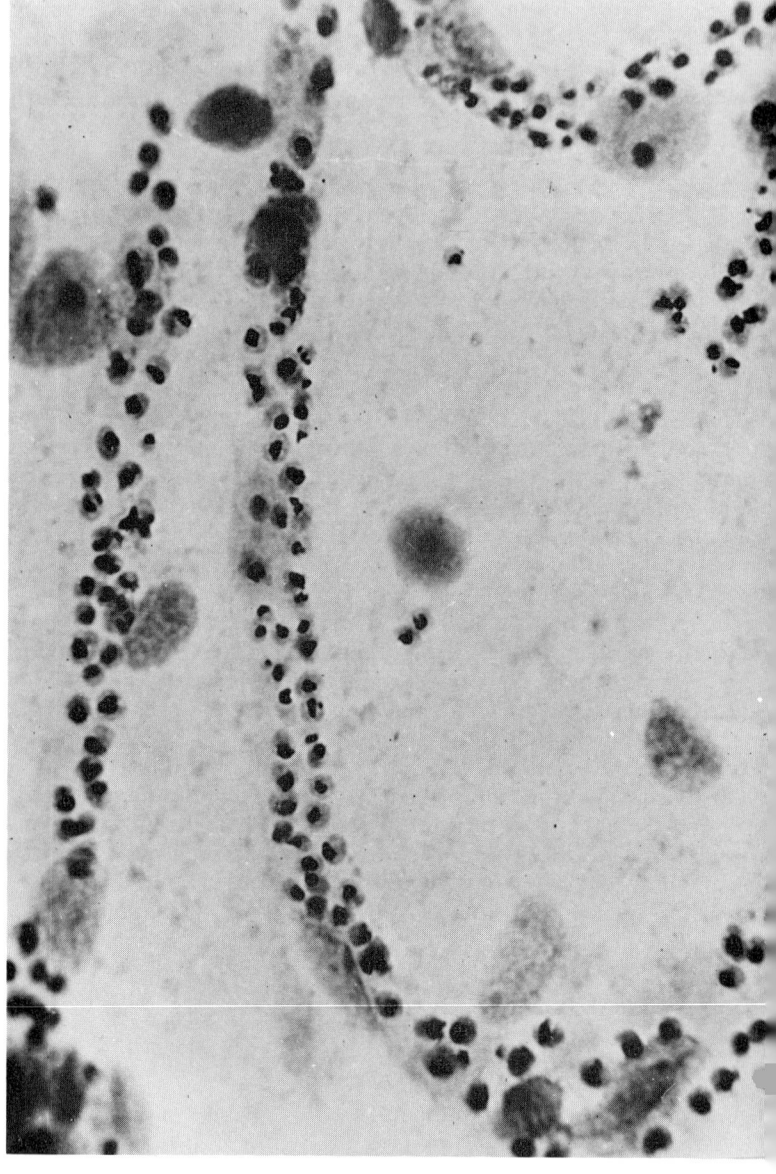

Fig 11 Blockage of capillaries of the brain by parasitised erythrocytes in a case of fatal *P. falciparum* malaria. Magnification × 650 (Wellcome Museum of Medical Science)

ring haemorrhages around the blocked arterioles and numerous petechial haemorrhages in the sub-cortical white matter of the cerebrum, brain stem and cerebellum; (3) Necrotic lesions in midzonal brain tissue with a peripheral reaction of small glial cells ('malarial granuloma') around an occluded capillary. (Fig. 12)

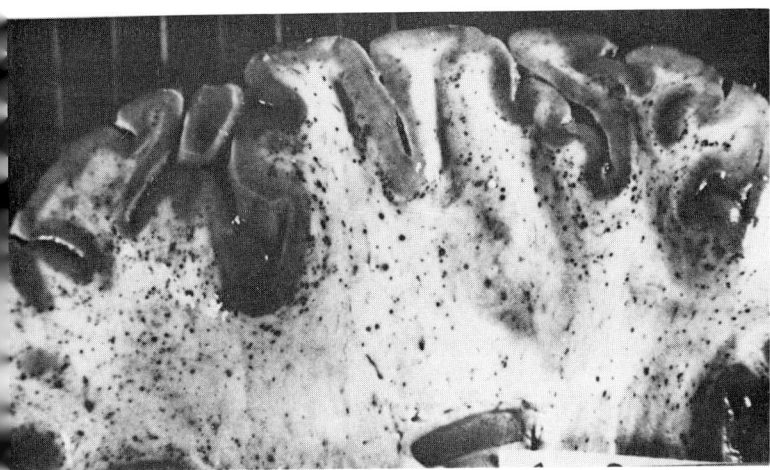

Fig 12   Diffuse petechial haemorrhages in the white matter of the brain. Oedema, vascular congestion, peri-vascular haemorrhages and thrombosis of capillaries by clumps of parasitised erythrocytes. (Dr Gabriel Toro, National Institute of Health, Bogotá, Colombia)

The physiopathology of these changes is very complex. It has been demonstrated that obstruction of the circulation in the capillaries of the brain occurs before the 'plugging' by infected red blood cells takes place. There is an early alteration of the endothelial permeability with escape of proteins to the perivascular spaces. Recent studies suggest that the antigenic challenge of *P. falciparum* produces a form of hyperergic reaction of the central nervous system with various stages of vasculomyelinopathy. This may explain the beneficial effects of corticosteroids for the treatment of cerebral malaria.

The spleen is always affected in malaria. The main change is that of congestion, but later the organ becomes dark from the accumulation of pigment in parasitised cells in the capillaries and sinusoids. Parasitised and apparently normal cells and also haemozoin granules are seen in the pulp histiocytes and sinusoidal lining cells. Pigment is also seen free or in giant phagocytic cells. Other findings are diffuse cellular hyperplasia, dilated sinuses and occasional thrombi in capillaries and foci of necrosis in the splenic pulp. On long exposure to the infection the connective tissue is increased.

The liver is swollen and dark in colour. The Kupffer cells are large, numerous and contain pigment. Capillaries are distended with macrophages, parasitised cells and pigment. Degeneration and necrosis in the centro-lobular regions are commonly seen. This is probably due to local anoxia as a result of stagnation of local circulation. While in the acute phase of malaria haemozoin shows a diffuse distribution in the Kupffer cells of the liver, in repeated infections followed by an immune response haemozoin is concentrated in the Kupffer cells of the periportal tract.

In kidneys any severe *P. falciparum* infection causes congestion and punctate haemorrhages in the cortex and medulla. Acute diffuse glomerulonephritis has been described, but is transient. In the *nephrotic syndrome* associated with *P. malariae* there are focal hyalinising lesions of the tuft of the glomerulus and segmental endothelial cell proliferation. Thickening of capillary walls of the basal membrane is due to the deposition at this site of antigen-antibody complexes. This has been revealed by fluorescent antibody tests on sections of affected kidneys.

Bone marrow changes are similar to those seen in the spleen but less marked. There is erythroblastic hyperplasia with large eosinophilic normoblastic cells.

There may be intense localisation of the parasites in any part of the *gastro-intestinal tract* leading to local oedema, haemorrhages and even ulceration.

The placenta shows an enormous concentration of *P. falciparum*. Developing and mature schizonts are numerous in the intervillous spaces, especially next to the stratum spongiosum, and there is much pigment within the fibrin masses occasionally surrounding degenerate villi. There is an increase of histiocytes in the maternal side of the placenta. The effect of the infection of the placenta is often seen in the low birth-weight of the baby.

Clinical pathology

The clinical pathology in an attack of malaria is mainly related to the effect of the blood and blood-forming organs. There is always some poikilocytosis, polychromasia, and other signs of anaemia. Leucocytosis may occur in the early stage and be followed by leucopenia and monocytosis. The polymorphonuclear count shows a shift to the left. The platelets are diminished and there is some depletion of coagulation factors. However intravascular coagulation is relatively rare and occurs as a late phenomenon. A reticulocyte response follows the treatment. Total plasma proteins are reduced with an alteration of the albumin/globulin ratio. As a result of destruction of red blood cells there is an increase of urobilinogen in the urine. Blood sugar levels rise during pyrexia. The erythrocyte sedimentation rate is generally increased.

Clinical evidence showed that there is no direct relationship between the number of parasites found in the peripheral blood and the course of cerebral malaria.

Transient increase in serum creatinine, blood urea nitrogen and reversal of the urinary sodium/potassium ratio are frequently reported.

If dysfunction of the liver occurs (in falciparum malaria) there is bilirubin in the plasma and urine. The van den Bergh reaction is indirect or direct depending on the liver damage. Hepatic function tests may show some deviation from the normal; cerebro-spinal fluid pressure is raised and protein increased in severe falciparum infection.

Albumin, red blood cells, hyaline and granular casts may be present when acute renal dysfunction develops; chloride concentration is low whenever renal tubules have been damaged.

The volume of urine must always be recorded to ensure the early diagnosis of oliguria. The presence of haemoglobin in urine of patients with *P. falciparum* infection does not always imply an abnormality of renal function. It means that consequent on the rapid lysis of erythrocytes the plasma haptoglobin levels have been exceeded and that free haemoglobin or the products of its breakdown are being excreted by the kidney. Decreased production of urine does not necessarily lead to overt uraemia in malaria: the acute renal insufficiency is a functional abnormality leading to derangement in electrolyte balance and other symptoms.

It should be emphasised that the whole clinico-pathological picture of the malaria infection is of great complexity. This was presented in a masterly way by Maegraith who pointed out that while the malaria parasite initiates the disease process, the subsequent events depend on many internal and external factors, including functional humoral and cellular responses as well as the nutritional state of the host.

Thus the dynamics of the blood circulation are disturbed, the blood flow in the liver, kidneys and other organs is slowed down, the medullary and cortical blood supplies to the adrenal glands get out of balance, there is interference with the absorption through the intestinal wall. There are upsets in the endocrinal equilibrium and in the general metabolism. Pharmacologically active substances including kinins[1] affect the permeability of the vascular endothelium leading to further changes of the blood flow and subsequent anoxia.

---

[1] A number of mammalian proteinaze enzymes known as kallikreins have important biological properties. Found in plasma, tissues and urine they act, when activated, on the alpha-globulin to form kinins, such as bradykinin, which have been implicated in inflammatory conditions and in shock. Kinins are hypotensive, they increase capillary permeability and cause the release of biologically active substances such as catecholamines, histamine and prostaglandins. They are also involved in blood coagulation, fibrinolysis and the activity of the complement.

Studies of simian and rodent malaria have shown the biochemical and structural damage inflicted on the liver and kidney cells by various soluble factors circulating in the blood. The respiration and oxidative phosphorylation of mitochondria isolated from these cells are inhibited and there are marked defects in their organellae.

Altogether the whole circulatory hormonal and metabolic balance of the body is disturbed and the effects of this, at first transient may eventually become irreversible and lead to the characteristic pathological effects seen in the tissues of individual organs.

IMMUNE RESPONSES IN MALARIA

Malaria immunity may be defined as the state of resistance to the infection brought about by all those processes which are involved in destroying the plasmodia or in limiting their multiplication. It also comprises the factors which modify the effects of the invasion of the organism by malaria parasites and aid in the repair of damaged tissues.

There are two types of immunity, natural and acquired. *Natural immunity* to malaria is an inherent property of the host, a refractory state or an immediate inhibitory response to the introduction of the parasite, not dependent on any previous infection with it. An example of such a state is the innate resistance of man to avian or rodent plasmodia. Another example is the relative refractoriness of persons of African origin to the infection with *P. vivax*. Both innate and acquired immunity ultimately depend on the genetic constitution of the host.

It has been postulated that the relative insusceptibility of West African and American blacks to infection with *P. vivax* is due to the extreme rarity of Duffy group blood determinants (Fy^a and F^b) in these populations, while they are common in other racial groups. This suggests that these determinants may be erythrocyte receptors for *P. vivax*.

Other genetic aspects of resistance to some types of malaria infections should be considered here. The high incidence of the abnormal haemoglobin S (Hb S or sickle cell haemoglobin) in many parts of the world, but particularly in Africa, was difficult to explain since this genetic defect is often lethal in its homozygous expression (SS) as in sickle cell anaemia, though apparently relatively harmless in its heterozygous expression (AS), which results in the sickling of erythrocytes when the oxygen tension is low. The similarity of the geographical distribution of haemoglobin S (HbS) and holoendemic falciparum malaria was striking and it has been suggested that the maintenance of the high frequency of HbS in the population might be due to the selective advantage that the heterozygote enjoyed against the adverse effects of *P. falciparum* malaria. Such hypothesis of balanced polymorphism of this genetic abnormality is now generally accepted. This means that a high gene frequency for a harmful mutant is maintained in some parts of the world by a strong selection pressure. HbS appears to protect infants against the lethal effects of falciparum malaria: this accounts for the frequency of this abnormality in Africa. The mechanism whereby the sickle-cell haemoglobin partially protects its bearer from the severe effects of falciparum malaria is not fully understood, but it appears that the malaria parasites do not grow well in HbS containing erythrocytes; moreover the infected erythrocyte which shows a tendency to sickling when the oxygen tension is lowered is disposed of faster by the macrophages and other cells of the reticulo-endothelial system.

There is no clear evidence that other genetic variants of haemoglobin such as HbC, HbF (fetal), thalassemia or HbE in South-East Asia confer a protection against falciparum malaria.

It has also been postulated that the genetic deficiency of an enzyme – the glucose-6-phosphate dehydrogenase (G6PD) – also exerts a protective effect against severe infection with *P. falciparum*. This red cell enzyme defect appears to be harmless unless the red cells are challenged in some way, usually by the exposure to various drugs (including sulphonamides and primaquine). G6PD deficiency is inherited as a sex-linked trait with full expression in males. There are many variants of this enzymopathy. The evidence of the protective effect of G6PD deficiency against malaria of heterozygotes is not as strong as for haemoglobin S, but generally accepted. It appears that this effect is evident in females heterozygous for the X-linked G6PD gene.

The mechanism by means of which a genetic characteristic of the erythrocyte of the host can increase a natural resistance to malaria is complex. Three possibilities have been envisaged: (1) Intracellular factors of the red blood cell can affect penetration of the merozoite: (2) The same factors can impede the intracellular development of the parasite: (3) Parasitised cells can be more readily removed from the circulation by the action of the lymphoid-macrophage system. From the available evidence the presence of G6PD deficiency may be related to the first two mechanisms while in the case of haemoglobin S the third mechanism is more likely.

The study of immune responses in malaria has made remarkable progress during the past few years and only a few essential points of this rapidly growing discipline can be given here.

Acquired immunity may be either active or passive. Active immunity is an enhancement of the defence mechanism of the host as a result of a previous encounter with the pathogen. *Passive immunity* is conferred by the pre-natal or post-natal transfer of protective substances from mother to child or by the injection of such substances contained in the serum of immune persons. There is evidence of such *congenital (or neo-natal) immunity* in new-born babies of highly immune mothers in endemic malarious areas of the world. The protection acquired by a host against subsequent reinfection with the homologous strain of the relevant species of the malaria parasite and maintained for variable periods of time is known as *residual immunity*.

In endemic areas where transmission of malaria continues throughout the greater part of the year the population develops and maintains a high degree of immune response while at the same time allowing the nearly permanent presence of small numbers of malaria parasites in many subjects. This state of resistance in a previously infected host often coupled with asymptomatic parasitaemia is known as *premunition*. Such a state of collective immunity is slowly acquired so that infants and young children may suffer severely and many of them die. Those, however, who survive to the adult age show little evidence of adverse effects of the attenuated infection.

The immunity acquired following an infection with any of the four species of human malaria parasites is species-specific. This means that a degree of protection acquired against one species of plasmodium may not be effective against parasites of the different species. Moreover there is evidence that some strains of parasites of one species may have a different antigenic composition from other strains and thus the immune response may be strain-specific.

Immunity in malaria is directed against the asexual erythrocytic forms of the parasite but not necessarily against sporozoites, pre-or exo-erythrocytic forms or gametocytes.

In addition to the immunological consequences of infection by some distinct strains within one species of human plasmodia there is a probability that the malaria parasite may undergo changes in its antigenic structure and so evade the immune defences of the host. This antigenic variation has been demonstrated in simian malaria but its existence in human infection has not been proved.

The physical basis of malaria immunity depends on the activity of both *humoral and cellular factors*, though the physiological condition of the host also plays some, albeit little known, part.

The humoral factors are represented by *antibodies* which appear in the blood. These comprise opsonins, precipitins, agglutinins, but the most important protective antibodies are carried on the gamma-globulin fractions of the serum. The cellular factors are macrophages and other cells produced by the reticulo-endothelial (lymphoid-macrophage) system of the spleen, liver and bone-marrow which undergoes intense proliferation following the malaria infection. The phagocytic activity of these cells which dispose of a large number of parasites has been well recognised as one of the main mechanisms of

Pathology and Immunology of Human Malaria

defence. However, recently the interdependence of cellular and humoral factors has become better known.

Today the tendency is to view the immune response as an *integrated phenomenon*, the main points of which may need a brief explanation.

When an antigen enters the body, two types of immune response may occur, both of which depend upon circulating small lymphocytes. The cell-mediated response depends upon sensitised lymphocytes with antibody-like molecules on their surface. The humoral antibody response consists of the synthesis and release of immunoglobulins into the blood and tissue fluids.

The thymus gland consists of lymphoid and epithelial cells, and acts on primitive lymphocytes from the bone-marrow to make them immunologically competent. Such lymphocytes are known as T-cells and are responsible for cell-mediated immune responses. They also help the antigenic stimulation of B lymphocytes to be more effective. The term B lymphocytes is related to the bursa of Fabricius.

The bursa of Fabricius is situated in association with the terminal end of the gut in chickens. It is similar in structure to the thymus, and is derived from gut epithelium. The bursa is responsible for the development of immuno-competence in cells that will synthesise humoral antibody. The bursa equivalent in man has not been clearly defined, although lymphoid tissue associated with the gut, such as the tonsils or Peyer's patches, may fulfil this role.

Hence the two populations of small lymphocytes comprise T-cells that are dependent on the thymus and are responsible for cell-mediated immunity, and B-cells which depend upon the equivalent of the bursa in man and synthesise circulating antibody. T-cells have a smooth outer membrane, while B-cells have numerous surface projections. Immunoglobulins are demonstrable on the surface of B-cells, but not on T-cells (Fig. 13).

The evidence that T-cells have a significant immune function in human malaria is not strong and the results of studies on experimental animals must be interpreted with caution.

Plasmodial antigens are taken up by macrophages and probably modified in some way before they stimulate lymphocytes that are either thymus-dependent (T-cells) or thymus-independent B-cells. T-cells form the majority of circulating lymphocytes and are long lived. When stimulated by the modified antigen they undergo transformation to lymphoblasts which are cytotoxic to plasmodia and release soluble factors (lymphokinins). Some of these factors act on the B lymphocytes which are involved in antibody production. B-cells give rise to plasma cells which synthesise the immunoglobulins and antibodies. In addition to the T-cells and B-cells other substances such as the complement fractions are needed to produce the full immune response.

In the immune sequences that occur following a malaria infection the role of macrophages in spleen, liver and bone-marrow is the earliest feature but the process of conveyance of malarial antigens to T-cells and B-cells is still obscure.

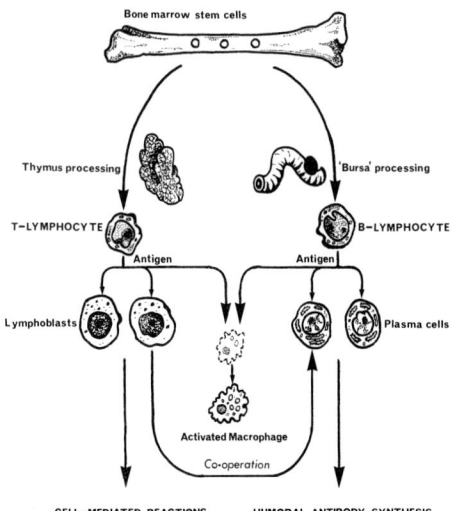

Fig 13 Diagram of two types of immune response by two populations of lymphocytes originating from the bone-marrow stem cells. (Modified from Roitt, 1971)

Two processes fundamental to the action of antibody are complement activation and phagocytosis by the polymorphonuclear neutrophils. Complement is a complicated chain of enzymes of which nine components and several side chains have been recognised. Complement is activated when it becomes attached to antibody already combined with the antigen. It seems that one of the actions of an activated complement is the lysis of cell walls bearing the antigen to which the antibody is fixed.

Malaria antibodies have been detected in sera of infected persons thanks to the availability of indirect fluorescent antibody test and immunoprecipitation or other techniques.

The gammaglobulin fraction of serum contains five types of immunoglobulin, IgG, IgM, IgA, IgD and IgE. Structurally, antibody consists of two heavy and two light peptide chains linked by disulphide bonds. Each major type of heavy chain gives rise to one distinct class of immunoglobulin.

IgG antibodies (7S antibody type) represent the most effective immunoglobulin in internal body fluids, particularly in extravascular situations where it binds with micro-organisms, thus ensuring that their phagocytosis is enhanced. A complex of bacteria or other pathogens plus IgG adheres to phagocytes which have specialised surface receptors for IgG. IgG is believed to cross the placenta to provide a major line of defence against infection in the neonatal period.

IgA appears in saliva, tears, nasal fluid, sweat, colostrum and secretions of the lung and intestine. It is thus a major defence for exposed surfaces against micro-organisms. IgA is synthesised locally by plasma cells.

IgM (19S antibody type) antibodies are efficient agglutinating and cytolytic agents. They appear early in the immune response to infection and are largely confined to the blood stream.

IgD was recognised through the analysis of a myeloma protein. Its antibody activity is not clear.

Only very low concentration of IgE immunoglobulin are present in the serum; these antibodies are probably bound to mast cells with release of vasoactive amines. This process is responsible for hay fever when patients with an allergy come into contact with pollen. The physiological role of IgE is not certain, but the serum level rises after infection with helminths.

The synthesis of the various immunoglobulins proceeds at different rates. The IgM response occurs early, and tends to fall off rapidly. IgG antibody builds up over a longer period of time, but on secondary challenge the acceleration is faster and at a much higher titre. The same probably holds for IgA. These immunoglobulin classes provide the main defence against foreign antigens. Feed-back mechanisms limit antibody production after antigenic stimulation has ceased. The simplest explanation is that the antibody blocks the antigenic determinant needed for lymphocyte stimulation, but many other factors are undoubtedly involved.

Specific activity of malarial antibody has been confirmed in various degrees in all three immunoglobulins: IgG, IgM and IgA. No specific malarial antibody activity has been detected in IgD and IgE immunoglobulins.

Prolonged exposure to malaria results in high serum levels of IgG which contains protective substances; they seem to have their antiplasmodial effect at the time of schizogony of the parasite when the merozoites escape from the erythrocyte. The role of IgM in malaria infection is little known, though it is possible that it is particularly important in young children.

Studies made in non-immune volunteers showed that serum concentrations of IgG, IgA and IgM rose shortly after the beginning of parasitaemia; IgG and IgM increased more than IgA, while IgG immunoglobulin persisted longer.

Although the specific protective anti-plasmodial factor forms only a small part of the IgG immunoglobulin it can be transmitted passively by the injection of a large amount of the IgG fraction of immune human serum. Moreover, in sera from African newborn, who possess some transient resistance to malaria infection, the IgG immunoglobulin transmitted from the immune mother across the placenta was present in considerable amount.

The four species of human plasmodia have a number of common antigens. Within each species the antigens related to the developmental phase are also similar, but not identical. Precise information on the qualitative and quantitative antigenic differences that exist between species and between the phases of the life-cycle in one species still eludes us. The most complete information concerning antigenicity of a parasite is available for *P. falciparum* in which over 30 distinct antigens have been found by McGregor.

A number of soluble *antigen fractions* in *P. falciparum* infections have been identified, and classified into L (labile), R (resistant) and S (stable) on the basis of their susceptibility to heat. It seems that L and R antigens are of plasmodial origin. Each of the three classes of antigens has been subdivided into sub-groups on the basis of other factors.

In vitro studies have shown that the antigens increase in number and amount as the parasite matures. Sera from patients with severe *P. falciparum* infections contain mainly S-antigens and more rarely R-antigens: L-antigens have not been recovered from sera.

The working of protective immunity to malaria is seen best in holoendemic areas of tropical Africa. Although infection of the placenta is frequent, congenital malaria is rare because of the prenatal transfer of specific IgG antibodies from the maternal blood across the placenta. Such passively acquired immunity is transient and after the first year of life many young children have high parasitaemia; severe clinical illness leads to a high fatality rate. In older children clinical illness is less common while enlarged spleen and parasitaemia remain prevalent; in adults parasitaemia becomes infrequent and of low density; clinical illness is rare; palpable spleen enlargement is uncommon.

Antibodies are found in high prevalence and titre in sera from newborn infants. In the early months of life antibodies decay and their titre becomes low. Around the third year of life, in response to infection, the prevalence and titre of antibodies rise slowly to a peak and maintains a high level in older age-groups. Such age-related pattern of antibody profiles in various populations forms a valuable method for the assessment of malaria endemicity and for evaluation of the efficacy of malaria control activities.

IMMUNOPATHOLOGY

A number of pathological conditions related to malaria infection are recognised today as being the consequences of immune response to the infection.

Anaemia. The degree of anaemia following the plasmodial infection is greater than can be explained by simple destruction of erythrocytes by parasites. The mechanism of such an effect is not clear, but two possibilities exist: (a) production of a toxic factor or auto-antibodies to the erythrocytes; (b) adherence of circulating antigen-antibody complexes to uninfected erythrocytes and haemolysis through the effect of the complement. However, neither the presence of a toxic haemolysin nor a respective antibody could be demonstrated in sera of children with acute malaria and anaemia. It seems that the main factor responsible for such anaemia is the direct destruction of infected erythrocytes by malaria parasites and increased erythro-phagocytosis of normal cells by the lymphoid-macrophage system. Nevertheless, the evidence of a complement mediated cell destruction cannot be dismissed. Even after complete clearance of malaria parasites a degree of haemolysis continues for about a month.

Nephropathies. Immune complexes play an important part in the pathogenesis of adverse effects of malaria infections on the kidneys. Two main types of lesions have been observed in man and have also been demonstrated in experimental animals: (1) Acute and reversible lesions typical of *P. falciparum* infections with relatively mild clinical symptoms[1] and (2) Chronic and progressive lesions characteristic of *P. malariae* infections and generally with severe symptoms.

In the acute forms of glomerulonephritis and nephrotic syndrome which occur during the course of *P. falciparum* infections, renal biopsies show deposits of immunoglobulins (mainly IgM), complement and malarial antigen. These immune complexes clear relatively rapidly after proper antimalaria treatment. In the chronic progressive lesions, accompanied by persistent proteinuria, gradually deteriorating renal function and hypertension, the renal biopsies show the coarse and fine deposit of immunoglobulins (IgG, IgM), complement and *P. malariae* antigens in the glomerular capillary walls. Specific antimalarial treatment has little or no effect but fairly good responses to prednisolone, azathioprine and cyclophosphamide were reported in some cases.

Only some subjects with *P. malariae* infection suffer from 'quartan malaria nephrosis' characterised by heavy proteinuria, hypoalbuminaemia and pronounced oedema. Immunological studies showed that

---

[1] Severe renal failure with oliguria and retention of urea may occur in patients with heavy infections of *P. falciparum*. The pathogenesis of such lesions is probably similar to that of blackwater fever.

this condition is consistent with the hypothesis that glomerular damage is due to a deposition of specific antigen-antibody complexes in the glomeruli; this effect continues probably as a result of auto-immune response to damaged tissue.

Tropical splenomegaly syndrome (T.S.S.). This is the term for the presence of very large spleens of undetermined aetiology in an endemic malarious environment. Alternative terms are *'big spleen disease'* or *'idiopathic splenomegaly'*. Cases of T.S.S. have been reported from Nigeria, Sudan, Uganda, Zambia, Zaïre, some other African countries, Viet-Nam and New Guinea.

The syndrome is seen most often in young adults. Together with the grossly enlarged spleen there is an enlargement of the liver with a degree of portal hypertension. The patient usually has anaemia, leucopenia and thrombocytopenia. The IgM level is high and this is almost always associated with a high malaria antibody titre. There is lymphocytic infiltration of the hepatic sinusoids and periportal fibrosis.

The diagnosis of tropical splenomegaly is by exclusion of some specific disorders causing a grossly enlarged spleen (typhoid, chronic brucellosis, schistosomiasis, kala-azar, hepatic cirrhosis, sickle cell anaemia), but also chronic lymphatic leukaemia and malignant lymphoma. There is no evidence of any genetic pre-disposition and the real cause of this syndrome is obscure, though the presence of endemic malaria is a common background picture of the environment. However, only a small proportion of people exposed to malaria develop T.S.S., so that several additional factors are involved. Some patients, but by no means all, respond to long-term treatment.

It is possible that in this syndrome there is an overproduction of IgM together with a non-specific mitogenic effect of malaria parasites on the splenic tissue.

Immunosuppressive effect of malaria

It has been recently observed that malaria may suppress some immune responses. Thus field studies in West Africa showed the partial suppression of antibody responses to tetanus toxoid, or to Salmonella typhi (O antigen only) and this suggests a defect in macrophage processing of antigens. Experimental studies on rodent malaria suggest that acute malaria has an enhancing effect on the infection with the Moloney lymphomagenic virus. These studies seem to support the hypothesis linking the frequency of Burkitt's lymphoma and the Epstein-Barr virus to malaria infection and its suppressive effect on the antibody response to some viruses. Malaria may also act at a cellular level, causing hyperplasia of the lymphoid-macrophage system suitable for proliferation of the Epstein-Barr virus.

Malaria, by affecting the normal immune response to unrelated antigens may have a profound effect on the health of children in the tropics. Moreover the infection may be followed by serological changes which in temperate climates are related to connective tissue disease (*e.g.* rheumatoid factor – an antiglobulin to IgG). The usual indicators of auto-immune disease must be interpreted with caution in malarious areas.

IMMUNISATION AGAINST MALARIA

Early work on the immune response to malaria infection of experimental animals and man led to the studies on the possibility of producing a malaria vaccine, similar in action to the principle of immunisation against bacterial diseases. It was intended to base it on the development of attenuated strains of plasmodia capable of stimulating immunity to virulent strains. Attenuated forms of malaria parasites of experimental animals have been prepared by various methods. Among these one should mention exposure of plasmodia to physical effects, including UV light and irradiation, passage through unusual hosts, action of drugs or immune serum and *in vitro* cultivation.

Promising results were obtained in avian and rodent malaria; the attenuated plasmodia conferred some degree of resistance on the host so that a challenge of the experimental animals with non-attenuated parasites resulted in lower parasitaemia, longer survival and in some cases significant protection from otherwise fatal infection.

During the past ten years an immense amount of scientific work was devoted to the problem of immunisation against malaria and only a brief review of the present state of knowledge can be given here.

It is obvious that the complex cycle of development of malaria parasites in man and in the mosquito offers several points for immunological interference with the multiplication of plasmodia in man and with their transmission through the Anopheles.

Blocking of sporozoite entry into the body or prevention of growth of the tissue phase in the liver; interruption of asexual development in the erythrocytes; elimination of gametocytes or interference with their infectivity to the mosquito. Any of these stages may lend itself to the prospective vaccine just as each stage responds to the action of specific antimalarial drugs.

It was desirable that the effect of the new immunological weapon should extend to all four species of malaria parasites of man even though *P. falciparum* causes the highest mortality and morbidity.

Following on successful experiments with vaccination of rodents using sporozoites of *P. berghei* an attempt was made to develop a vaccine for the human *P. falciparum*. This was done by x-ray irradiation of large numbers of infected mosquitos, which then were fed on human volunteers over a period of months. When challenged by non-irradiated infected Anopheles, some of the volunteers were protected against the infection. This artificially induced active immunity lasted for three months and was species-specific or homologous viz. gave no protection against *P. vivax.*

In contradistinction to the work on the sporozoite vaccine which was attempted recently on human subjects, most of the experimental studies on vaccination against erythrocytic forms of plasmodia was done on monkeys using *P. knowlesi* although lately *P. falciparum* was also used.

Already in the 1940s a vaccine consisting of killed erythrocytic forms of *P. knowlesi* emulsified in Freund's complete adjuvant (a complex mixture of killed mycobacteria emulsified in water and oil) showed some protective effect in rhesus monkeys. More recently it was shown that merozoites isolated from an *in vitro* culture of *P. knowlesi* and combined with Freund's complete adjuvant produced, after injection into rhesus monkeys, not only a high degree of protection lasting for over a year, but also an effect against the antigenic variants of *P. knowlesi*. A further important step was a successful vaccination of Aotus monkeys using *P. falciparum* merozoites in conjunction with Freund's complete adjuvant.

Some newer studies showed that the use of an antigen composed of a mixture of asexual trophozoites and micro- and macrogametocytes produces anti-gamete antibodies which blocked the sexual development of the malaria parasite within the body of the mosquito that fed on immunised animals. Thus such mosquitos are not infected and are not capable of further transmission of malaria.

These important steps in the development of a prospective vaccine against human malaria were recently followed by a striking success of Trager in the USA who achieved a continuous *in vitro* culture of the human *P. falciparum*. This opens the way to the preparation of large amounts of antigen against the most virulent form of malaria infection of man.

However the practical obstacles on the way to a fully successful, potent and safe malaria vaccine are very considerable.

The difficulty in obtaining large quantities of attenuated sporozoites from infected mosquitos is evident. Secondly, the immunity achieved is shortlived and does not always extend to the erythrocytic infection of different strains or other species of plasmodia.

Problems facing the merozoite based prospective vaccine are not less difficult. The success achieved in monkey malaria requires the use of an adjuvant different from Freund's complete formula, which has serious side effects in man. Furthermore, we need better understanding of the role of the new adjuvants in the complex immune process involving humoral and cellular factors, which act together in the body defences against the infection. Since there are no satisfactory experimental animals that can be regularly infected with *P. falciparum* the testing of the prospective vaccine on human subjects presents daunting technical and ethical issues.

The practical problems facing the development of either the sporozoite or the merozoite-gametocyte vaccine are still formidable. Although the scientific advances of applied immunology have opened now possibilities for prevention and cure of malaria the final goal is not yet within our reach, though it gets closer every year.

MALARIAL HAEMOGLOBINURIA (BLACKWATER FEVER)

Malarial haemoglobinuria commonly known as blackwater fever is essentially a syndrome of acute intravascular haemolysis accompanied by haemoglobinaemia and haemoglobinuria, occurring typically in individuals who have experienced repeated and severe attacks of falciparum malaria. It is characterised by an abrupt onset, passage of dark red or almost black urine, vomiting of bile-stained fluid, jaundice, early prostration and a high mortality. It is known in other than English speaking countries under various names such as fièvre bilieuse hémoglobinurique, Schwarzwasser Fieber, Vomito negro etc. It is likely that many descriptions of this syndrome in the past were confused with yellow fever and with severe attacks of 'bilious remittent' malaria.

Few morbid conditions have been the subject of so many conjectures as blackwater fever. The literature dealing with the subject is voluminous, but most of the known facts regarding its nature, aetiology and prophylaxis were established or confirmed by Stephens and Christophers as the result of their classical researches in West and Central Africa at the beginning of this century. At that time and for many years afterwards blackwater fever was a cause of high mortality and disability among British and Asian expatriates in that region. Stephens and Christophers showed that the syndrome was brought about by exposure to severe and long-continued malarial infection, which induces a condition of unstable equilibrium in the blood, so that quinine or any other determining factor can precipitate an attack; the type of malaria most frequently associated with it was that produced by *P. falciparum*. They deduced from these findings that the most effective method of preventing the disease was to institute vigorous malaria control measures. Much of the pathology of blackwater fever was elucidated more recently by Maegraith.

The condition is comparable (if not identical) with an exacerbation of intravascular haemolysis seen sometimes in severe malaria due to *P. falciparum* although in typical cases of blackwater fever parasites may be scanty or absent in the peripheral blood.

Epidemiology

Broadly speaking the geographical distribution of blackwater fever corresponds with that of holo- and hyperendemic falciparum malaria. In south-east Asia it was common in the foothill tracts where transmission of malaria is possible throughout the greater part of the year; but it was never met with in the north-west plains of India, which have a short transmission season, and are visited periodically by widespread regional malaria epidemics of great severity. Similarly the condition is found in many parts of tropical Africa, while in North Africa it is extremely rare.

Blackwater fever does not occur outside the geographical distribution of malaria, except in individuals who have been infected elsewhere. Its occurrence is related to conditions favouring the transmission of the disease throughout the greater part of the year. Conversely, the disappearance of blackwater fever is one of the earliest indications of successful control of malaria in such regions. Non-immune immigrants are the most frequent victims of the disease, which, though not unknown, is comparatively rare among indigenous populations of highly malarious countries. Age and sex have no bearing on the incidence of blackwater fever, though it is less common in children.

There has been a marked reduction in the incidence of blackwater fever in tropical Africa in recent years, probably because of the regular drug prophylaxis now widely adopted and since the use of synthetic antimalarials has replaced the quinine prophylaxis.

Pathogenesis

The general theory is that following repeated attacks of malaria and the consequent destruction of red blood cells an auto-immune factor is formed which induces haemolysis. It has been suggested that the presence of the parasite changes the antigenic structure of individual erythrocytes and stimulates the production of antibodies which in conjunction with the complement lead to haemolysis. The fact is that in any autoimmune mechanism auto-antibodies might be detectable by the usual antiglobulin Coombs test. However, such antiglobulins were only rarely found in malarial anaemia.

The predisposing factors of blackwater fever are, as mentioned before, repeated infections with *P. falciparum*. Among the precipitating factors exposure to cold, excessive physical exertion and other stresses such as over-indulgence in alcohol have been cited; the last named very likely owes its notoriety to the neglect of regular drug prophylaxis and other antimalarial precautions. Irregular therapeutic and suppressive dosage with antimalarial drugs, particularly quinine, is an important factor in many cases. It should be remembered that quinine has a slight haemolytic action and some persons have an individual intolerance of this drug.

Pathology

The most striking phenomenon in blackwater fever is the rapid and severe haemolysis of both parasitised and unparasitised erythrocytes. This may occur only once or may recur spasmodically at intervals of hours or days. Occasionally the initial haemolysis is continuous and overwhelming and may cause death from extremem anaemia. In less severe forms the destruction of erythrocytes is often very rapid; sometimes a million or more cells per 1 μl are destroyed in the course of 24 hours.

The gross pathological picture is not unlike that seen in severe falciparum malaria but haemozoin is less marked in the reticulo-endothelial system and lesions in the central nervous system are uncommon. Heavy parasitaemia is rarely seen in the peripheral circulation. When the lysis of red blood cells occurs and the amount of free haemoglobin in the plasma exceeds 100 mg/100 ml (up to this concentration haemoglobin can be bound by haptoglobins which constitute a major portion of alpha-globulins) other mechanisms come into play. Some haemoglobin combines with albumin to form methaemalbumin which is found in the serum, but the unbound haemoglobin passes through the glomerular membrane and appears in the urine. Bilirubin, both conjugated and unconjugated, shows raised levels in the blood.

Kidney function may be affected at any stage of the disease. About half the deaths in blackwater fever are attributable to renal failure. The fundamental lesion is a renal vaso-construction with a juxtaglomerular shunt at the junction of the cortex and medulla, rendering the cortex and peripheral glomeruli ischaemic and causing marked changes in the tubules. A combination of reduced glomerular filtration, excessive tubular reabsorption and possibly nephron blockage finally results in anuria. Usually there is first a reduction in urine concentration, indicating tubular dysfunction. Commencing failure is evidenced by a reduction in urinary output. Severe oliguria may be succeeded by anuria associated with symptoms of acute uraemia. Recovery from this stage is rare.

The macroscopic appearance of the kidneys varies considerably. When acute uraemia has supervened, they are swollen, slightly oedematous and pale or yellowish-brown, depending on the amount of pigment present. The cortex is usually pale in relation to the medulla, in which there is some degree of congestion. This may be intense, but is often irregular and tends to affect particularly the region of the cortico-medullary junction and tips of the pyramids.

Histological changes are present in some degree in the kidneys even in cases when uraemia and anuria were not notable features. The changes are similar but less marked than in anuric cases and presumably arise from the same pathogenic process. There are few changes to be noted in the glomeruli. Some of them may be congested and there are occasionally haemorrhages into the tufts, but this is unusual. Amorphous hyaline material is usually present in the capsular space. The cortex is pale and relatively bloodless. The vessels in the medulla are irregularly congested and there are often haemorrhages into the interstitial tissue and sometimes into the tubules. Degenerative and necrotic lesions of the epithelial cells are frequent and are particularly marked in the distal convoluted tubules and the upper reaches of the ascending loops of Henle. In some cases the degenerating cells contain granules and globules of acidophilic hyaline or granular material. When haemorrhage has occurred into the lumen, the tubule is filled with erythrocytes.

Changes in the cortical tubules arise from local ischaemia and consequent anoxia, and the dysfunction thus produced is responsible for the changes in urinary concentration. The degree of tissue damage depends on the ultimate local tissue anoxia produced, together with the associated toxic effects of general anoxaemia resulting from anaemia and of the passage of haemoglobin and its products.

As emphasised by Maegraith, the importance of the concept, that the renal changes develop primarily from vascular phenomena, lies in the realisation that the process is basically a reversible one and independent of the reaction of the urine. Thus the former hypothesis of tubular blockage by haemoglobin precipitated by acidosis and the consequent suggestion of alkaline therapy is unfounded.

When the kidney tubules are involved there is some reduction in urine concentration. The chloride and urea concentrations are both low. In some cases the passage of unconcentrated urine is associated with polyuria; in the more severe forms with oliguria. It should be noted that measuring the specific gravity of the urine is not a reliable guide to its concentration, since high values will be obtained if haemoglobin or albumin is present.

The liver shows evidence of damage ranging from granular fatty change to advanced necrosis or atrophy. These changes particularly affect the cells in the central zone of the lobule; the more peripherally placed cells may be apparently unaffected or at most show some fatty change. The central vein and tributary sinusoids are widely dilated, and if lysis has not been too severe, are congested and filled with erythrocytes. Similar lesions are seen in many other conditions often associated with peripheral vascular failure. The pathological changes are thus not specific to blackwater fever.

Anaemia is of varying degree. The red cell count is often in the neighbourhood of one million or fewer erythrocytes per μl in severe cases. There are no obvious changes in the appearance of the red cells. Malaria parasites are detectable in less than 30% of cases after haemolysis has begun. In cases in which haemolysis has been severe it is unusual to find parasites; they are more likely to be found in the early stages before lysis has become extensive. The red cell count rises roughly in proportion to the loss of circulatory volume and the haemoglobin percentage with it. The count at any particular time may thus bear little relation to the true state of cell destruction. Biochemical changes in the blood depend on the associated organ syndromes. In nearly all cases the urea nitrogen concentration is raised, in uraemic cases to a very high level. Total blood and plasma chloride concentrations are usually low, especially after severe vomiting. Haemoglobin may often be detected in the blood during the lytic phase; sometimes bile pigments may be present in considerable excess. The van den Bergh reaction is usually indirect or biphasic, occasionally direct.

Vascular failure frequently occurs in blackwater fever and in fatal cases contributes materially to the pathological picture. The renal and hepatic anoxia described above may occur in shock and in 'crush syndrome'. Other features, such as the widespread capillary haemorrhages and stasis of the small blood vessels of the brain, often described in blackwater fever, are probably associated with general peripheral vascular collapse.

Clinical picture

There is usually a history of residence in the holo- or hyperendemic area of several months or more during which the patient has experienced repeated attacks of falciparum malaria, with symptoms of persistent headache, pains in the back and limbs and general ill-health between the attacks.

The onset of the syndrome proper is usually abrupt, with headache, nausea, vomiting of bile-stained fluid, severe pains in the loins and marked prostration. There is often a rigor, and the temperature usually rises to 38.9°C or 39.4°C (102°F or 103°F) or higher and is generally either continuous or remittent. Sometimes the temperature becomes intermittent with repeated rigors and heavy sweating between exacerbations of fever, and occasionally hyperpyrexia may develop. In other cases, in which shock develops, fever may be absent throughout.

Haemolysis may occur once only during the course of an attack or may recur spasmodically, at intervals varying from a few hours to several days, with clear intervals in between. In the haemolytic phase destruction of red cells may proceed very rapidly. Occasionally haemolysis becomes uncontrollable and overwhelming, but in other cases it may be mild.

In the haemolytic phase the urine contains varying proportions of oxyhaemoglobin and its derivatives, chiefly methaemoglobin, and is typically dark red to almost black from the onset, the colour depending on which pigment predominates. Oxyhaemoglobin is bright red and methaemoglobin brown; the former is in excess in alkaline urine, the latter in acid urine. As the lysis abates, each specimen of urine becomes less pigmented until finally clear. Albumin is present in high concentration throughout the lytic period, but when the pigment clears, the albumin usually disappears.

During haemoglobinuria there is always a thick greyish brown deposit in the urine containing hyaline and granular casts, amorphous epithelial debris and haemoglobin pigments. The urine passed during and for some days subsequent to haemolysis is unconcentrated so far as its electrolytes are concerned, although its specific gravity may be high. Its reaction may be acid, neutral or alkaline.

In the developed stage of the attack the patient is typically restless and anxious with a varying degree of dyspnoea and collapse. Prostration is marked from the onset, except in very mild cases, but the patient remains fully conscious till late in the illness, when he may pass into delirium or coma. Nausea and vomiting are common and are often very severe and intractable. Jaundice is a cardinal symptom and may appear a few hours after the onset of the attack. Pain in the epigastrium is sometimes very severe. The liver enlarges and the edge becomes palpable and often extremely tender. Severe hepatic failure may be accompanied by intractable hiccup, which is regarded as a bad prognostic sign. Petechial haemorrhages in the gums are sometimes present. The faeces are frequently watery and may contain bile.

In severe cases, and sometimes after an apparently mild lysis, the patient collapses and passes into a state of medical shock. The face is drawn and anxious, the eyes sunken, the skin inelastic and pale but usually moist. Restlessness and anxiety increase and death frequently occurs from peripheral vascular failure.

Diagnosis. The appearance of haemoglobinuria associated with a febrile paroxysm and rigor followed by severe anaemia in a subject who has been exposed to falciparum infection is highly suggestive of blackwater fever, particularly if accompanied by jaundice and vomiting.

Haemolysis may be induced in some subjects by quinine in the absence of malaria, but this is mild and unaccompanied by fever or serious symptoms. The 8-aminoquinoline class of drugs or sulphones may also precipitate haemolysis in persons with G6PD deficiency. This may occur in up to 20% of the populations of some parts of the world and a drug-induced haemolytic anaemia due to this enzyme deficiency must be excluded before a diagnosis of blackwater fever can be confirmed. Paroxysmal haemoglobinuria and favism may be excluded by careful consideration of the patient's history. Haemoglobinuria must be distinguished from haematuria due to schistosomiasis or Weil's disease, and from intense bilirubinuria. Spectroscopic and simple urinary tests should enable the differentiation from these conditions to be made without difficulty.

The liver dysfunction in blackwater fever with hepatic enlargement, tenderness and intense jaundice, especially in the temporary absence of haemoglobin from the urine may make diagnosis from Weil's disease, yellow fever or infectious hepatitis somewhat difficult. The absence of malaria parasites in the blood does not necessarily exclude blackwater fever.

Treatment. Owing to the excessive blood destruction associated with blackwater fever there is always grave risk of cardiac failure. Hence the first essentials in treatment are careful nursing and absolute rest. Oral or intravenous glucose should be given freely and every effort made to control vomiting. To counteract the restlessness of mind and body parenteral phenobarbitone, chlorpromazine or other sedatives and tranquillisers are recommended.

Vascular failure should be treated by intravenous plasma, followed if necessary by intravenous balanced salt solution, with isotonic glucose. The daily fluid intake should not be excessive, and should be adjusted to the urinary output.

If the erythrocyte count is below 2 million per µl blood transfusion is required. Great care is needed in cross matching red blood cells and serum of the donor and recipient. The volume of blood given must be adjusted to the degree of haemolysis. Prednisolone phosphate may help in containing the haemolysis; the daily dosage is 40 to 60 mg. Antimalarials are rarely required during the crisis but if the parasites are present chloroquine or proguanil should be given; quinine should preferably be avoided, but need not be excluded.

Renal failure must be considered when the daily volume of urine is less than 400 ml and the plasma urea concentration more than 100 mg per 100 ml. To determine this threshold it is necessary to record from the beginning the 24-hour output of urine, the volume of each specimen, its specific gravity (which can be low) and also the plasma urea concentration. The intake of fluids, electrolytes and protein must be watched. When the plasma urea concentration reaches 170–200 mg per 100 ml renal dialysis must be considered, especially if the patient had excessive fluid administration. If renal dialysis cannot be done peritoneal dialysis should be substituted using 6.3% dextrose with 0.56% sodium chloride and 2.6 mEq. potassium per litre.

The mortality rate varies greatly in different areas and is generally stated to be from 10 to 40%; but under unfavourable circumstances, such as during military operations, it may be very considerably higher than this. More than half the fatalities result from the renal failure; most of the others from hepatic or vascular failure.

The prognosis after recovery from an acute attack is good, but there is always a danger of further attacks if the subject is exposed to reinfection with *P. falciparum*.

Chapter 5

Diagnostic Methods in Malaria

A definite diagnosis of malaria infection is established on the finding of parasites in the blood. Malaria must be suspected in all cases of fever in endemic areas or in persons who have been exposed to the infection when visiting a tropical country even after spending a few hours at an exotic airport.

Tentative antimalarial treatment may be advisable when facilities for blood examination are not available or if a laboratory report cannot be obtained immediately. Even in this case, however, a blood slide should be taken for subsequent examination, before the treatment is administered. Failure to control the fever by carefully supervised administration of an adequate drug tends to exclude malaria as the cause of the disease unless resistance to a specific antimalarial is suspected.

Malaria may be confused with any other fever; a careful history and examination may reveal those in which symptoms and signs provide a firm basis of differentiation – respiratory and intestinal infections, tonsillitis and meningitis; the latter may occasion difficulties for several days, but an examination of the cerebro-spinal fluid permits a definite diagnosis. Surgical conditions such as a middle ear infection, an abscess or cellulitis usually direct attention to the affected part. A urinary infection is often misdiagnosed as malaria until the urine is examined. Even more difficult are the initial periods of fever in many virus diseases before the rash and other symptoms appear: measles, small-pox, chicken-pox, influenza, poliomyelitis and yellow fever. In fact, some of the virus infections do not cause distinctive physical signs and do not admit of a precise diagnosis on clinical grounds. In cases of continued fever, especially if there is no response to antimalarial therapy, there exist many possibilities: tuberculosis in all its manifestations, typhoid, typhus, liver abscess, urinary infections, endocarditis, brucellosis, relapsing fever, trypanosomiasis, kala-azar, severe blood disorders and rapidly growing tumours.

The diagnosis of malaria is always a matter of clinical judgement; it cannot be merely a matter of uncritically reading a laboratory report, however essential that examination may be. Sound judgement is a supreme virtue in the face of several apparently contradictory facts. Thus the detection of a few parasites in a blood film of a semi-immune indigenous child demonstrates the presence of infection, but it does not necessarily determine the actual disease for which medical aid was sought; this may vary from pneumonia to a fractured femur. On the other hand, many non-immunes take antimalarial drugs prophylactically and this (in the case of a breakthrough of malaria) considerably reduces the chance of detecting malaria parasites in the blood. A thorough search of one or several thick blood films should demonstrate parasites in such cases although occasionally the diagnosis of 'clinical malaria' appears justified, especially if fever rapidly subsides after the appropriate treatment. A similar situation is created if antimalarial drugs are given several hours before the examination of the blood. At this stage only the rapid disappearance of all clinical signs lends specious confirmation to the probable diagnosis. Non-immunes appear more ill in the presence of a scanty parasitaemia than do partially immunes who often appear to tolerate with relative equanimity a heavy parasite load. At all times one has to bear in mind the significance of the laboratory report, having regard to the time when the blood film was prepared and the relation to drug administration. One should also remember that many technical mistakes can arise in the long chain of events between the taking of the blood slide and the report on its examination.

The formerly advocated method of 'provocation' by sub-cutaneous injection of 0.5 ml of 1:1000 solution of adrenaline, which was supposed to produce a contraction of the spleen and the appearance of parasites in the blood, is of no value for the diagnosis of malaria and may be dangerous when used in patients with high blood pressure. This view has been recently confirmed by studies on malaria in Viet-Nam.

BLOOD EXAMINATION FOR MALARIA PARASITES

The only certain means of diagnosing malaria infection is the detection of the *Plasmodium* by microscopical examination of the blood. This examination should be a routine procedure in medical practice not only in all malarious areas, but also in non-malarious countries whatever may be the symptoms or primary diagnosis, if the patient was travelling abroad within a year.

The main reason for this is that the clinical picture of malaria may be of infinite variety; this infection may also occur as a result of blood transfusion from an infected donor or it may be a complicating factor of other diseases. One should remember that the presence of malaria parasites in the blood is a sign of *infection* but not necessarily a cause of the *disease*; persons who have resided for many years in malarious areas may have scanty malaria parasites in their blood but the symptoms which made them see the doctor may be due to a different cause.

Preparation of blood films

For malaria blood films use perfectly clean 25 mm × 75 mm (1" × 3") glass slides that are free of grease and scratches. Blood may be obtained from the ear lobe or (preferably) from the 4th finger of the left hand. In infants the big toe is best. The skin should be cleaned with ether or methylated spirit and be completely dry before being punctured with either a sterile Hagedorn needle or a special pricker (Microlance) or an improvised one. Squeeze the finger gently until a blood drop exudes (Fig. 14).

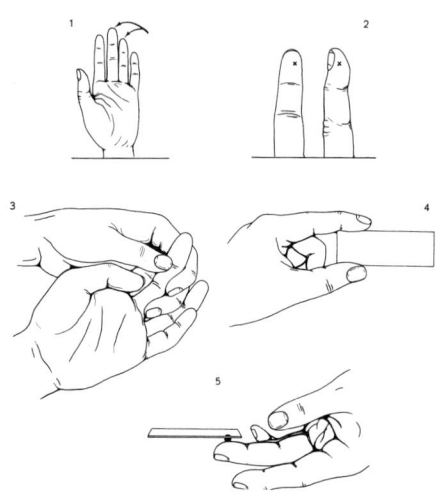

Fig 14 Details of correct technique of blood collection for a thin or thick blood film.
1. The second or third finger of the left hand is generally selected. 2. The site of the puncture is the side of the ball of the finger, not too close to the nail bed. 3. If the blood does not well up from the puncture, a gentle squeeze will bring it up. 4. The slide must always be grasped by its edges. 5. The size of the blood drop is controlled better if the finger touches the slide from below. (WHO, 1961)

For a thick film touch the drop of blood with a glass slide held above the blood drop and then after reversing the slide spread the blood evenly with a corner of another slide to make a square or a circular patch of a moderate thickness that will just allow one to read through it. Keep the slide horizontal while drying and protect it from dust and flies (Fig. 15).

For a thin film the drop of blood should be smaller than for the thick film. Apply the smooth edge of another clean glass slide to the drop of blood at an angle of 45°, touch the drop of blood till it spreads along the

Diagnostic Methods in Malaria

edge. Push the spreader forwards keeping it at the same angle. Dry the thin film by waving it in the air. A properly made thin film should consists of an unbroken layer of single red blood cells with a 'tongue' not touching the edge of the slide (Figs 16, 17).

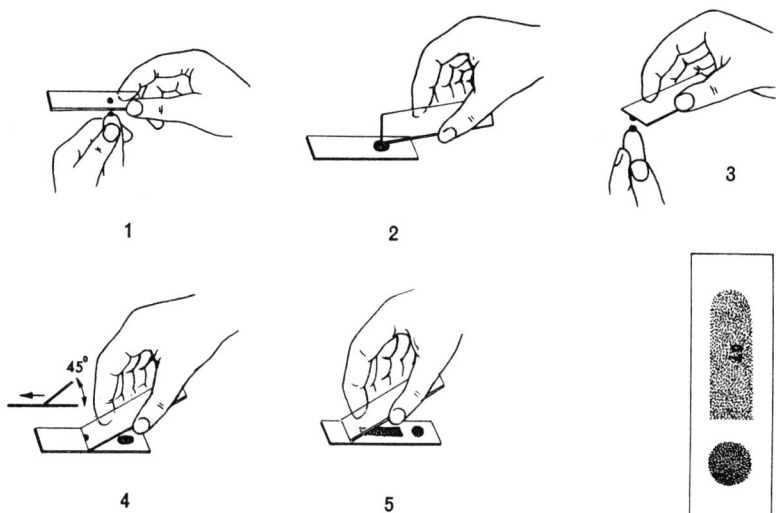

Fig 15 Preparation of a thin and thick blood film on the same slide.
1. The drop of blood is touched with a clean slide. 2. Spread the drop of blood with the corner of another slide to make a circle or a square about 1 cm². 3. Touch a new drop of blood with the edge of a clean slide. 4. Bring the edge of the slide carrying a drop of blood to the surface of the first slide, wait until the blood spreads along the whole edge. 5. Holding it at an angle of about 45° push it forward with a rapid but not too brisk movement. 6. Write with a pencil the slide number on the thin film. Wait until the thick film is quite dry. (WHO, 1961)

Thin and thick films may be taken on the same slide. Blood films may be stained with Leishman's or with Giemsa stain, the second being preferred in the tropics. A rapid method of staining thick films is that of Field's, using buffered, isotonic Romanowsky stain with a counterstain by eosine (Figs 18, 19).

Detailed instructions for preparation of stains will be found in manuals by Wilcox (1960), Shute and Maryon (1966) or other books (*see references*). Only the most important methods are given here.

Giemsa stain. The stock solution of Giemsa stain is easily prepared from Giemsa powder available commercially.

Giemsa powder (Azure B type)	3.8 g
Glycerol, pure	250 ml
Methyl alcohol (certified pure)	250 ml

The stain is prepared best by mixing alcohol and glycerol and then adding gradually small quantities of powder in a porcelain mortar and grinding until most of the powder is dissolved. Some residue may

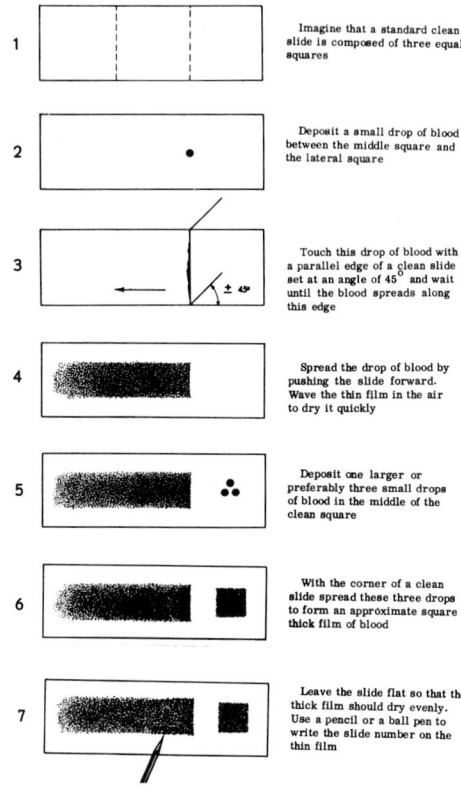

Fig 16 Preparation of thin and thick blood film on the same slide (alternative method). (WHO, 1961)

remain and by leaving the mixture for about a week without filtering, the maximum amount of the stain will be absorbed. The prepared stock solution can then be filtered and should be kept in a bottle of hard glass with a close-fitting ground-glass stopper and away from the sunlight.

Stock solutions of Giemsa may be purchased commercially, but some brands seem to be better than others.

Dilutions of Giemsa stain. Stock solutions of Giemsa stain must always be diluted by mixing an appropriate amount of it with distilled neutral or slightly alkaline water. The water for dilution can be kept at a standard degree of alkalinity, by using phosphate buffer salts. A buffer solution which gives a pH of 7.2 is prepared as follows:

Potassium dihydrogen phosphate KH_2PO_4	0.7 g
Disodium hydrogen phosphate Na_2HPO_4	1.0 g
Distilled water	1 litre

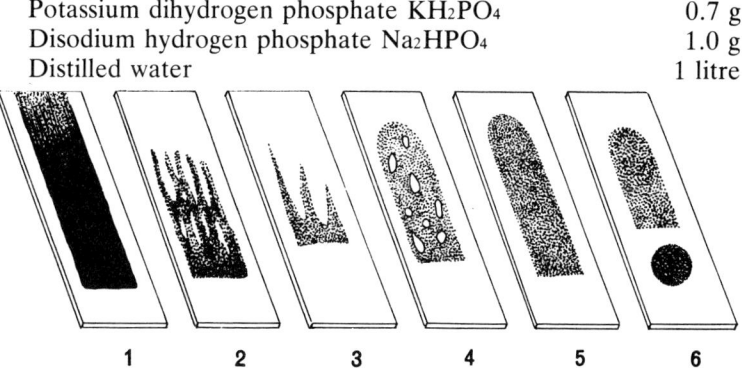

Fig 17 Common faults of a thin blood film.
1. Too much blood – the end of the thin film is lost and the film itself is too thick. 2. Old, devitrified slide or the blood was clotting when the film was made. 3. Uneven contact of the spreader or the edge of the spreader ragged. Film too short. Too little blood. 4. Greasy slide. 5. Good thin film. 6. Thick and thin film on the same slide. (WHO, 1961)

This solution should be tested after its preparation to make sure that its reaction is correct. It remains stable for a long time provided that it is kept in a well stoppered bottle of neutral glass.

Tablets of phosphate buffer salts can be obtained commercially for 100 ml or 1000 ml of water.

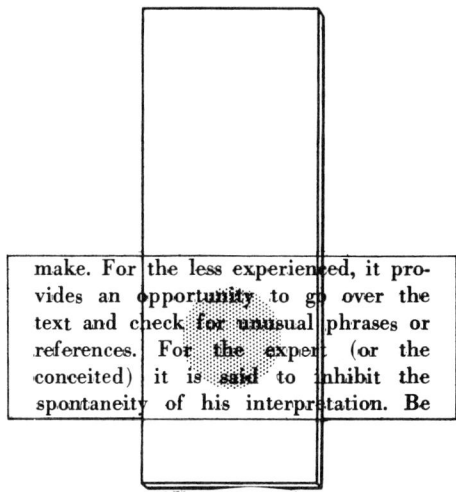

Fig 18 Correct thickness of a thick blood film. (WHO, 1961)

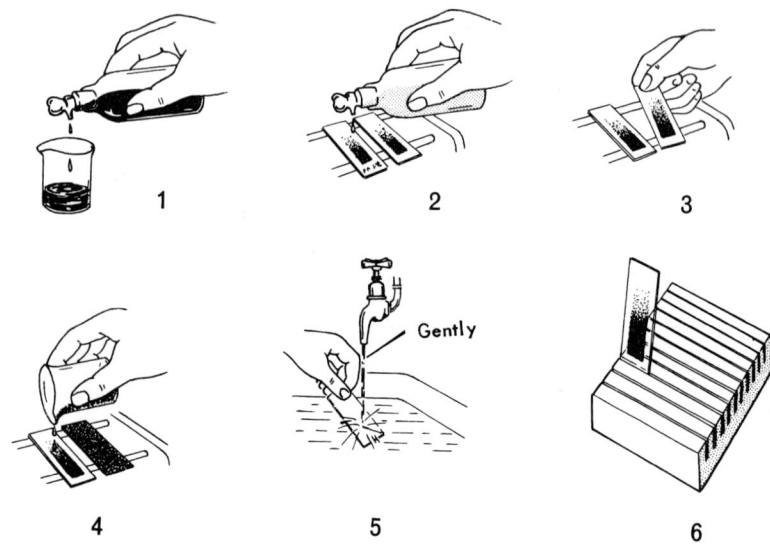

Fig 19 Staining a thin blood film with Giemsa stain.
1. Prepare the staining solution by diluting the Giemsa stock solution with buffered water in a small beaker. The best solution for reasonably fast staining is 2 – 3 drops of Giemsa to each ml of water. One slide requires about 3 – 4 ml of the diluted stain. 2. Fix the thin film by pouring a few drops of methyl alcohol for a few seconds. 3. Pour off the alcohol and pour on the diluted stain before the film is dry. 4. Stain for 20 – 30 minutes. 5. Do not pour off the stain but flush off and rinse by holding the slide in a large container with tap water or under a gentle stream of tap water for 10 – 15 seconds. 6. Place the slide on end in the slide rack to dry. (WHO, 1961)

Technique of staining thin films using Giemsa stain (Fig. 19)
1. The thin film should be fixed in absolute methyl alcohol for 30 seconds. This can be done simply by immersing the film in methyl alcohol or by putting a few drops on it by means of a pipette.
2. The staining solution must be freshly prepared by mixing 5 ml of stock solution with 100 ml of buffered water. For one or two slides less staining solution is adequate providing that it will contain 5% of stock stain.
3. Transfer slide to staining solution or pour it on the slide lying flat on two glass rods. Stain for 20–30 minutes.
4. Flush slide with tap water and stand upright to dry.

Technique of staining thick films using Giemsa stain
1. The thick film should be dry (but not by heating the slide). If it is to be stained within one hour of taking it, then it can be gently heated on top of a microscope lamp for a few minutes.

2. The staining solution must be freshly prepared by diluting 5–7 ml of stock solution of Giemsa to 100 ml of distilled water adjusted to neutral or to pH 7.2 when using phosphate buffer as above.
3. The single slide with the blood film can be stained either horizontally or vertically in a staining trough. In the first case cover the whole slide without any previous fixation with the diluted stain and allow to act for 20–30 minutes.
4. The slide is then gently flushed with distilled water (tap water may suffice) care being taken not to wash the blood film away.
5. Stand the slide upright to dry.

Technique of staining thick films with Field's stain (Fig. 20). This rapid method gives excellent results when the technique is carefully followed. It can be used only for thick films on single slides.

1. The Field's stain consists of two solutions:

    Solution A
Methylene blue (medicinal)	0.8 g
Azure I	0.5 g
Disodium hydrogen phosphate (anhydrous)	5.0 g
Potassium dihydrogen phosphate	6.25 g
Distilled water	500 ml

    Solution B
Eosin	1.0 g
Disodium hydrogen phosphate (anhydrous)	5.0 g
Potassium dihydrogen phosphate	6.25 g
Distilled water	500 ml

    If the anhydrous salt is not available, then crystallised sodium phosphate, $Na_2HPO_4 + 12H_2O$ can be used, at 12.6 g.

2. The phosphate salts are dissolved first in separate containers and the stain is added to each container. Leave the appropriate solutions for 24 hours and filter. Keep in separate bottles for subsequent use.
3. The Field's method of staining requires the use of three wide mouth staining jars, about 40 mm in diameter and 100 mm long. Jar No. 1 is filled with staining solution A, jar No. 2 is filled with distilled and buffered water, jar No. 3 is filled with staining solution B.
4. The technique of staining individuals slides is as follows:
    (a) Dip the slide for one second in solution A.
    (b) Wash off the stain from the back of the slide with a stream of tap water.
    (c) Dip the slide in the buffer solution in jar No. 2 until the excess of the blue stain has left the film.
    (d) Dip the slide for one second in solution B.
    (e) Wash off the stain with a gentle stream of tap water.
    (f) Stand the slide upright to dry.

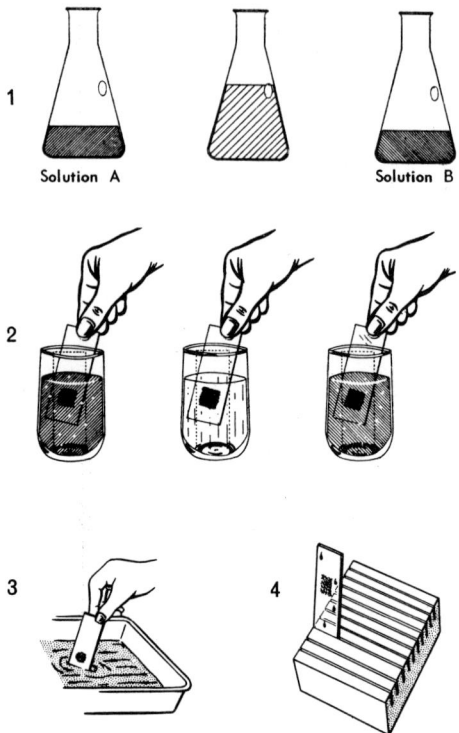

Fig 20 Staining a thick blood film with Field's rapid stain.
1. Prepare three containers with solution A, water and solution B. 2. Dip the blood film into solution A and count slowly up to five (about 2 – 3 seconds). Remove and wash in a beaker with distilled water or suitable tap water, counting slowly up to 10 (4 – 6 seconds) or until the stain ceases to run from the slide and film. Dip into solution B and count up to two (1 second). 3. Remove and again wash, waving gently in tap water and counting slowly up to 10. 4. Place on slide rack to dry. (WHO, 1961)

Examination of blood films. The thick film method, which concentrates by a factor of 20–40 the layers of red blood cells on a small surface, is in practised hands by far the best for general clinical use.

The parasites are easily detected in the thick film but they may be more difficult to identify than in a thin film. This is due to the fact that

Diagnostic Methods in Malaria 85

the red blood cells are not visible, as a result of haemolysis subsequent to staining an unfixed film. The only elements that are seen in the film are leucocytes and the parasites. However the appearance of the latter is somewhat altered because of de-haemoglobinisation and slow drying in the course of preparation of the film. Thus the young trophozoites appear as incomplete rings or spots of blue cytoplasm with a detached red chromatin dot. In late trophozoites of *P. vivax* the cytoplasm may be fragmented and Schüffner's stippling may be less obvious; the band forms of *P. malariae* are less characteristic. However, the schizonts and gametocytes of these species retain their usual appearance and the same goes for the crescents of *P. falciparum*. Pigment granules undergo little change in the thick film. The interpretation of the parasites seen in a thick film requires some experience, which can be easily acquired by studying first the morphology of parasites in a thin film and then searching for corresponding forms in a thick film. As mentioned before the thick film is a time saving method which reveals even scanty infections within a short time. (Fig. 21)

Although the thick film is recommended as a routine method it may be supplemented by taking a thin film which could be of value when the correct identification of some parasite species (e.g. *P. ovale*) is of importance. Thin and thick films may be taken on the same slide. For staining these double films Giemsa is the best method. The thin film must be fixed with methyl alcohol, but care should be taken to leave the thick film untouched by this fixing agent. Standard practice requires that the thick film should be examined for at least 5 minutes (corresponding to approximately 100 microscopic fields under oil immersion); thin films must be examined for 15–20 minutes before a negative report can be issued. In doubtful cases repeated blood films must be taken every 4 hours and examined. In severe infection with *P. falciparum* such repeated examinations are necessary to assess the response of the parasite to treatment. It is advisable to have some indication of the density of parasitaemia by counting the mean number of parasitised erythrocytes in relation to an arbitrary (such as 10 000) number of red blood cells (there are on the average between 300 and 500 red blood cells in a microscope field under oil immersion but this depends largely on the optical system used and its magnification) or the average number of parasites per microscope field. A more precise method consists of counting the number of parasites and leucocytes in a thick film until several hundred of the latter have been enumerated. If a total white blood cell count of the patient's blood is made the ratio of parasites to leucocytes will give the number of parasites per μl or mm^3 of blood. This is known as the *parasite count*.

For designation of the relative parasite count a simple code from one to four crosses is often used by laboratory technicians. For the usual magnification between 500 and 600 times this is as follows:

+   1–10 parasites per 100 thick film fields
++   11–100 parasites per 100 thick film field
+++ 1–10 parasites per one thick film field
++++ more than 10 parasites per one thick film field

For all parasite counts the use of a hand operated tally counter is necessary. It should always be remembered that examination of 100 thick film fields corresponds to the average volume of only about 0.2 mm^3 of blood. Thus the part played by chance factors in the microscopic diagnosis of malaria infection must be recognised. The chance

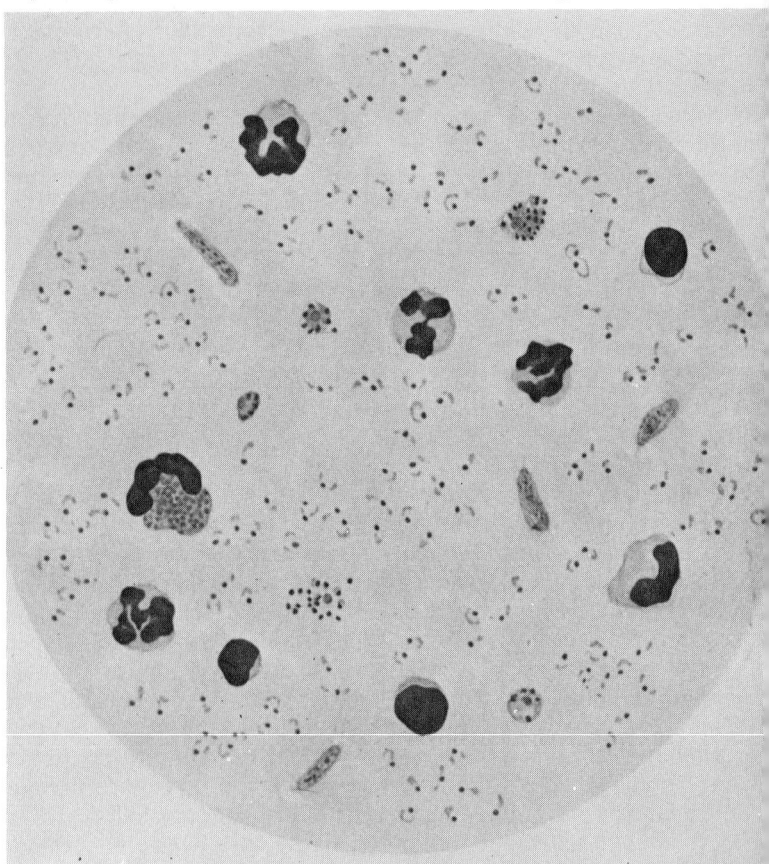

Fig 21 Heavy infection with *P. falciparum* in a thick blood film stained by Giemsa Romanowsky. Magnification × 650.
Note: Four 'crescents' of *P. falciparum* and several developing and fully grown schizonts. Also one eosinophil, four poly-nuclear leucocytes, one large and three small lymphocytes. The field is studded with hundreds of trophozoites of *P. falciparum*. (Wellcome Museum of Medical Science)

factor rises as the true number of parasites in a unit blood decreases. Thus in doubtful cases it is desirable to increase the time devoted to the examination of a single blood slide and if necessary to take several blood slides at proper intervals of time.

Based on the examination of 100 microscopic fields under oil immersion, with a magnification of 500–600 times, the numerical threshold at which malaria parasites can be detected by an experienced technician in well stained blood films is about 200 parasites per mm^3 if a thin film technique is used; for a thick film the threshold is lower – about 10–20 parasites per mm^3 of blood – but here the experience of the microscopist is an important factor. Some authors have recommended the examination of smears from the bone-marrow, obtained by sternal puncture, as a supplementary diagnostic method when malaria parasites cannot be found in peripheral blood. This method has no advantage whatsoever over the usual blood examination. For post-mortem examinations, if death from malaria is suspected and no full autopsy can be carried out, a specimen can be obtained from a puncture of the spleen or brain. For the latter specimen a large-bore needle can be pushed through the supra-orbital plate into the brain and a smear, obtained by suction, should be spread on the slide, fixed, and stained in the usual way.

Some reports, stating that numerous parasites of *P. falciparum* in all stages of development could be found in bloodless exudate from scarified skin of African children, have been consistently disproved by competent parasitologists.

Technical details for microscopical examination of blood films are outside the scope of this book and can easily be found elsewhere (*see references*). Whenever possible a binocular microscope with a substage illumination should be used in preference to a monocular instrument. Nevertheless, in experienced hands a good monocular microscope is perfectly adequate for routine work. The use of a wide angle eye-piece to obtain a better coverage of the microscopic field of an oil-immersion is of great value and thoroughly recommended.

Care should be taken, when examining the thick film, not to confuse artifacts or blood platelets with malaria parasites. In doubtful cases blood films should be sent to the nearest competent laboratory for confirmation of diagnosis.[1]

Diagnostic characters of human malaria parasites as seen in a well stained thick film are given in Tables 2 and 3.

The best illustrated guide for staining and identification of human malaria parasites in thick and thin blood films is undoubtedly that of Aimée Wilcox, 'Manual for the Microscopical Diagnosis of Malaria in Man' (1960). The colour plates of this manual are of an excellence that has been rarely surpassed. Moreover the price of this booklet is well below the cost of other similar or more ambitious publications.

Table 2

Appearance of malaria parasites in a thick blood film (mainly after Russell et al. (1963))

Stage	*Plasmodium vivax* (and *ovale*)	*Plasmodium malariae*	*Plasmodium falciparum*
Early trophozoite	Fairly numerous; irregular cytoplasm; fairly large single chromatin bead; often mixed with later stages.	Few; more regular cytoplasm; medium size single chromatin bead; segmenters present occasionally.	Often very numerous; delicate cytoplasm; small, sometimes double chromatin bead; no other forms usually present except perhaps crescents.
Half-grown trophozoite	Great irregularity of cytoplasm which tends to scatter away from single chromatin bead; few small granules of pigment.	Regular compact deep blue cytoplasm around single chromatin bead; pigment forms early and tends to concentrate.	Not common in peripheral blood; regular cytoplasmic ring, broken ring, and comma patterns; single and double chromatin bead.
Late trophozoite	Considerable cytoplasmic scatter and irregularity; chromatin bead often isolated; fine granular pigment with moderate dispersion and often isolated from cytoplasm; other stages usually present; Schüffner's stippling sometimes seen as a pink halo.	Numbers generally few, older stages present; rounded compact cytoplasm often obscuring chromatin; scattered pigment relatively abundant.	Not in peripheral blood except in very heavy infections; solid, irregularly rounded; chromatin indistinct; pigment concentrated.
Early schizont or pre-segmenter	Large amount of cytoplasm loosely covering abundant chromatin which is beginning to segment; pigment granules discrete and lightly concentrated in one or two areas; Schüffner's stippling often seen as a pink granular	Smaller and not so numerous; some scatter of cytoplasm and segmentation of chromatin; pigment in small separate granules.	Seldom in peripheral blood, but if so will be associated with numerous typical ring forms; irregular, fairly compact, dark staining; pigment fused in a single mass.

Mature schizont (segmenter)	8–16, usually 12–14 merozoites; relatively large size, early vacuole formation; pigment granular and clumped; other stages often present.	6–12, usually 8 merozoites, each with vivid purple, ovoid head of chromatin; early vacuole formation; pigment compact clump of granules.	Very rare in peripheral blood; 12–24 or more merozoites, fairly uniform ovoid or round chromatin beads; merozoites grouped or scattered; pigment a single dark mass.	
Gametocyte	Round or oval, relatively large, with fairly uniform cytoplasm somewhat frayed at edges, small rodlet-shaped pigment, irregularly scattered, abundant chromatin, more diffuse in males.	Rounded, compact, with abundant peripheral pigment in round granules; single chromatin mass often obscured and more diffuse in males.	When mature and normal has distinctive crescentic shape, females longer and more slender with central pigment and chromatin; males fatter and paler, with scattered pigment and diffuse chromatin, coarse grains of pigment.	

Note: In properly stained thick films the erythrocytes are lysed and invisible, except for a cloudy, bluish background. Nuclei of white blood cells stain deep mauve, while clumps of platelets are pink. The parasites show a dull red or magenta-coloured nucleus and light blue cytoplasm. Species differentiation of very young forms of parasites is often impossible. In *P. vivax* and *P. ovale* infections stippling is usually present. Gametocytes of *P. falciparum* ('crescents') are distinctive but in slowly dried films they are rounded up and can be then confused with schizonts or gametocytes of *P. malariae*.

While in vivax, quartan and ovale malaria all stages of development of malaria parasites can be usually found in the peripheral blood in falciparum malaria the schizogony takes place in the internal organs and normally only early trophozoites ('ring') appear in the blood. In very infections with *P. falciparum*, the appearance of schizonts is a danger signal.

Table 3

Differential characteristics of infected erythrocytes and human plasmodia in stained thin films

CHARACTERISTICS	P. falciparum	P. vivax	P. ovale	P. malariae
Infected erythrocyte enlarged	–	+	±	–
Infected erythrocyte not enlarged	+	–	±	+
Infected erythrocyte oval, crenated margin*	–	–	+	–
Infected erythrocyte decolorised	–	+	+	–
Infected erythrocyte, Schüffner's dots* *(stippling)*	–	+	+	–
Infected erythrocyte, Maurer's dots*	+	–	–	–
Multiple infections in erythrocytes*	+	Rare	–	–
Parasite, all forms in peripheral blood	–	+	+	+
Parasite, large coarse rings	–	+	+	+
Parasite, double chromatin dots*	+	Rare	–	–
Parasite, accolé forms*	+	Rare	–	–
Parasite, band forms*	–	–	+	+
Parasite, crescentic gametocytes	+	–	–	–
Number of merozoites	8–24	12–24	8–12	6–12

* Not invariable but suggestive when seen.

Various more or less refined methods have been used to improve and facilitate the conventional ways of examining stained blood slides under the microscope. These methods vary: centrifugation of heparinised blood specimen, staining of the blood slide with fluorescent stains (fluorochromes) have been used, but the results were only moderately good in relation to the complexity of techniques involved.

While the thick film is usually the standard method for examination of blood for the presence of malaria parasites the thin film may be needed for identification of *P. ovale* or some infections in which scant parasites in early stages of development cannot provide the diagnostic clues. Moreover, the thin film method routinely used in hospital laboratories for differential counts of various types of white blood cells may occasionally and surprisingly reveal the presence of malaria parasites in the erythrocytes. The diagnostic criteria of malaria parasites of the four species are essentially the same in thin as in thick blood film although at times the distortion of plasmodia in the unfixed thick film adds to the difficulties faced by the beginners. Moreover the examination of the thin film may be much slower especially if the parasites are scanty but it has one advantage, namely the preservation of the shape and details of the infected red blood cell, and this may be of value in doubtful cases when the identification of the species of the plasmodium causes some difficulty. (Fig. 22)

In view of this an additional table indicating the characteristic changes of the infected red blood cells may be of value (Table 4).

SEROLOGICAL TESTS

Serological methods of diagnosis of malaria have become of practical value since 1962 when the technique of indirect fluorescent antibody (IFA) test was introduced. *The homologous antigen* used in this test consists of a film of human malaria parasites of a given plasmodial species and preferably erythrocytic schizonts obtained from man, from an infected *Aotus* monkey or from an *in vitro* blood culture. It seems that the use of cultured parasites of *P. falciparum* offers now a most convenient and stable source of antigens from different strains of this plasmodial species without the previous laborious adaptation to susceptible monkeys.

Heterologous antigens of lesser specificity are malaria parasites of monkeys (*P. brasilianum, P. cynomolgi, P. fieldi*) which have a wider range of antigenic determinants. The anti-human sera may be polyvalent (for all immunoglobulins) or monovalent (for IgG or IgM only); these sera must be conjugated with fluorescein isothiocyanate as a marker. The blood can be collected after a finger prick in a capillary tube, for subsequent separation of serum, or it can be collected on filter paper and dried before an eventual elution using physiological saline. There are a number of modifications of the test itself, which indicates the presence of an immune response to a malaria infection and not necessarily the synchronous presence of malaria parasites. The test is of particular value for epidemiological studies and for tracing asymptomatic infections in blood donors. High titres (1:200 and over) point to a recent infection and the use of an appropriate human antigen points to an infection with one of the species of human plasmodia. Generally fluorescence at a dilution of serum of over 1:20 is regarded as a positive test (Table 5).

The indirect haemagglutination (HA) test is also used and lends itself more as a field method since it does not require the special fluorescent microscope. In this test glutaraldehyde stabilised tanned sheep cells are sensitised with the specific antigen obtained from an *Aotus* monkey infected with *P. falciparum* or another human plasmodium. The sensitised and control cells can be lyophilised and remain stable under field conditions. This test has been used for epidemiological surveillance and for detection of remaining foci of malaria.

Immuno-precipitation techniques (double gel diffusion tests) have been used mainly for identification of antigens formed in the course of

Table 4

Changes in the red blood cells infected with human malaria parasites as seen in the thin blood film

	P. vivax	P. malariae	P. falciparum	P. ovale
Infected cell	Larger than normal, paler, often slightly distorted. Schüffner's dots present in nearly all infected cells except for very young rings. Multiple infection by several parasites not uncommon. Pigment brownish in short scattered rods.	About normal size or slightly smaller. Stippling not seen by normal staining. No multiple infection or erythrocyte, as a rule. Pigment seen even in early stages, dark granules rather than rods, often seen at the periphery of the cell.	Normal in size. Multiple infections of erythrocyte very frequent. Some cells yellowish, seem to have a thicker rim (brassy cells). No Schüffner's stippling but irregular clefts (Maurer's dots) may be seen in overstained films. Pigment granular with tendency to coalesce. In gametocytes (crescents) the outline of erythrocyte barely seen.	Many infected erythrocytes enlarged and definitely oval in shape while the parasite is round or elongated. The outline of infected cells often ragged (fimbriated). Schüffner's dots prominent at all stages of the parasite. Pigment brownish similar to that of *P. vivax*.

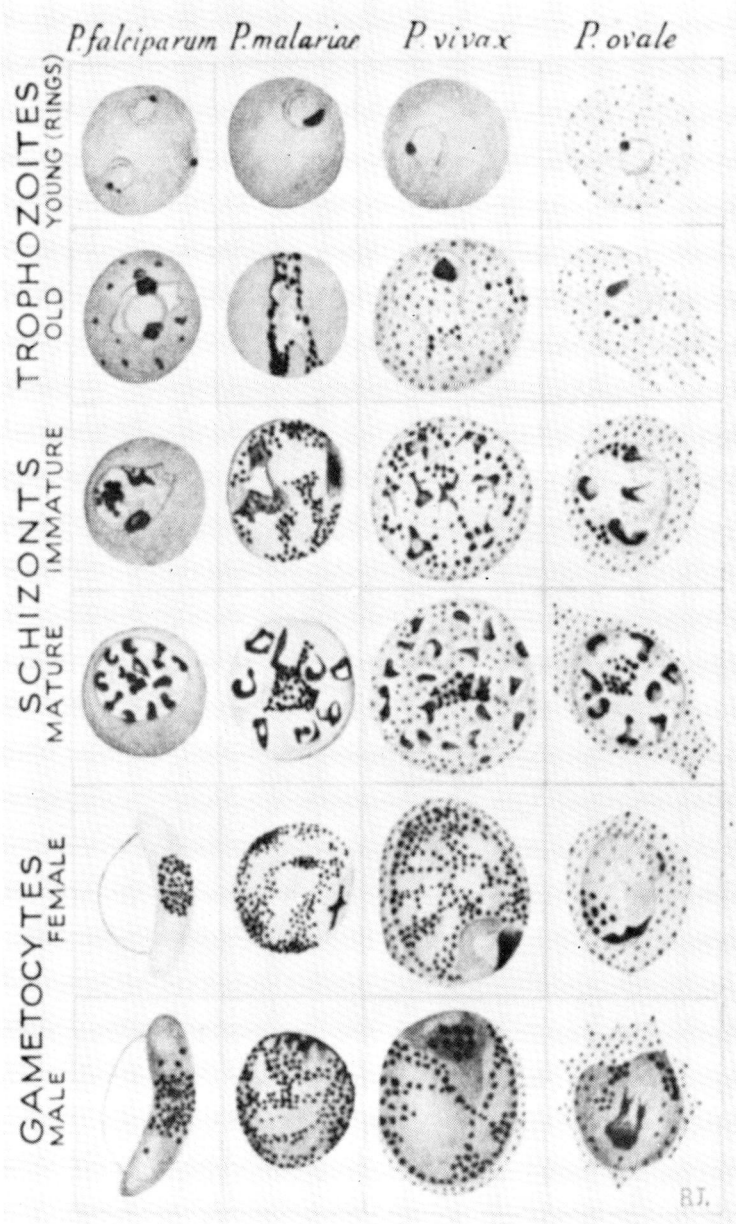

Fig 22 Morphological characteristics of erythrocytic stages of four species of human plasmodia. Magnification × 2000. (From C. A. Hoare 1949)

Table 5

Serological tests commonly used for detection and measurement of malaria antibodies

Test	Current application	Source of antigens	Antibodies identified	Sensitivity
Immuno-precipitation	Epidemiological studies and research	Erythrocytic schizonts and soluble antigens	IgG, IgM	Poor
Immuno-fluorescence (IFA)	Epidemiological studies, research and aid to diagnosis	Erythrocytic schizonts	IgG, IgM and IgA	Good
Indirect haemagglutination (HA)	Epidemiological surveys	Erythrocytic schizonts		Good[1]
Enzyme linked immuno-sorbent assay (ELISA)	Epidemiological studies and aid to diagnosis	Erythrocytic schizonts		Good[2]
Radio-immuno assay	Research	Soluble antigens		Good[3]
Merozoite inhibition in culture	Research	Merozoites from erythrocytic schizonts		Good[4]

Note: Complement fixation tests are obsolete and have not been included in this table.

[1] This test can be performed with simple equipment and permits the study of large numbers of sera under field conditions. It is however difficult to standardise. Antibodies are detected some time after parasitaemia becomes patent.

[2] Requires small quantities of antigen and is easy to perform without expensive equipment.

[3] Very sensitive for detection of antibodies at low concentration but expensive and not suitable for field use.

[4] Used only for the detection of protective antibody.

infection, although the study of the antibody response was also investigated by this method. The test is highly sensitive but is used as a research tool rather than as a diagnostic method.

ELISA test. An enzyme-linked immuno-sorbent assay (Elisa) test has been introduced recently for epidemiological studies. A base of a plastic tube or plate is coated with a soluble antigen. The serum containing antibody is incubated in the coated tube and the excess of antibody is removed. The anti-antibody specific globulin labelled with the appropriate enzyme is then added to the tube and the excess of it removed. The enzyme substrate is then added and its change of colour is proportional to the antibody concentration in the test serum. The actual enzyme widely used was alkaline phosphatase conjugated with antihuman globulin; paranitrophenyl phosphate was used as an indicator of the enzyme reaction.

Tests of immunofluorescence, immuno-haemagglutination, immuno-precipation and the enzyme-linked immuno-sorbent method have been used widely for the detection and measurement of antibodies in response to the malaria infection. Each of these tests has its advantages and limitations;not one of them is able to distinguish the protective from non-protective antibody. Recently other tests using *in vitro* growth of malaria parasites have been developed and these are of promise for the detection of true protective antibodies; the methods employed are based either on the uptake of labelled aminoacids by the growing parasites or they measure the capacity of merozoites to reinvade erythrocytes.

Appraisal of the value of serological tests

As mentioned previously, the serological tests are of limited use for the diagnosis of acute malaria, since they become positive only several days after the appearance of malaria parasites in the blood. Thus these tests cannot replace the simple and yet reliable technique of examination of the blood by an alert and experienced microscopist. Nevertheless, serological testing for malaria has now been recognised as an invaluable method in epidemiological studies. For this purpose it is best to use the most practical and sensitive test available, because it will yield much information, providing that the possible disadvantages of non-specific positive reactions are recognised and assessed. It should be remembered that high sensitivity is sometimes obtained at a cost of low specificity of the test. In areas where malaria is or has been endemic, serology will be particularly useful for the following aims: (1) Establishment of age-specific indices of malarial endemicity, (2) Assessment of changes in the degree of malaria transmission, (3) Delineation of malarious areas and of foci of transmission. Whenever possible the serological and parasitological information should be collected and evaluated together. In areas where malaria is not endemic serological tests can be of use for the following purposes: (1) Screening of blood donors, (2) Exclusion of diagnosis of malaria in patients with symptoms such as pyrexia and with negative results of blood examination for plasmodia, (3) Case-detection and identification of the species of malaria parasites when other methods failed. The present serological tests suffer from the general disadvantage that the methods of collection of serum or plasma, as well as the selection of antigens and techniques of various tests, are not standardised, so that comparison of results between them is subject to caution. The simple technique of collection of blood on filter paper for the indirect fluorescent antibody test (IFA test) is as follows:

Collection of capillary blood on paper for serology[1]

1. Whatman No. 3 chromatography paper cut into strips of about 14 × 9 cm should be stored in self-sealing polythene bags, each containing up to ten pieces. For use in humid climates it is preferable, before cutting them into strips, to soak the sheets of paper in 1/10 000 Thiomersal (Merthiolate), to act as a fungicide, and to allow them to dry thoroughly.
2. A finger or ear lobe is cleaned. Ensure that cleaning fluid, if used, has dried. A *deep* prick is made and drops of blood are allowed to fall on to the paper, so that the skin does not touch the paper. Collect a minimum of 2 to 3 spots of *not less than* 50 μl each from every subject. If necessary several drops of blood may be allowed to fall on top of each other on the same spot of the paper and to soak in until the spot is about 1 cm in diameter. Let each of the drops spread out on its own. Up to five sets of blood samples from different subjects can be put on one piece of paper. Ensure that each set is clearly marked with reference number.
3. Papers should be protected from dirt and flies, e.g., by standing on their sides inside a covered bowl. Allow to dry thoroughly at room temperature or by holding in *gentle* heat – not more than 37°C. Under field conditions this is often not practicable on the spot. The partially dried papers are then taken back to the laboratory, preferably within a few hours, where they are thoroughly dried and then sealed in the polythene bags. The bags are stored as soon as possible in a refrigerator (4°C) or preferably deep freeze (−20°C or less). Under these conditions specific immunoglobulins are probably stable for at least several months. So long as the papers are *well dried* the bags can probably be kept at ambient temperature for several weeks without serious degradation of the immunoglobulins.
4. At the serological laboratory a calibrated paper punch is used to cut out circles of paper containing the equivalent of 50 μl of blood. When eluted in 0.4 ml of diluent this will give an approximate 1/16 dilution of serum.
5. Slightly greater precision, of doubtful value for most survey work and taking more time, may be obtained by taking up measured amounts of 50 μl of blood in a pipette or capillary tube and expelling these on to a paper. (This obviates the need for a calibrated punch when the processing of the blood samples takes place in the laboratory.)

---

[1] Instructions according to the technique used by Dr C. C. Draper of the Ross Institute, London School of Hygiene and Tropical Medicine.

Chapter 6

The Anopheles Vector

Human malaria can be transmitted only by anopheline mosquitos. In addition to transmitting malaria, anophelines also transmit filariasis and some viral diseases, but other mosquitos are more important as vectors of the two latter infections.

The Anopheles belong to the order of *Diptera*, sub-order *Nematocera*, family *Culicidae*, sub-family *Culicinae* and tribe *Anophelini* in the zoological classification. Within the tribe *Anophelini* the genus Anopheles has several sub-genera (Fig. 23).

There are about 400 species of Anopheles mosquitos throughout the world, but only some 60 species are important vectors of malaria under natural conditions. Natural susceptibility or resistance of

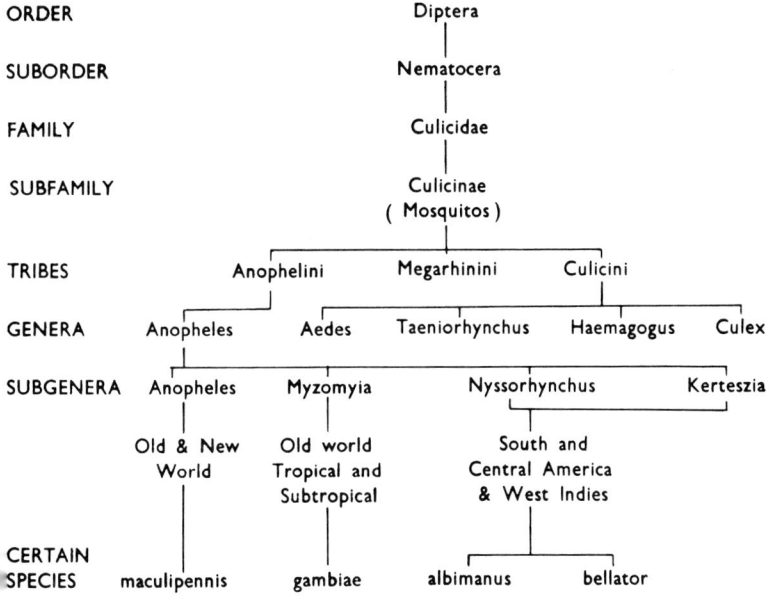

Note: It is customary to omit the subgeneric name when referring to a species e.g. Anopheles maculipennis, and Anopheles gambiae, except in strictly systematic work.

Fig 23 Classification of mosquitos.

Anopheles to infection with a defined species of malaria parasite is largely unexplained though it is certainly related to biochemical processes in the body of the mosquito and to its nutritional requirements.

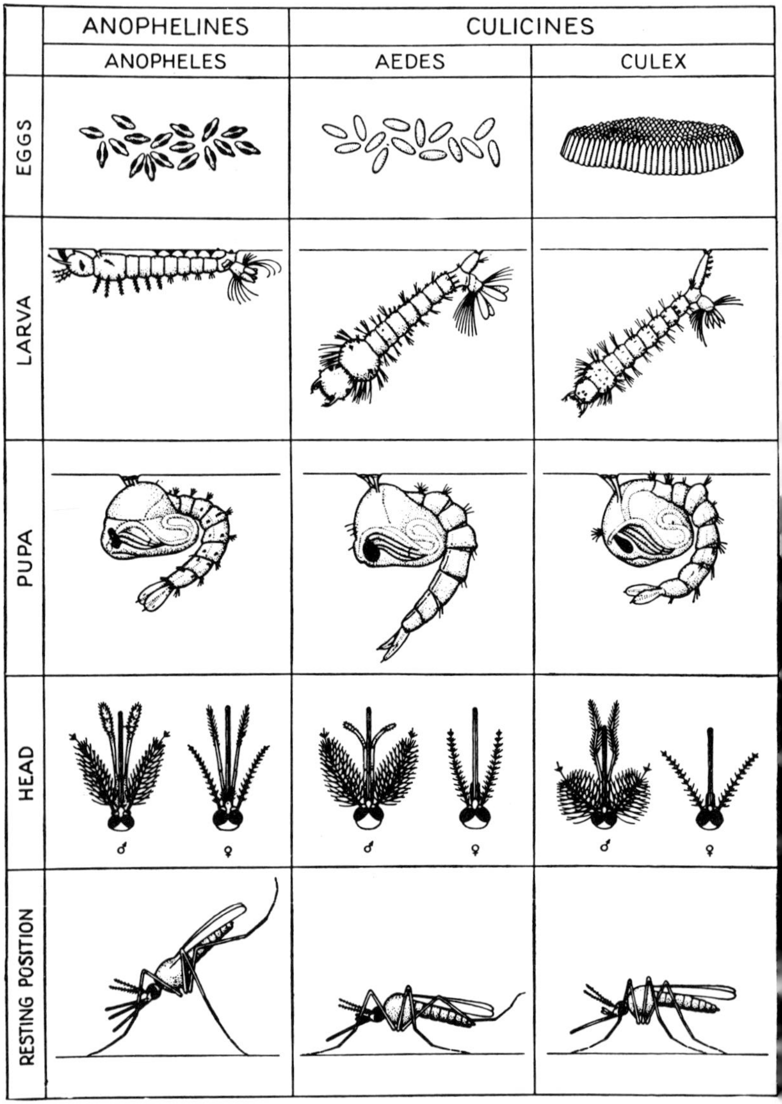

	ANOPHELINES	CULICINES	
	ANOPHELES	AEDES	CULEX
EGGS			
LARVA			
PUPA			
HEAD	♂ ♀	♂ ♀	♂ ♀
RESTING POSITION			

Fig 24 Differentiation of Anopheles, Aedes and Culex mosquitos at various stages of their development. Note the length of palpi in female Anopheles in comparison with other tribes of mosquitos. (Wellcome Museum of Medical Science)

The Anopheles Vector

Among the main factors determining whether a particular species of Anopheles is an important vector the frequency of its feeding on man (in preference to animals) is of particular relevance. The other factors are the mean longevity of the local population of an anopheline species and its density in relation to man. Thus a particular species of Anopheles may be an important vector in one area of the world and of no importance in another area.

Although Anopheles mosquitos are most frequent in tropical or sub-tropical regions they are found in temperate climates and even in the Arctic during the summer. As a rule Anopheles are not found at altitudes above 2000–2500 metres.

A large area of the Pacific Ocean roughly bounded by, and including, New Zealand, the Galapagos Islands, Hawaii, Midway Island, Palau Island, the Caroline Islands, the Gilbert Islands, Samoa, Fiji and New Caledonia is free from Anopheles mosquitos and there is no indigenous malaria within this area.

ANATOMY AND PHYSIOLOGY OF ANOPHELES

The external morphology of both female and male Anopheles provides the criteria for recognising both the genus and the species of these mosquitos. The successive stages of growth and metamorphosis of the mosquito are the egg, larva, pupa and finally the adult or imago (Fig. 24).

Anopheline eggs
These are about 0.5 mm in length, boat-shaped and provided with tiny air-filled floats that allow them to remain on the surface of the water. The frill, separating the 'deck' of the egg from the rest of it, is more or less continuous. They are laid singly by the female Anopheles on the type of water preferred by a particular species. The pattern of grey exochorion on the surface of the brown egg, its shape and size are useful for species differentiation. The site chosen by the Anopheles for egg laying and subsequent development of the larvae is known as the breeding place or *larval habitat*.

Anopheline larva
The larvae hatch from the eggs as small 'wrigglers' and have a distinct head, thorax and abdomen, the latter composed of 9 segments (Fig. 25).

The thorax is broader than the head or abdomen and somewhat flattened. It has several groups of hairs that are useful in identifying the species, but there are no other special structures.

The abdomen is long and subcylindrical. Its first 7 segments are similar, but the eighth and ninth are considerably modified. The eighth

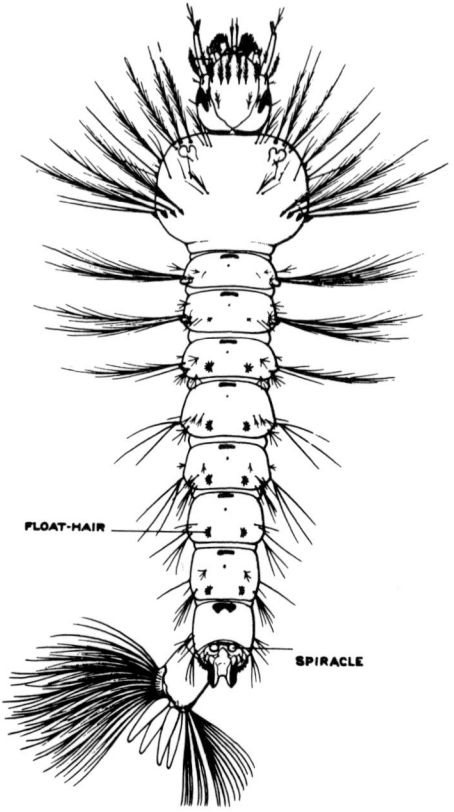

Fig 25 Larva of an Anopheles mosquito. (Wellcome Museum of Medical Science)

segment bears the respiratory apparatus, which in anophelines consists of paired spiracular openings while there is a prominent air tube in the other groups. The ninth segment is out of line with the other segments and bears 2–4 tapering membranous appendages commonly known as anal gills. Each of these sections is provided with hairs, which are useful for distinguishing different species of Anopheles. The larvae have conspicuous mouth brushes which sweep food particles into the mouth. In feeding at the surface the head of the larva turns through 180 degrees. The body of the larva lies parallel to the water surface; on the upper side of the abdomen it has a row of conspicuous *palmate* or *float-hairs*. In contradistinction to Culicine larvae those of Anopheles have no breathing syphon but two spiracular openings leading to the tracheae. Like all mosquito larve those of Anopheles undergo three successive moultings (*ecdyses*) during their growth, when they shed their chitinous skins. These successive moults separate the life of the larva into 4 stages or instars. At the end of the fourth stage the larva changes into a pupa (Fig. 26).

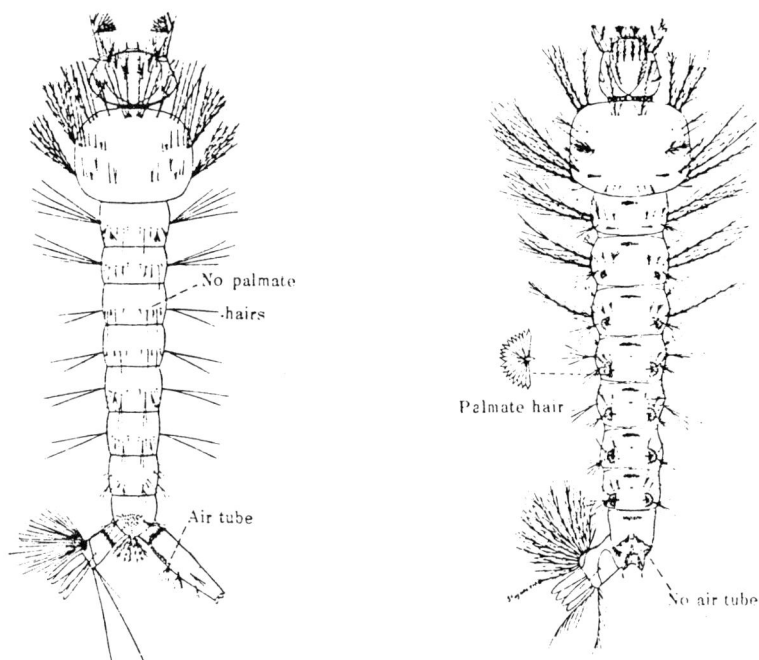

Fig 26 Morphological differences between larvae of Culex or Aedes mosquitos (left) and larvae of Anopheles (right).
Note: In Anopheles absence of breathing syphon (air tube); presence of float or palmate hairs on abdominal segments. (WHO, 1972, 'Vector control in international health')

Anopheline pupa

This has a superficial similarity to that of other mosquitos though it differs from them in several details such as lateral hairs on the abdomen. The pupa differs greatly from the larva in shape, the front part, consisting of the head and thorax, being considerably enlarged and enclosed in a sheath; on the upper surface is a pair of respiratory trumpets. The abdomen comprises 8 freely movable segments with a pair of paddles at the tip. Pupae do not feed during their aquatic existence and come to the water surface to breathe through their short respiratory trumpets.

Adult Anopheles

The head, thorax and abdomen of an adult Anopheles (*imago*) are shown in Fig. 27. The head with its prominent compound eyes has a

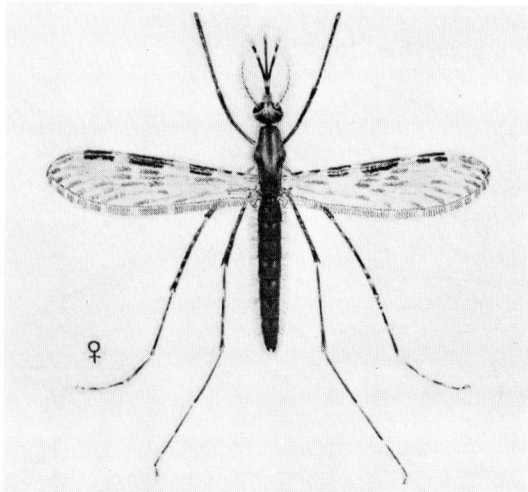

Fig 27 Female specimen of *Anopheles gambiae*, the most important vector of malaria in the African tropical areas. (Wellcome Museum of Medical Science)

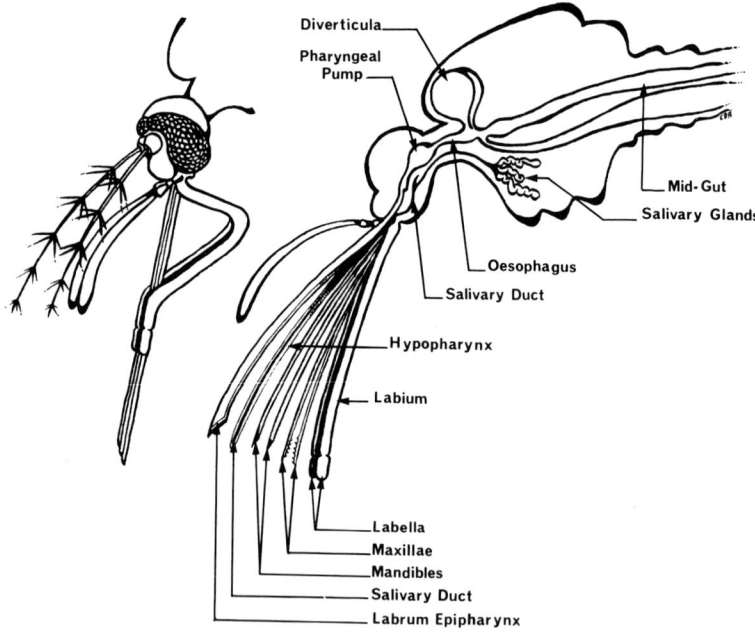

Fig 28 Anatomy of the proboscis of female Anopheles mosquito.

pair of *antennae* which are plumose in the male and sparsely feathered in the female. The *palpi* situated on both sides of the *proboscis* are about as long as the latter in male and female Anopheles while in the Culicine mosquitos the female palpi are short. The proboscis in the female is a composite structure that includes the *labium*, a pair of *labellae*, the *labrum*, the *hypopharynx* (leading to the pharyngeal pump) and a pair of toothed *mandibles* and *maxillae*. The latter serve to penetrate the skin of the animal on whose blood the female Anopheles feeds (Fig. 28). The thorax with its rounded *scutellum* carries a pair of *wings* and a pair of *halteres*. The wings of Anopheles have a characteristic venation.

The abdomen has eight similar segments each with a dorsal plate or *tergite* and a ventral plate – *sternite*; the last terminal segment is modified into *terminalia* for mating, and in the female also for ovipositing. Each of the six legs has a *femur*, a *tibia and* a five-segmented *tarsus* (Fig. 29). The arrangement and colour of the scales on the veins of wings and on palpi and legs of Anopheles are important for the identification of species. Most anophelines rest at an angle while culicines usually rest with the abdomen parallel to the resting surface.

Internal anatomy of anopheles

Certain internal structures of the adult anopheline mosquito are important for a study of malaria transmission (Fig. 30).

There are two *salivary glands* situated in the forepart of the thorax above the forelegs. Each gland consists of three lobes; the two outer ones are long while the central one is short. A duct from each lobe immediately unites with the others to form the right and left ducts; these in turn unite to make one main salivary duct. Near the base of the hypopharynx there is a salivary pump.

The *alimentary canal* consists of three main parts: the fore-, mid- and hindgut. Inside the head are the pharynx and oesophagus forming the foregut. The *pharyngeal pump* causes liquid food to be sucked through the food channel in the labrum which finds its way through the oesophagus into the midgut. Near the posterior end of the oesophagus two tubes lead off to a pair of *dorsal diverticula*. About the same place a ventral tube leads to a *ventral diverticulum*. When fed on liquids other than blood the liquids pass to the diverticula particularly the ventral one; when fed on blood the food passes directly to the midgut and stomach. Digestion of the blood-meal takes place in the expanded portion of the *midgut*, the 'stomach', where important changes in the malaria parasite also occur. Five *Malpighian tubes* open into the hindgut at the junction with the midgut; these have an excretory function. At the distal extremity of the hindgut is the *rectum*, the inner walls of which are furnished with six rectal papillae. In the female the anus lies between the *cerci* and the postgenital plate.

In the male Anopheles the pair of *testes* occupy the posterior part of the abdomen; each testis has a short duct which leads to a central ejaculatory duct leading to a complex structure of external male genitalia with its central *phallosome* and two prominent *claspers*.

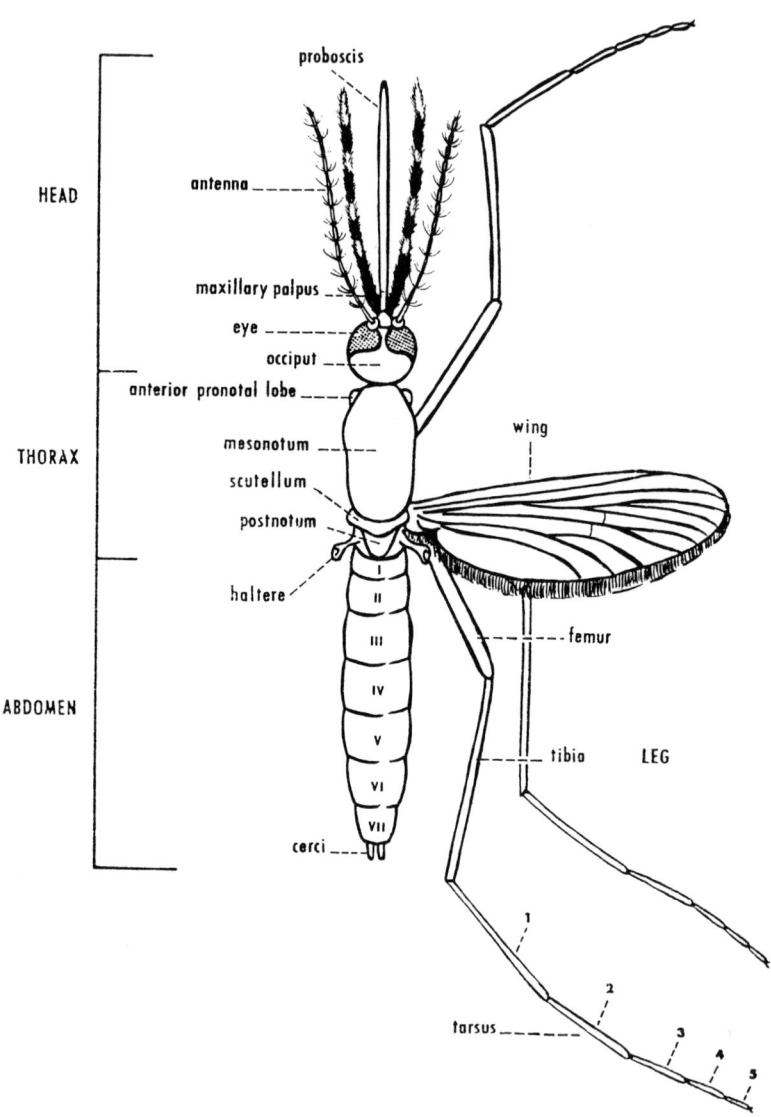

Fig 29 General anatomy of a female Anopheles mosquito. (Modified from WHO, 1972, 'Vector control in international health')

In a newly emerged female the *ovaries* lie under the 4th and 5th tergites, but in a gravid one they occupy a large part of the abdominal cavity. An *oviduct* from each ovary leads to a *common oviduct*, the distal portion of which is expanded to form the *atrium* into which the sperm duct opens. This duct comes from a single round *spermatheca* in which are stored the spermatozoa introduced by the male during copulation of Anopheles. Five stages in the structure and development of the ovaries are of value in assessing the age of the Anopheles in malaria studies.

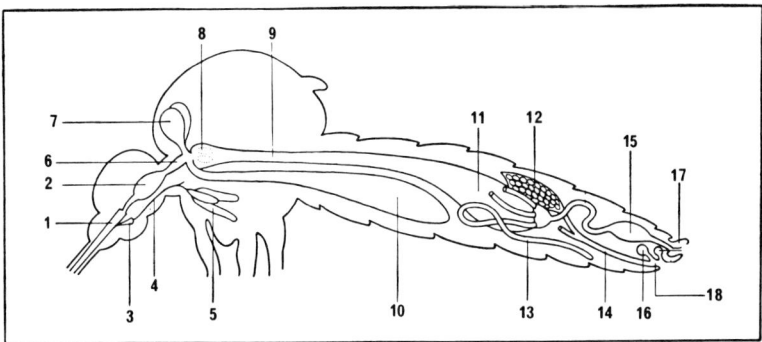

Fig 30 Schematic diagram of the internal anatomy of a female mosquito. (Redrawn from Marshall, 1928)
1. pharynx; 2. pharyngeal pump; 3. salivary pump; 4. salivary duct; 5. salivary glands; 6. oesophagus; 7. dorsal diverticula; 8. proventriculus; 9. midgut; 10. ventral diverticulum; 11. stomach; 12. ovary; 13. Malpighian tubules; 14. oviduct; 15. rectum; 16. spermatheca; 17. cerci; 18. atrium.

Determination of the age of female mosquitos is of importance for full understanding of the epidemiology of malaria and for assessment of the efficacy of anti-anopheline measures, most of which aim at shortening the average lifespan of the population of the malaria vector. Physiological age is determined from the fine structure of ovaries which indicate the number of gonotrophic cycles undergone by a female mosquito. By means of age-grading, it is possible to determine the age composition of the mosquito population and to find out the proportion of females which lives long enough to transmit the malaria infection.

A number of age-grading methods were formerly used. The earliest one classified the age of the mosquito by the degree of wear of the wing; later methods were based on such physiological characteristics as the presence of a 'mating plug', fertilisation, and enlargement of the ampulla of the common oviduct. At present two methods, developed by Soviet entomologists, are increasingly used:
1. A simple technique for distinguishing between parous and nulliparous female anophelines by examination of the tracheoles of the

ovaries permits an assessment of the nulliparous-to-parous ratio, from which the probability of survival of mosquitos and therefore their average longevity can be calculated.

2. A more elaborate technique is based on the dissection of the ovaries to count the number of dilatations left in the ovarioles subsequent to each ovulation and oviposition. The number of dilatations usually corresponds to the number of gonotrophic cycles, and this gives more direct evidence of the physiological age of the females.

The larva of Anopheles has a dorsal heart and tracheae, a simple alimentary canal, an aorta, and a nerve cord. Two salivary glands situated in the thorax are of importance since their cells contain polytene chromosomes, the pattern of which makes possible the identification of some closely related species. This method opened new ways for the science of cytotaxonomy and mosquito genetics.

Systematic classification of genera and species of Anopheles mosquitos is based on their morphological characters at all stages of their development but mostly on adults and larvae. Various keys for the identification of species have been prepared, usually for a well defined geographical area. The use of these generally binary keys is obvious as shown in Figs. 31 and 32.

DISTRIBUTION OF ANOPHELES

The following six zoo-geographical regions of the world have been generally recognised:

1. *Palaearctic Region:* comprising the whole of Europe and North Africa, Asia north of 30°N including the Japanese islands, northern Arabia including Iraq, Iran and Afghanistan.
2. *Oriental Region* all of southern Asia, Indonesian islands, Philippines and Taiwan.
3. *Australasian Region* comprising Australia, Tasmania, New Zealand, the islands of New Guinea and also Micronesia, Polynesia and the Hawaiian islands.
4. *Afro-tropical Region* (formerly known as '*Ethiopian*'): all of Africa south of the Sahara including Malagasy island, Seychelles, Mauritius and Reunion.
5. *Neoarctic Region:* northern Mexico and the north of North America.
6. *Neotropical Region:* from central Mexico to southern Argentina including the Caribbean islands.

Table 6 gives the list of the most important species of Anopheles, vectors of human malaria. The former classification of Anopheles into primary and secondary vectors is uncertain and arbitrary. 'Secondary' vectors are supposed to be species of Anopheles in the relevant area which, after the elimination of the 'primary' species responsible for

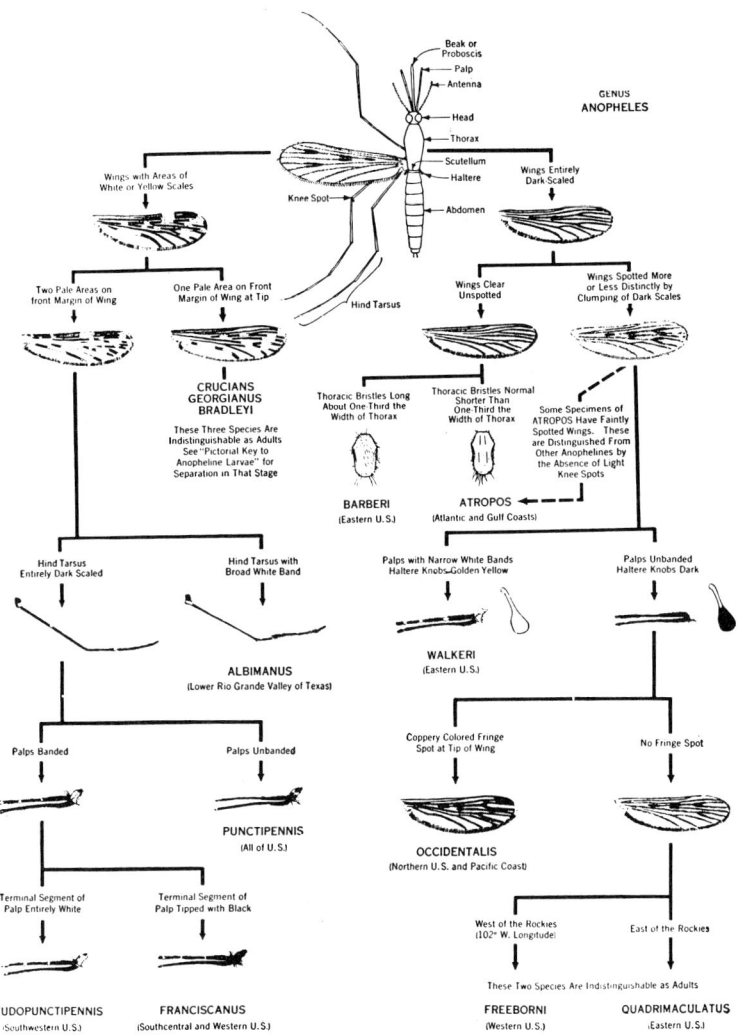

Fig 31 Example of the use of a taxonomic key for identification of a species of adult female Anopheles, according to a pictorial guide valid for the USA. (From 'Malaria Control in Impounded Waters', 1945, by courtesy of the Superintendent of Documents, US Government Printing Office, Washington DC)

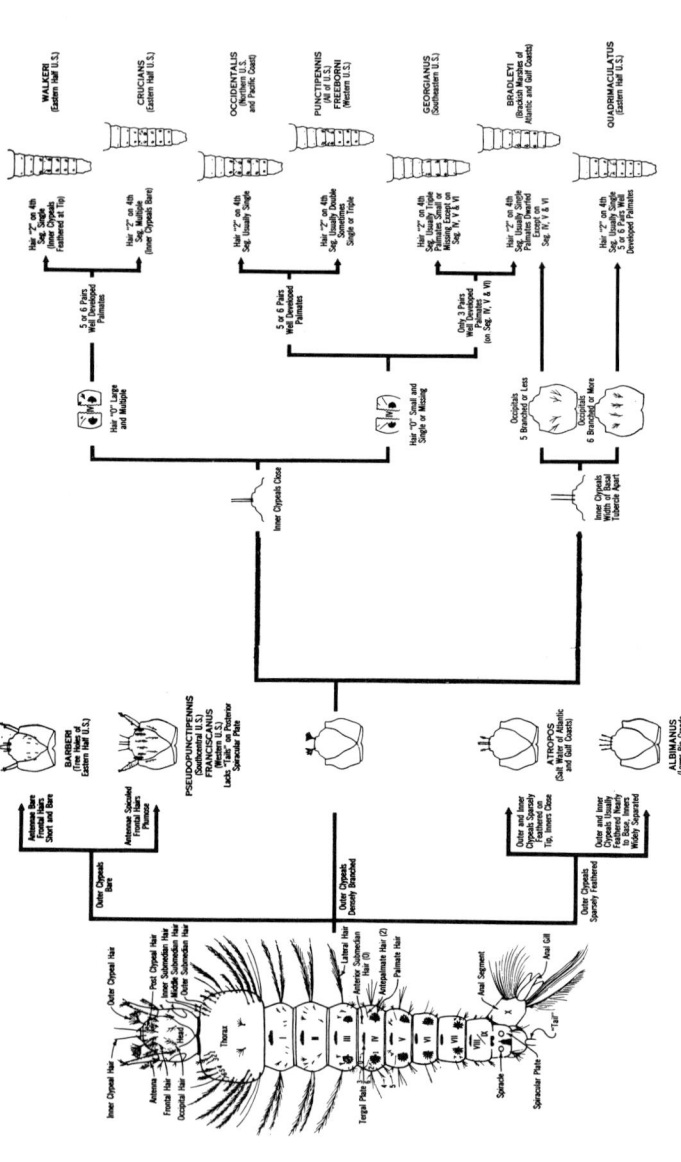

Fig 32 Example of the use of a taxonomic key for identification of a species of anopheline larva, according to a pictorial guide valid for the USA. (From 'Malaria Control in Impounded Waters', 1945, by courtesy of the Superintendent of Documents, US Government Printing Office, Washington DC)

endemic malaria, were able to maintain a degree of transmission of the infection, at least in a part of the area. The term 'secondary' vector may have also been used to describe Anopheles species of some importance during a certain season or in certain localities. In the incrimination of the main vectors of human malaria the dissection of wild caught

Table 6

Species of Anopheles vectors of primary importance in the transmission of malaria

A. aconitus Dönitz, 1902	A. maculatus Theobald, 1901
A. albimanus Wiedemann, 1821	A. maculipennis Meigen, 1818*
A. albitarsis Lynch Arribalzaga, 1878	A. mangyanus (Banks), 1906
A. annularis van der Wulp, 1884	A. melas Theobald, 1903
A. aquasalis Curry, 1932	A. messeae Falleroni, 1926
A. atroparvus van Thiel, 1927	A. minimus s.l. Theobald, 1901
A. aztecus Hoffman, 1935	A. moucheti s.l. Evans, 1901
A. balabacensis Baisas, 1936	A. multicolor Cambouliou, 1902
A. barbirostris van der Wulp, 1884*	A. nigerrimus Giles, 1900
A. bellator Dyar & Knab, 1908	A. nili (Theobald), 1904
A. campestris Reid, 1962	A. nuñez-tovari Gabaldon, 1940
A. claviger (Meigen), 1804	A. pattoni Christophers, 1926
A. cruzi Dyar & Knab, 1908	A. pharoensis Theobald, 1901
A. culicifacies Giles, 1901	A. philippinensis Ludlow, 1902
A. darlingi Root, 1926	A. pseudopunctipennis Theobald, 1901*
A. farauti, Laveran, 1902	A. punctimacula Dyar & Knab, 1906
A. fluviatilis James, 1902	A. punctulatus Dönitz, 1901*
A. freeborni Aitken, 1939	A. quadrimaculatus Say, 1824
A. funestus Giles, 1902	A. sacharovi Favre, 1903
A. gambiae Giles, 1902*	A. sergenti (Theobald), 1907
A. hispaniola (Theobald) 1903	A. sinensis Wiedemann, 1828
A. hyrcanus sinensis Wiedemann, 1828	A. stephensi s.l. Liston, 1901
A. jeyporiensis s.l. James, 1902	A. sundaicus (Rodenwald), 1926
A. koliensis Owen, 1942	A. superpictus Grassi, 1899
A. labranchiae Falleroni, 1926	A. umbrosus s.l. (Theobald), 1903
A. letifer Sandosham, 1944	A. varuna Iyengar, 1924
A. leucosphyrus Donitz, 1901	A. vestitipennis Dyar & Knab, 1906

Note: According to the International Code of Zoological Nomenclature, in writing the full scientific name of a mosquito the genus may be abbreviated to one or more letters but should always start with a capital letter. The name of the species must not be capitalised, even if it is derived from an author's surname. In precise description the surname of the author who first described and named the species is added without an intervening comma; the year of the publication is separated from the previous word by a comma. If the new name of the species replaces a name given to it originally then the present author's name is given in brackets.

Some names of species given in Table 6 refer to groups of Anopheles that have been subdivided into sub-species and varieties; this is indicated by the abbreviation s.l. (*sensu lato*).

Some species which are now known to represent complexes of sibling species are indicated by an asterisk.

Anopheles for the presence of plasmodial infection (with oöcysts or sporozoites) played an important part in the past. Today it is known that some anopheline species not normally associated with human habitations might be vectors of plasmodia of monkeys, rodents and other animals. Thus the previous interpretation of the vectorial importance of all species of Anopheles is based today on extensive epidemiological and entomological studies.

The concept of sibling species and species complexes has introduced an additional difficulty into the classification of Anopheles species considered as main vectors of malaria but the list given in Table 6 is not greatly different from the one given by Russell (1952) or Russell *et al*. (1963). True enough, over the past decade there have been some changes in this list because of splitting of species complexes of *A. barbirostris*, *A. gambiae*, *A. punctulatus*, *A. umbrosus* and others. The new trends in systematics of Anopheles attach more importance to biological and not only to morphological concept of species. This is of relevance to the malariologist as it helps him to understand the vagaries of relationship between some anopheline populations within a species complex and the transmission of malaria. Nevertheless the existence of sibling species or polymorphic species, the behaviour pattern of which influences their role as a vector, complicates what formerly appeared to be a simple problem.

Few of the species listed in Table 6 are vectors of human malaria over the whole area of their geographical distribution.

This is not only due to the fact that the inherent susceptibility of Anopheles to infection with human plasmodia varies somewhat in relation to the species of malaria parasite and its strain. The reasons for such 'susceptibility' (or not) to malaria infection are still not fully understood in biochemical or other terms. Numerous external factors such as temperature, humidity, etc., influence the development of the mosquito and its protozoan parasite.

Various species of Anopheles have well defined behaviour characteristics and this often determines the distribution of malaria. Thus in addition to climatic conditions, other factors affecting the breeding, feeding and survival of Anopheles must be taken into consideration in any control programme based on anti-mosquito measures.

The natural distribution of main vectors of malaria can be given broadly for the 12 epidemiological zones of malaria according to the classification by Macdonald. These are shown, together with the main vector species in Table 7 and Fig. 33.

Some important vectors of malaria have a very definite pattern of distribution over large areas. This is shown on the example of the Indian subcontinent on Fig. 34. The close relationship between various ecological zones within a relatively small area and the prevalence of certain species of Anopheles of West Malaysia is indicated in Fig. 35.

Table 7

Twelve epidemiological zones of malaria and some of the important vectors

Zone	Extension	Main malaria vectors
1 North American	From the Great Lakes to southern Mexico	*A. quadrimaculatus, A. freeborni* with *A. albimanus* as an incidental vector
2 Central American	Southern Mexico, the Caribbean islands, fringe of the South American coast	*A. albimanus, A. aquasalis, A. punctimacula, A. darlingi, A. aztecus*
3 South American	Most of the South American continent irregularly beyond the Tropic of Capricorn	*A. darlingi, A. aquasalis, A. pseudopunctipennis, A. bellator, A. cruzi*
4 North Eurasian	With the Palaearctic region excluding the Mediterranean coast of Europe	*A. atroparvus, A. sacharovi, A. maculipennis, A. messeae.* To the east *A. pattoni, A. sinensis*
5 Mediterranean	Southern coast of Europe, north-western part of Africa, Asia Minor and east beyond the Arab Sea	*A. labranchiae, A. sacharovi, A. superpictus, A. claviger, A. hispaniola, A. messeae*
6 Afro-Arabian	Africa north and south of the Tropic of Cancer including central part of the Arabian peninsula	*A. pharoensis, A. sergenti, A. multicolor, A. hispaniola, A. gambiae* (in part)
7 Afro-Tropical (formerly 'Ethiopian')	Southern Arabia, most of the African continent, Madagascar and the islands south and north of it	*A. gambiae* complex, *A. funestus, A. rufipes, A. moucheti, A. nili, A. pharoensis, A. d'thali*

Zone	Extension	Main malaria vectors
8 Indo-Iranian	North-west of the Persian gulf and east of it including the Indian sub-continent	*A. sacharovi*, *A. superpictus*, *A. culicifacies*, *A. stephensi*, *A. fluviatilis*, *A. annularis*
9 Indo-Chinese Hills	A triangular area including the Indo-Chinese peninsula, the north-western fringe beyond the Tropic of Cancer	*A. minimus*, *A. leucosphyrus*, *A. balabacensis*
10 Malaysian	Most of Indonesia, Malaysian peninsula, Philippines and Timor	*A. leucosphyrus*, *A. balabacensis*, *A. sundaicus*, *A. maculatus*, *A. sinensis*, *A. umbrosus*, *A. aconitus*, *A. philippinensis*, *A. minimus flavirostris*, *A. barbirostris*
11 Chinese	Largely the coast of mainland China, Korea, Taiwan, Japan	*A. sinensis*, *A. pattoni*, *A. sacharovi*
12 Australasian	Northern Australia, the island of New Guinea and the islands east of it to about 175° east of Greenwich, but excepting the malaria-free zone of the South Central Pacific	*A. koliensis*, *A. punctulatus*, *A. farauti*, *A. annulipes*, *A. bancrofti*

Notes:
1. The malaria-free zone of the south-central Pacific includes New Caledonia, New Zealand, the Caroline Islands, Marianas, up to Hawaiian islands, east to Galapagos and Juan Fernandez and rejoining the southern tip of New Zealand.
2. This table represents only a crude approximation of the distribution of most important vectors of malaria. For indication of generic and sub-generic relationships of confirmed and suspected vectors of malaria Russell *et al*. (1963) 'Practical Malariology' should be consulted.

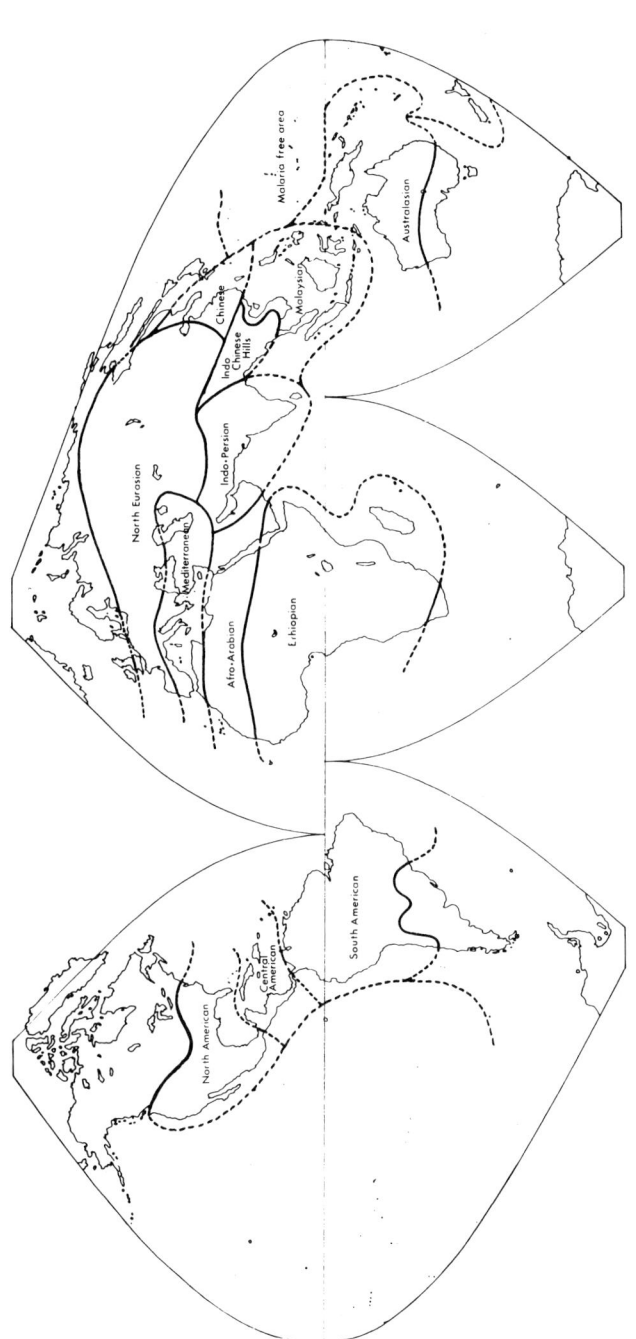

Fig 33 Twelve epidemiological zones of malaria according to the classification by Macdonald (1957).

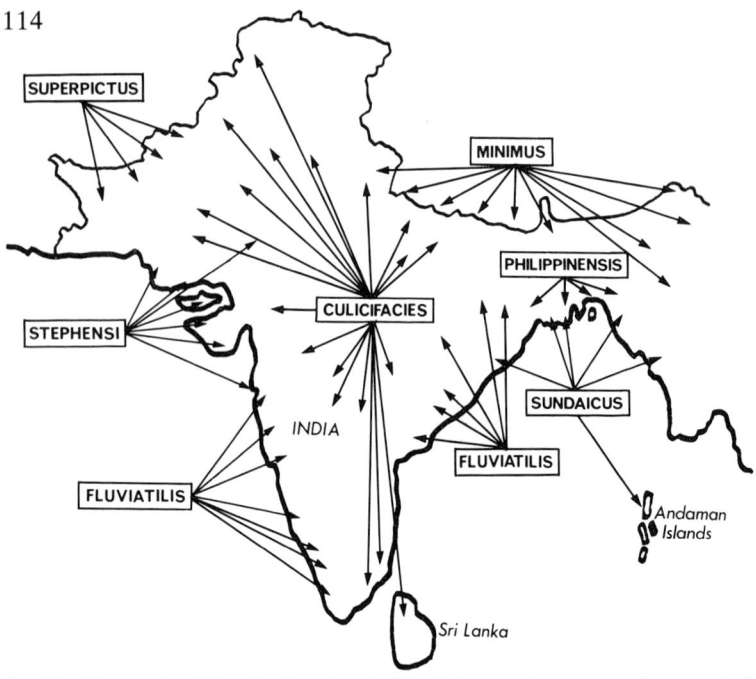

Fig 34 Geographical distribution of main Anopheles species, vectors of malaria in the Indian subcontinent. (From G. Covell, in Boyd, M.F. 1949)

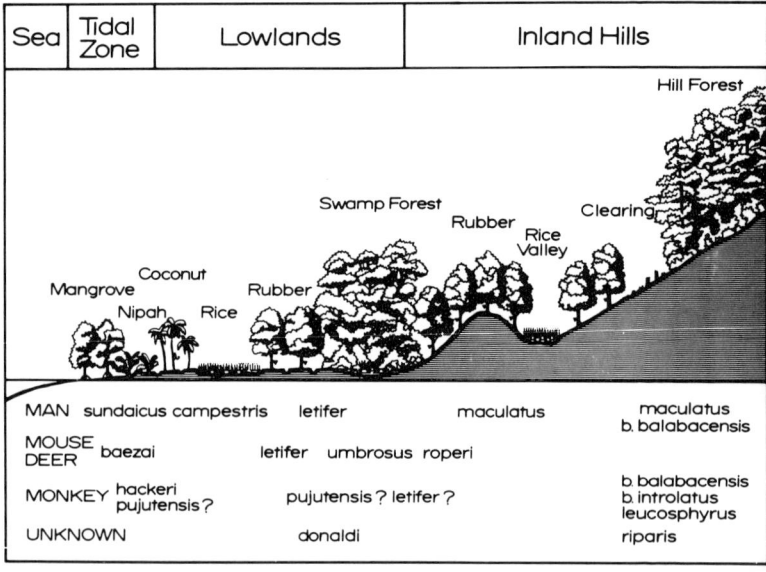

Fig 35 Ecological distribution of habitats of several species of Anopheles in a coastal area of West Malaysia. (Sandosham, 1965)

The Anopheles Vector

NATURAL HISTORY OF ANOPHELES

The male Anopheles feeds exclusively on nectar and fruit juices while the female feeds primarily upon blood. The mating of many species is preceded by the formation of swarms by the males. These occur during twilight and often at a certain light incidence. Males are apparently attracted to the females by their higher wing-beat frequencies. Copulation is usually initiated in flight. It is probable that the females of most species receive sufficient sperm for all subsequent egg batches from a single mating. In overwintering females, the sperm remains in the spermatheca for several months. Immediately after copulation a mating plug is produced in the genital chamber. This is believed to be formed by a secretion from the male accessory gland. The females of most species require at least two blood-meals before the first batch of eggs can develop. In subsequent cycles from the blood feed to oviposition a batch of eggs generally develops after each blood-meal. Eggs are always deposited in or near water, the number per batch varying between 100 and 600. Successive egg batches tend to decrease in size and may also show seasonal variation.

Adult female Anopheles normally feed on the blood of warm-blooded animals (Fig. 36). The amount of blood ingested by the female

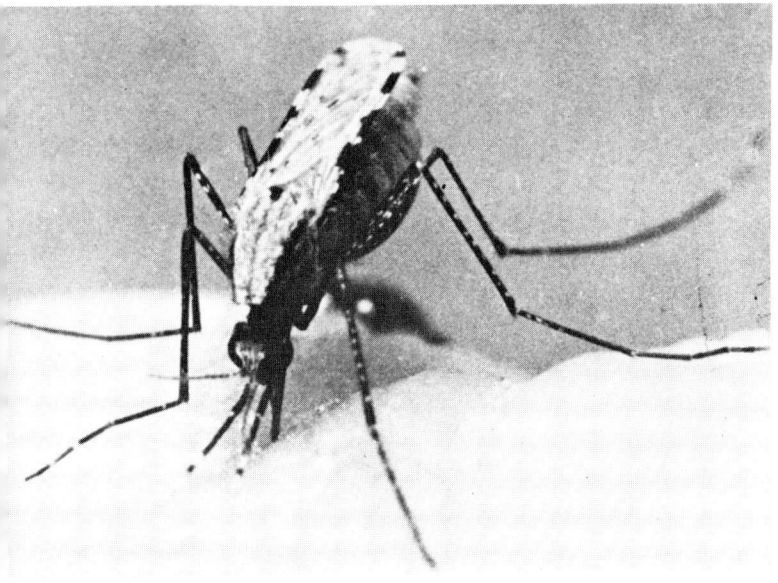

Fig 36 Female of *Anopheles gambiae* in the act of feeding on man. (Wellcome Museum of Medical Science)

mosquito depends largely on her own size and climatic conditions. It ranges between 1.3 and 3.0 µl and approximates to the weight of the mosquito. Blood contained in the stomach undergoes some concentration through excretion of plasma and is digested in one to a few days depending on the environmental temperature. The contents of the salivary glands are injected during the process of blood-sucking and this serves as an irritant, to increase the flow of blood to the capillary vessel, perforated by the biting apparatus of the mosquito. When the environmental temperature drops below a certain threshold females of some species of Anopheles undergo a process of hibernation during which they develop fat bodies, stop feeding and producing eggs. This process, known under the name of *gonotrophic dissociation*, may also occur in tropical Anopheles during the period of drought. The period of reproductive inactivity is the *diapause*.

Newly laid eggs usually require an incubation period of 2–3 days before they hatch, although in some species of Anopheles eggs may remain dormant for 16 days or even longer on wet mud; when flooded, such dormant eggs hatch within 3–4 minutes. However, anopheline eggs cannot survive after desiccation, though some species are more resistant in this respect.

Anopheline larvae are easily recognised by their appearance as they float horizontally on the surface of the water and feed by means of their mouth-brushes which sweep the floating particles towards the mouth. The larva moves by sharp jerks and if disturbed sinks below the surface.

After the third moult the fourth instar Anopheles larva develops into a comma-shaped, still aquatic pupa. Pupae do not feed but are nevertheless extremely active and respond quickly to all external stimuli. They dive into the water but soon rise again to the surface, where they breathe through their respiratory trumpets. After 2–4 days, depending on the temperature and other factors, the pupal skin splits dorsally and the adult insect (or *imago*) emerges. The process of emergence (or eclosion) takes a few minutes and if its outcome is successful the mosquito may rest for some time on the pupal cases to harden its wings before flying away.

The duration of the cycle from the egg to the adult Anopheles may vary between 7 days at 31°C, and 20 days at 20°C. Each species has its own optimum range of temperature.

When the adult (imago) emerges from any one batch the sexes are equal in number but the males appear first. The period from one egg-laying (oviposition) to another is known as the *gonotrophic cycle*. Its duration varies between 2–4 days in relation to the species of Anopheles and to environmental conditions, especially temperature.

The length of life of adult Anopheles depends on their internal characteristics such as greater vigour of some larger species but even more so on external factors among which temperature, humidity, presence of natural enemies etc. are the most important. When the mean temperature is over 35°C or the humidity less than 50% the longevity of Anopheles is drastically reduced, unless they find more favourable conditions in the microclimate of their resting places. The average duration of life of a female Anopheles under favourable climatic conditions is certainly over 3–4 weeks and occasionally much longer. Males live less long than the females and often not more than a few days.

Larval habitats

Collections of water which provide habitats for anopheline larvae may be temporary or permanent, natural or man-made. There is great diversity in the types of habitat utilised by the various species. This is due to the number of factors involved in the selection of sites by ovipositing females. The factors concerned include exposure to sunlight, temperature, salinity, organic content and other factors. Russell's classification of larval habitats (breeding places) of mosquitos is convenient and has been generally adopted:

1. Permanent or semipermanent standing fresh water
1.1. Large open marshes or marshy parts of lakes
1.2. Small ponds, pools, borrow-pits, stagnant canals and ditches
1.3. Spring fed pools, springs, and seepages from higher contours
1.4. Standing water in the fields (rice fields, plantations)
1.5. Open wells
1.6. Swamps and pools in the forest

2. Transient fresh water collections
2.1. Open pools in the fields or stagnant stream beds
2.2. Cattle hoof prints, pools in cart tracks, etc.

3. Permanent or semipermanent running fresh water
3.1. Open streams with vegetation
3.2. Stream beds running over gravel
3.3. Flowing water in canals and ditches
3.4. Streams in forests or plantations

4. Container habitats
4.1. Rock holes
4.2. Tree holes
4.3. Plant axils and epiphytic water-bearing plants
4.4. Discarded containers, natural and artificial (tins, tyres, coconut shells etc.)
4.5. Crab holes and cracks in the mud (fresh or brackish water)

118   *Essential Malariology*

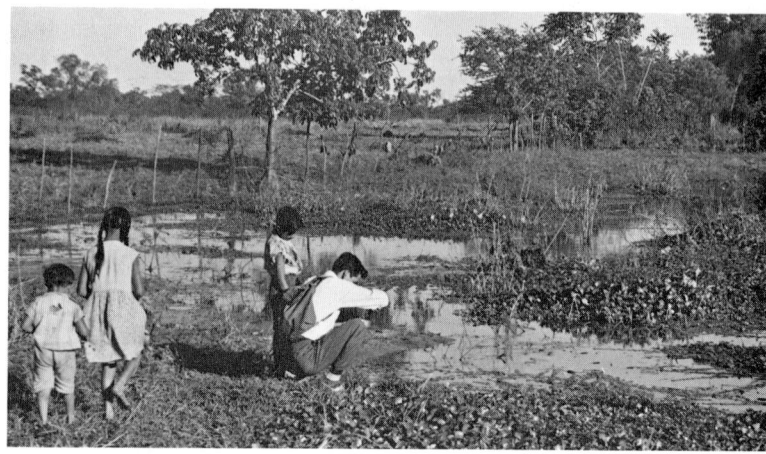

Fig 37 A typical larval habitat (breeding place) of *A. albimanus*, one of the main vectors of malaria in Mexico and Central America. (WHO photograph by M. Rude)

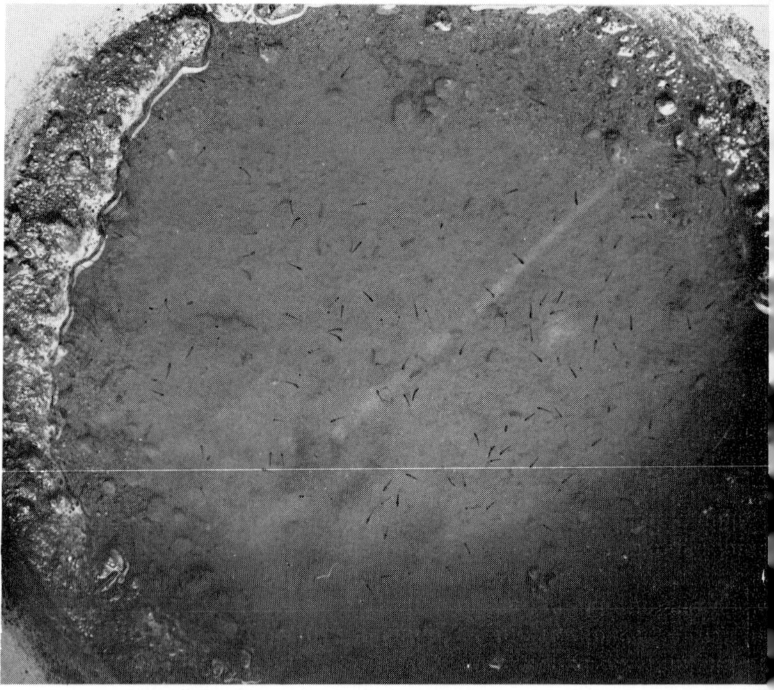

Fig 38 A typical habitat (breeding place) of *A. gambiae*, the major vector of malaria in tropical Africa. Note the hundreds of larvae on the surface. (WHO photograph by D. Henrioud)

5. Brackish water
5.1. Marshes, ponds and swamps (not tidal)
5.2. Tidal swamps
5.3. Small collections of brackish water

Larval habitats are commonly found in association with emergent vegetations, such as grass, or mats of floating vegetation or algae (Fig. 37.)

Artificial containers, such as pots or tubs, are generally unsuitable for most anopheline species although *A. stephensi* in India is often found in cisterns, wells, tin cans, earthenware pots, and other man-made receptacles. Some species readily breed in temporary rain pools and in small puddles of water, such as those found in the imprints of animals' hooves (Fig. 38). Large expanses of open water free from vegetation seldom support anopheline larvae, although breeding may occur in quiet pools and pockets of relatively still water along the grassy margins of lakes, streams, and rivers.

Man-made malaria is a term applied to many of man's activities which produce breeding places suitable for malaria-carrying mosquitos and so favour the incidence of the disease. Untouched mangrove swamps are often innocuous until man fells the trees and interferes with the natural line of drainage by constructing roads and railways. Riverine deltas are also often harmless until man creates breeding places and alters the watertable by erecting embankments to reclaim land for agriculture or building without providing proper drainage.

Irrigation works are frequently to blame in this matter, chiefly by a failure to provide adequate drainage facilities, thus predisposing to waterlogging. Other causes of 'irrigation malaria', are defective sluice-gates, badly maintained irrigation ditches, seepage from canal banks and beds, borrow-pits, and lack of a planned or controlled system of field channels. One of the commonest faults in road and rail construction is the improper placement of culverts. They tend to be either too high, so that water is held up on the upper side of the embankment; or too low, so that water remains in the bed of the culvert itself. Another common source of mosquito breeding is the line of borrow-pits commonly found alongside roads and railways. Breeding places are also often produced during the course of building construction, especially in connection with docks and other large works in urban areas of the tropics.

Seasonal fluctuations.

At the onset of the cold season some species are killed off. They may then be found only at lower altitudes where temperatures are still suitable. In other species the males only are killed off and the females seek shelter from cold (*hibernation*). Before they hibernate a last meal of blood is taken which, instead of helping in the formation of eggs, goes to make fat on which the females live while hanging immobile in their winter quarters. Before the females arrive at a hibernating place some species, in subtropical areas, may indulge in a long prehibernation flight, which is much longer than their normal one, extending to as much as 12 miles, e.g. *A. sacharovi* in Syria. In complete hibernation the female mosquitos remain torpid until the coming of the warm season. In some species only a partial hibernation occurs, and the females emerge occasionally from their winter quarters to have another feed in order to renew their store of fat, after which they return. In other species the winter is passed in the larval stage, e.g. *A. claviger* (northern Europe). Another seasonal effect is *aestivation*, seen in the hot dry season of some countries, where the female seeks to avoid the intensely dry atmosphere by remaining in a cool damp place until the dry spell is over.

Seasonal changes such as temperature, rainfall and humidity have an obvious effect on the anopheline population and thus also on the incidence of malaria. Some unusual events may give rise to major effects. Thus in 1958 in Ethiopia an excessive rainfall combined with high temperature resulted in high breeding activity of *A. gambiae* followed by an epidemic of malaria with three million cases and 150 000 deaths. On the other hand, a severe drought in south-western areas of Sri Lanka (Ceylon) contributed to an excessive breeding of *A. culicifacies* in 1934–35 and resulted in a severe epidemic of falciparum malaria.

Behaviour pattern of adult Anopheles

The adult female often takes its first blood-meal the night after it emerges from the pupal stage. Feeding occurs, almost without exception, between dusk and dawn, but anophelines may feed during daylight hours in densely shaded woodland or dark interiors of shelters and houses. The feeding habits vary greatly; some species prefer a non-human host and will feed on animals even if a human host is available, and the converse may be true of other species.

The readiness of Anopheles mosquitos to feed at a particular time of darkness depends to some extent on environmental conditions but the biting cycles of many species of mosquitos are so constant in different and yet comparable conditions that they reflect some basic phenomena of general biology characteristic for a particular species.

The facts involved in the location of a given human or animal host are still very little understood. A number of stimuli attract the female Anopheles to its host; among them temperature, moisture, colour, smell and carbon dioxide tension are of importance. Some individuals are particularly attractive to mosquitos while others are much less so.

There are also different degrees of attractiveness by different animals.

The terms '*anthropophilic*' or '*zoophilic*' have been used for certain species of Anopheles to indicate, respectively, a supposed preference for feeding on man or on domestic animals. It must be understood that such terms are relative, since many Anopheles species are ready to feed on alternative hosts when the favourite one is not available.

The origin of the ingested blood in the stomach of a freshly engorged mosquito can be determined by the use of precipitin tests. In practice the important answer that the results of such tests give is whether the blood was of human or of animal origin. The proportion of Anopheles giving a positive precipitin reaction for human blood is '*the human blood index*'; such an index is a valuable pointer to the importance of an Anopheles species to act as a vector of human malaria.

Resting places are frequently inside houses; female mosquitos commonly enter a house after dark, take a blood-meal, and then, being heavily engorged with blood, fly to a near by wall or ceiling where they normally rest during daylight. The mosquitos may rest on clothing hanging on a wall, on the back or underside of pieces of furniture or pictures, etc. The females frequently prefer the lower portions of the interiors of houses where temperatures are lower and the humidity is higher.

Some species seek secluded natural resting places such as clumps of vegetation, hollow trees and logs, large exposed tree roots, and holes or crevices in rocks and soil.

It is obvious that house-resting is of special importance in relation to control methods using residual insecticides. Generally speaking the daytime resting place is dark and with a degree of humidity that provides a tolerable microclimate for the mosquito. Natural resting places outside the houses are important as they may yield samples of the mosquito population, less biased than human habitations or animal shelters and not affected by the toxic action of the insecticide. This is the reason why entomologists use artificial resting places for collecting mosquitos in some treated areas.

The behaviour characteristics of Anopheles species may be artificially grouped, according to their feeding habits and their relationship to man, into three kinds; *domestic*, those which come into houses and rest there after feeding; *wild*, those which will only feed outside and never enter houses; and *intermediate group*, those which may feed in houses and leave at once. The feeding and resting habits of adult anopheline mosquitos have been intensely studied and special terms are used in relation to the pattern of behaviour. They are: (a) *endophily*, the habit of remaining within a man-made shelter throughout the whole or a definite part of the gonotrophic cycle. Food may be sought within or without a man-made structure; (b) *exophily*, the habit of spending the greater part of the gonotrophic cycle out of doors.

Food may be sought within or without a man-made structure; (c) *endophagy*, the habit of obtaining the blood-meal within a man-made structure; (d) *exophagy*, the habit of seeking the blood-meal out of doors. Some species fail to conform to a rigid pattern, for example, *A. fluviatilis* (India) in the second half of its gonotrophic cycle rests outside until oviposition, and *A. aquasalis* in Trinidad, though strictly exophilic, leaving a house immediately after a meal, feeds as much indoors as outdoors.

Since all these characteristics are of great importance in control programmes, the habits of the vector species must be well understood by teams engaged in malaria control or eradication.

Flight range

Anopheles mosquitos are not usually found more than two or three kilometres from their breeding places in any large number. Normally the females disperse further than the males. However, strong seasonal winds may carry Anopheles up to 30 km from their main breeding place and various other factors may greatly influence the average flight range of some species. Generally tropical Anopheles have a shorter flight range than mosquitos present in temperate climates.

Dispersal by flying is known as active dispersal, whereas passive dispersal means carriage by any other means than the insects' own wings; this may be wind, aeroplane, train, truck and ship, and may result in Anopheles being found very many miles from their place of origin.

Generally speaking, the control of anophelines within two kilometres of docks, parking sites for aircraft or other systems of transportation, and storage areas where migrating mosquitos may rest, should provide adequate protection.

For the study of Anopheles dispersal or flight range adult mosquitos may be marked with different colours of fluorescent powders. The newer methods consist of adding radioactive phosphorus or strontium compounds to the aquatic medium in which the larvae grow. The emerging adults are radioactive and this can be recognised by the conventional physical or photographic methods.

Anopheles species complexes

Early in the present century it was recognised that within a species group of some Anopheles there are forms with some biologically and morphologically different characteristics. The practical implications of this phenomenon became more obvious at the end of the First World War when the return of troops to Europe from some extremely malarious areas resulted in highly localised outbreaks of indigenous malaria instead of widespread epidemics that could be expected from the known distribution of potential mosquito vectors. This situation of *anophelism without malaria* remained puzzling until the discovery of some subtle differences in groups of Anopheles within one apparently single species.

The detection of 'long-winged' and 'short-winged' forms of *Anopheles maculipennis* in the Netherlands and their association with fresh and brackish water of their breeding places provided the first clue. Other studies in Italy resulted in the discovery of forms of *A. maculipennis* that could be separated on the basis of their egg markings. Further studies of behaviour patterns of these groups and their reproductive compatibility showed that within the *A. maculipennis* species there are at least five sibling species and two sub-species, all of them forming the *A. maculipennis* complex.

The practical importance of this work was the clear evidence that the different species within the *A. maculipennis* complex differ in their feeding and other habits and thus in their ability to transmit malaria. It follows that those which are not involved in the transmission of the infection can be largely ignored in control activities.

More recently the pioneering work carried out in Italy demonstrated the value of studying the structure and the banding patterns of chromosomes in the salivary glands of Anopheles for identification of sibling species. These cytotaxonomic methods were concentrated at first on the polytene or giant chromosomes found in various tissues of insects but most clearly seen in salivary glands. The banding pattern of polytene chromosomes is constant, corresponding to the gene sequence. In addition to the banding pattern there are other characters or changes of the chromosome structure such as inversions, translocations, deletions etc.

Further studies were based on crossing experiments to determine the genetic compatibility of various groups and the sterility or otherwise of hybrids. For this purpose it is necessary to colonise separate groups of Anopheles in cages in laboratory conditions. Where mass cage matings between separate groups is impossible crossing can be obtained by an artificial forced mating technique. This involves the presentation of genitalia of an anaesthetised female to those of a male Anopheles whose head was cut off just before, thus inducing a reflex action of copulation and fertilisation. Using this technique it has been possible to cross species which will not mate in cages.

These and other cytotaxonomic and cytogenetic methods were soon extended to other species of Anopheles and especially to *A. gambiae*, the most important malaria vector in Africa.

Until 1956 *A. gambiae* was considered a single species with some dark or light varieties breeding in fresh or salt water. A vast amount of research on this group has shown that *Anopheles gambiae* is a complex of at least six species. Four of these six species have been given the provisional names of species A, B, C and D; the other two (*A. melas* and *A. merus*) are salt water species, usually found near the coast. The

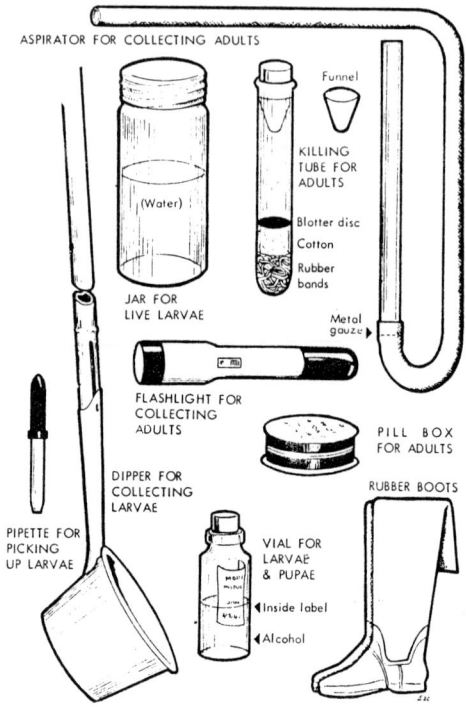

Fig 39 Basic equipment for collection of larvae and adults of mosquitos in the field. (WHO, 1972 'Vector control in international health')

first two are extremely efficient vectors of malaria throughout tropical parts of the African continent. Species C has only been found in south-east Africa, Ethiopia and Zanzibar: species D exists in a forest area of Uganda. The study of cross fertility within the *A. gambiae* species complex served as a basis for research on the possibility of mass release of sterile hybrid males as a method of genetic control of natural populations.

Among a few other Anopheles species complexes that of *A. punctulatus* of New Guinea and the surrounding area should be mentioned. Originally three species were recognised on morphological features, but recent laboratory studies have shown the presence of an unsuspected fourth.

The Anopheles Vector

ENTOMOLOGICAL METHODS

There are a number of techniques, either simple or elaborate, for collection of Anopheles in their aquatic stage or as adults. The main practical indications for these methods are mentioned in the section describing the purpose of a malaria survey, and only a few of these methods can be described here (Fig. 39).

For collection of mosquito eggs, larvae or pupae various scoops, ladles and dishes, preferably with a white enamel bottom, are used in the field. More elaborate equipment includes fine mesh 'larval nets'. The proper technique of dipping for anopheline larvae or pupae demands a fairly good knowledge of the type of water and aquatic vegetation preferred by malaria vectors (Fig. 40). Perseverance is just as important as proper clothing and footwear for muddy conditions.

Sketch-maps indicating the distribution of streams, swamps and other sources of flowing or standing water are needed to pin-point the location of larval habitats producing dangerous species of malaria vectors.

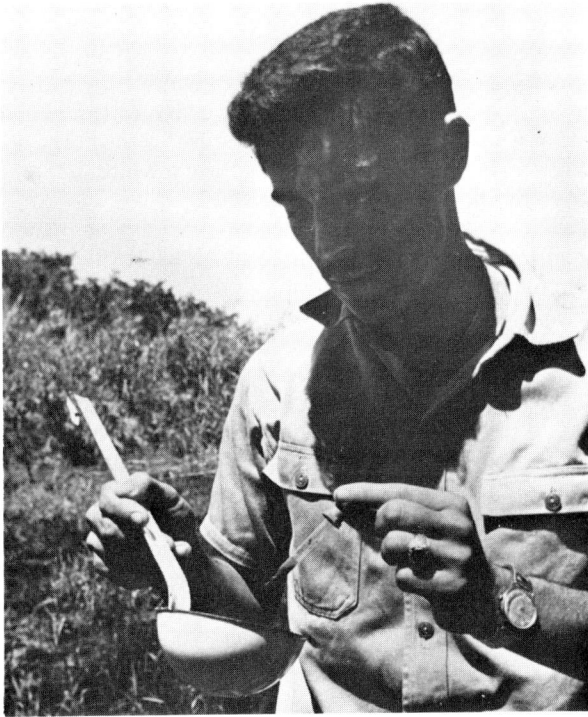

Fig 40 Method of collection of anopheline larvae in the field. (WHO photograph)

It may be pertinent here to quote P. F. Russell's dictum that 'sun-loving Anopheles are not effectively sampled by shade-loving personnel; nor can aquatic larvae be adequately scouted by dry-footed collectors'.

Live adult *Anopheles* are collected by simple 'tube catching' or by suction tubes. Various types of suction tubes are used. Fig. 39 shows the type of collecting equipment which is simple and generally adequate. It consists of a collecting suction tube (aspirator), a killing tube, pill boxes, cages (if live mosquitos are collected), field record forms, a pencil, an electric torch and a map. The killing bottle is made from glass or a plastic tube about 2.5 cm (1 inch) in diameter and 16.5–18 cm (6–7 inches) in length. The tube is filled to a depth of about 2.5 cm (1 inch) with finely chopped rubber bands or art gum; a sufficient quantity of chloroform is added to saturate the rubber. A disc of blotting paper or fine gauze is placed over the rubber. The tube is closed with a cork stopper. Such a tube remains effective for several weeks and can be recharged with chloroform when necessary.

Obviously this simple method of collecting adult Anopheles sheltering in houses or animal quarters suffers from many errors and depends not only on the time of day when the collection is made but also on the skill and reliability of the collector. An alternative, widely used and very convenient method of collection of dead Anopheles from human houses and animal shelters consists of spraying inside the closed room a pyrethrum-kerosene solution in the form of a coarse mist and retrieving the dead mosquitos from a white sheet, previously spread over the floor of the room or shed.

A large variety of other techniques have been developed for sampling mosquito populations. Captures at night on human volunteers exposed to the bites are one of the methods used; another method uses special traps with animal or human 'baits'; light-trap collections suitable for other mosquitos are generally unsatisfactory for collections of Anopheles. Naturally, none of these sampling techniques has a direct relationship to the actual mosquito population in the locality. Nevertheless each of these methods, used properly, gives some idea of the relative trends and enables us to establish an appropriate baseline. Thus the mean number of Anopheles females in relation to a dwelling unit such as a house or a room is known as the '*anopheline density*'.

Such sampling indicates which species of mosquitos are present in the locality and by the number of specimens collected in proportion to the number of houses or rooms visited it provides information on whether the control operations are effective. Regular sampling over long periods gives a meaningful set of data. Thus, it is important to establish sampling stations in the early part of the control programme and select them so that they reveal the situation over the whole area. In addition to the collection of adult mosquitos, regular sampling for larvae in known larval habitats is helpful for monitoring the control operations.

Identification of species of Anopheles collected in the field is of obvious importance since it permits the separation of harmless species from those that are important malaria vectors. For the proper use of entomological keys to larvae or adults of various species known to exist in an area, the knowledge of mosquito anatomy is necessary. Most of the characters mentioned in the keys can be observed with the aid of a good magnifying glass or a binocular microscope, but some larval details may require the use of the low power of a standard microscope. Generally, simple entomological keys are based on the appearance of female Anopheles; keys for males are much more difficult to compile because the markings on the palps and on wings are less characteristic or not so obvious. The principle of the use of binominal entomological keys is explained in Figs 31 and 32.

Malaria infection in Anopheles

The presence of an infection in Anopheles may confirm the importance of a given species as a vector of malaria. In relation to the cycle of development of plasmodia in mosquitos it is important to recognise the relevant stages in the stomach of the Anopheles (oöcysts) and in the salivary glands (sporozoites).

Dissection of the midgut of the female mosquito is not difficult though it requires some practice. It is far easier to carry it out than to describe in detail the successive stages of this operation. These are as follows:
1) Identify the species of the killed Anopheles and record its source of collection.
2) Remove the wings and legs.
3) Place a drop of normal (0.85%) saline on the glass slide and place the trimmed insect close to the drop, with the abdomen pointing towards the observer.
4) Under a low-power magnification of a dissecting microscope, using a dissecting cutting needle (Shute's needle) nick the chitinous skin at the sides of the abdomen between segments 6 and 7.
5) Holding the thorax with one needle, place the other needle across the tip of the abdomen and draw the abdominal contents out with a steady gentle traction, so that they touch the drop of saline.
6) When the contents, including the midgut, come out cut off the tip of the abdomen, the ovaries and the Malpighian tubes.
7) Transfer the loosened midgut into a fresh, larger drop of saline on the same slide. A hair may be inserted to prevent excessive pressure of the coverslip.
8) Place gently a small coverslip on the isolated midgut and examine

under a compound microscope for the presence of oöcysts. Use low power first and confirm under higher magnification. The oöcysts lie on the outer surface of the midgut and appear as clear round or oval bodies, containing distinct pigment granules. Larger, more mature oöcysts are 30–60 microns in diameter, they have lost the pigment and are filled with hundreds of sickle shaped sporozoites, which escape from the oöcyst when the latter is ruptured by a gentle pressure on the coverslip.

Dissection of salivary glands of the female mosquito may be carried out by two methods; that more commonly used proceeds by the following stages.

1) Place the trimmed Anopheles on its right side on a slide with a small drop of normal saline close to the neck.
2) With the left hand dissecting needle press gently on the thorax; place the right hand needle just behind the head and gently pull the head off.
3) The glands are usually dragged out attached to the head and show as small, sausage shaped, refractile bodies, 12–14 microns in length.
4) Cut the glands loose from the head and immerse them in the drop of saline on the slide.
5) Cover the glands with a small coverslip, rupture them by a gentle pressure and examine under high power for the presence of sporozoites.
6) The presence of sporozoites can be confirmed by removing the coverslip, inverting it on the slide, securing to it with a drop of Canada balsam and, after fixing with absolute methyl alcohol, staining it with Giemsa stain.

An Anopheles which, on dissection, shows oöcysts on the stomach wall is *infected*; when it shows sporozoites in the salivary glands, it is *infective*. The percentage of female Anopheles caught in nature showing sporozoites in the glands is the *sporozoite rate*. The percentage showing oöcysts on dissection of the midgut is the *oöcyst rate*. These rates should be related to some determined species, and the number of mosquitos dissected should be indicated. Information as to the source of capture (e.g., houses, stables, natural shelters) is important. In highly endemic areas considerable variation in the sporozoite rate may be due to seasonal increase or decrease of the mosquito population, and in such a case some statistical assessment of the significance of the rate is necessary.

Maintenance of laboratory colonies of some Anopheles for subsequent studies of the pattern of inheritance of insecticide resistance or the development of methods of genetic control became possible only ten years ago, when methods of artificial fertilisation of female Anopheles were introduced.

Chapter 7

Epidemiology of Malaria

Geographical distribution
Indigenous malaria has been recorded as far north as 64°N latitude (Archangel in the USSR) and as far south as 32°S latitude (Cordoba in Argentina). It has occurred in the Dead Sea area at 400 metres below sea level and at Londiani (Kenya) at 2600 metres above sea level or at 2800 metres in Cochabamba (Bolivia).

Within these limits of lattitude and altitude there are large areas free of malaria, which is essentially a focal disease, since the transmission of malaria depends greatly on local environmental and other conditions.

Malaria has a major place among the endemic tropical diseases. It has been estimated in the 1950s that the annual incidence of the disease was of the order of 250 million cases with 2.5 million people dying of malaria every year. The extent of endemic malaria has now greatly decreased as a result of eradication and control programmes carried out during the past quarter of a century. A more detailed account of the present situation is given in a different chapter of this book.

Epidemics of malaria, so common in the past, are now less frequent. One of the greatest epidemics of malaria in modern times struck the Soviet Union after the First World War; more than 10 million cases were reported in 1923–26, and there were at least 60 000 deaths. The Sri Lanka or Ceylon epidemic of 1934–35 caused nearly 3 million cases of malaria and 82 000 deaths; in 1938 the invasion of Brazil by *A. gambiae* was followed by an epidemic with over 100 000 cases and at least 14 000 deaths; in 1942–44 the same mosquito invaded lower Egypt and caused about 160 000 malaria cases and more than 12 000 deaths; in 1958 an epidemic of malaria in Ethiopia caused more than 3 million cases and 150 000 deaths; in 1963 there was an epidemic of malaria in Haiti, in the wake of the typhoon Flora, with 75 000 cases. In 1967 a serious resurgence of malaria in Sri Lanka greatly handicapped the progress of eradication of this disease from the island. Since 1973 there is a marked resurgence of malaria in several countries of southern Asia. In 1976 alone well over 7 million cases of malaria were reported from the Indian sub-continent.

P. vivax has the widest geographical range; it is prevalent in many temperate zones, but also in the sub-tropics and tropics. *P. falciparum* is the commonest species throughout the tropics and sub-tropics although it may occur in some areas with temperate climate.

P. malariae is patchily present over the same range as *P. falciparum* but much less common. *P. ovale* is found chiefly in tropical Africa, but also occasionally in the West Pacific.

Natural transmission of malaria infection occurs through exposure to the bites of infective female Anopheles mosquitos. The source of human malaria infection is nearly always a human subject, whether a sick person or a symptomless carrier of the parasite.

With the possible exception of chimpanzees in tropical Africa, which may carry the infection with *P. malariae*, no other animal reservoir of human plasmodia is known to exist. However, there have been a few cases of natural or accidental infection of man with some plasmodia of simian origin.

The alternation between the human and the mosquito host represents the biological *cycle* of transmission of the malaria parasite. The transmission of the infection by the mosquito from the human carrier (donor) to the human victim (recipient) represents the *chain* of transmission.

However, the infection may also be transmitted *accidentally*; this occurs not infrequently as a result of blood transfusion when the donor harbours malaria parasites. Drug addicts using the same hypodermic needle have been known to infect one another. *Congenital* infection of the newborn from an infected mother also occurs, but is comparatively rare.

Deliberate transmission of malaria was common during the first half of this century for malaria therapy of neurosyphilis. Other instances of deliberate infection refer to experimental trials of antimalarial drugs, when the disease is transmitted to volunteers. In both cases the transmission may be carried out either by injection of infected blood or by bites of infected mosquitos.

Natural transmission of malaria depends on the presence of and relationship between the three basic epidemiological factors: the *host*, the *agent* and the *environment*. Man is the vertebrate host of human plasmodia; the Anopheles mosquito is the invertebrate host. However, the latter may also be considered as the agent of transmission while the malaria parasite is the true agent of the infection. The environment should be considered from its three aspects: physical, biological and socio-economic (Fig. 41).

Host factors

Sex and age are not important factors with regard to the malaria infection, but children have generally a higher degree of susceptibility than adults. There are factors involved in the immune response: persons of African origin seem to have a greater innate immunity to some types of malaria than other races.

There are many epidemiological variables in the response of the human victim to the infection. There is evidence that in certain parts of the world the high frequency of haemoglobin S in the population is due to the evolutionary selection related to the fact that the presence of this haemoglobin has a mitigating effect on the severity of *P. falciparum* infections.

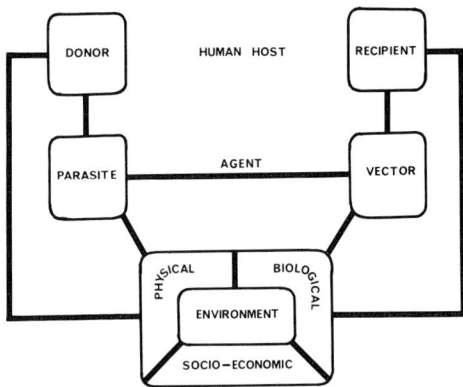

Fig 41 Epidemiological factors of host, agent and environment involved in the transmission of malaria.

It seems that persons with red blood cells negative to Duffy blood group determinants are relatively insusceptible to infections with *P. vivax*. There is also some evidence of the protective action of genetic deficiency of an enzyme (glucose-6-phosphate dehydrogenase) normally present in the erythrocytes.

Generally speaking, populations exposed continually to intense malaria in highly endemic areas develop a degree of immunity to the infection. Mosquitos derive the infection from an individual with parasites in his blood, but not necessarily from an individual with fever or other manifest signs of disease. When malaria is endemic a proportion of the population are usually carriers of gametocytes and this may be particularly the case amongst young children and infants.

Agent

Within each of the four species of human plasmodia, there are a number of strains which have different epidemiological and other features, although they are indistinguishable morphologically. Thus the European strains of *P. falciparum* are readily carried by *A. atroparvus* which is refractory to infection with African or Indian strains of this plasmodium. The pattern of relapse in West Pacific strains of *P. vivax* is different from the relapse pattern of vivax malaria occurring in other parts of the world. There are also considerable differences between the long incubation period of the disease caused by some North European strains of *P. vivax* and the short incubation period seen in infections by other strains of this plasmodial species. Finally several geographical strains of *P. falciparum* and *P. vivax* show different types and degrees of resistance to antimalarial drugs.

There are nearly 400 species of Anopheles of which some 60 are proved vectors of human malaria. However in each geographical area there are usually not more than three or four anopheline species that can be regarded as important vectors. To be an effective vector a species must be present in adequate numbers in or near human habitations. A species with a marked preference for human blood rather than for animal blood is a better vector. Finally the length of life of a mosquito is a paramount factor in malaria transmission; the latter varies in different places in relation to temperature and humidity. Thus the development of plasmodia in the Anopheles depends on a minimum temperature below which it does not occur, and above which the amount of transmission is dependent on this and other environmental factors.

There is a condition known under the term *anophelism without malaria*; this generally means the presence of Anopheles which cannot transmit the infection either because they are non-vectors, or because the plasmodia have been eliminated from the local population and importation of malaria from elsewhere is unlikely or is effectively prevented.

Environment

Variation in climatic conditions has a profound effect on the life of a mosquito and on the development of malaria parasites. Hence its influence on the transmission of the disease and on its seasonal incidence. The most important factors are temperature and humidity. Malaria parasites cease to develop in the mosquito when the temperature is below 16°C. The best conditions for the development of plasmodia in the Anopheles and the transmission of the infection are when the mean temperature is within a range of 20–30°C while the mean relative humidity is at least 60% (Fig. 42). A high relative humidity lengthens the life of the mosquito and enables it to live long enough to transmit the infection to several persons.

The association of malaria with rainfall in parts of the world where the latter is seasonal is due not only to greater breeding activity of mosquitos, but also to the rise in relative humidity and higher probability of survival of female Anopheles. Excessive rainfall or drought play an important part in production of regional epidemics of malaria.

Rainfall, which normally increases the amount of surface water, may have at times a negative effect on the amount of transmission of malaria. Excessive rainfall may transform small streams into rapid torrents and thus strand many larvae and pupae on the edges of the

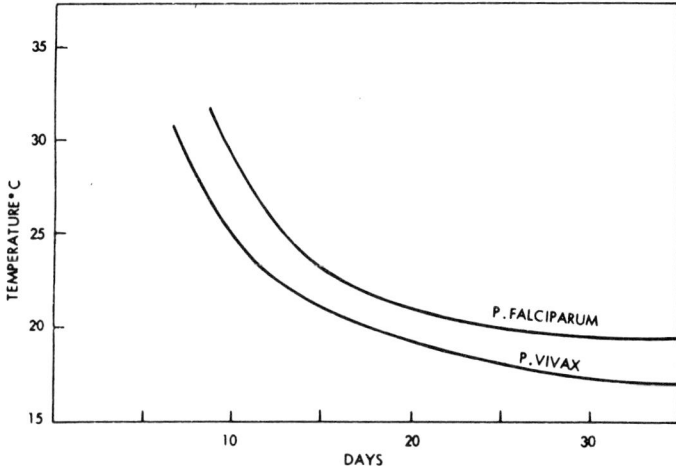

Fig 42 Duration of sporogonic (extrinsic) development of malaria parasites in Anopheles in relation to the environmental temperature. (Macdonald, 1957)

water channel. Conversely deficient rains in other parts of the world change many rivers into a string of pools in which certain Anopheles would breed in profusion. The latter occurrence was often observed in Sri Lanka, where severe epidemics followed the years of drought, resulting in greatly increased breeding of *A. culicifacies*. It is not only the amount of rainfall which is important but also its distribution over the month or the year. Russell proposed a formula for the distribution of rainfall:

$$\frac{\text{Total rainfall} \times \text{number of rainy days}}{\text{Number of days in the month}}$$

The presence of waterbearing plants (in which Anopheles breed) or the presence of cattle (on which some Anopheles feed) constitutes a biological factor of the environment. (Fig. 41)

Finally social and economic factors, such as sanitation, housing, occupation, poverty, etc., have an important effect since malaria is more prevalent in underdeveloped countries. The evidence concerning the susceptibility to malaria infection in relation to human malnutrition is inconclusive.

Various human activities may be conducive to dispersal of plasmodia or dangerous vectors of malaria to new areas of the world. In 1930 Brazil was invaded by *A. gambiae* from Africa probably transported by ships plying between Dakar and Natal in connection with the new air route. This resulted in a serious epidemic of malaria in north-

Table 8

Some characteristics of unstable and stable malaria (after Macdonald, 1957)

Characteristics	Unstable	Stable
Endemicity	Usually low to moderate; High endemicity may occur.	Very high endemicity common; low to moderate may occur.
Determining causes	Vector of low anthropophily and low to moderate longevity. Climatic conditions favourable for short periods of transmission.	Vector of high anthropophily and moderate to high longevity. Climatic conditions favourable for long periods of transmission.
Anopheline density (sufficient to maintain transmission)	High (1–10 or more bites per person/night).	Very low (as low as 0.025 bites per person/night).
Seasonal changes	Pronounced.	Not very pronounced, except for short dry season.
Fluctuations in incidence and predominant parasite	Very marked and uneven. Most often *P. vivax* as main parasite.	Not marked and related to seasons. *P. falciparum* prevalent parasite.
Immunity of the population	Variable with some groups of low immunity.	High, though varying in degree.
Epidemic outbreaks	Likely when climatic or other conditions suitable.	Unlikely to occur in the indigenous population.
Amenability to control or eradication	Not unduly difficult by imagicides and larvicides combined with chemotherapy. Daily anopheline mortality of 20–25% may be adequate for control of transmission.	Very difficult to control especially in rural areas. Eradication unlikely unless socio-economic conditions favourable. Daily anopheline mortality at least 50% for a degree of control.

eastern Brazil but an anti-mosquito campaign resulted in the eradication of *A. gambiae* from South America. In 1966 *A. stephensi* was recorded for the first time in Africa having been probably carried by aircraft from Saudi Arabia to Egypt.

Wars and large scale population movements whether of pilgrims or labour forces from endemic areas have often been a factor in the spread of malaria. The return of troops from malarious war areas to England during the First World War resulted not only in a high number of cases of imported malaria but also in an outbreak of local disease which caused nearly 500 cases of 'introduced' malaria among the civilian population. In the United States nearly 20 000 cases of imported malaria were reported during the period 1969–74, in soldiers returning from south-east Asia.

During the past decade the greatly increased speed and volume of human travel has resulted in large numbers of imported malaria in many countries. Problems of malaria imported or introduced into non-endemic countries by persons infected elsewhere have been dealt with in a separate section.

MALARIA IN THE HUMAN COMMUNITY

The term *endemicity* refers to a general statement indicating the amount or severity of malaria in an area or community. Any precise information on the degree of endemicity must be based on quantitative and statistical concepts.

Malaria is described as *endemic* when there is a constant incidence of cases over a period of many successive years. *Epidemic malaria* is a term which indicates periodic or occasional sharp increase in the amount of malaria in a given indigenous community.

A more general classification into *stable* or *unstable* malaria has been proposed. In *stable* malaria the amount of transmission is high without any marked fluctuations over the years, though seasonal fluctuations may exist. In *unstable* malaria the amount of transmission varies from year to year. In the first case the collective immunity is high and epidemics are unlikely; in the second case the collective immunity of the population is low and epidemics are possible (Table 8).

Malaria is *autochthonous* when contracted locally; it is *indigenous* when natural to an area or country. Malaria is *imported* when the infection was acquired outside the specified area. Secondary cases contracted locally but derived from imported cases are referred to as *introduced* malaria. Infections deliberately produced for the purpose of malaria therapy or caused accidentally (by blood transfusion or otherwise) are known as *induced* malaria.

Two types of measurement are commonly used for the assessment of the impact of the malaria infection on the community:

Incidence – describes the frequency of illnesses *commencing* during a defined period; it refers to the number of cases of disease or infection occurring per unit of population during a given time interval. *Prevalence* – refers to the number of cases of disease or infection *existing* in a population at any given time. Usually in morbidity statistics one should distinguish between 'period prevalence' (over a stated time) and 'point prevalence' (at a particular point in time). However, the difficulty of distinguishing between a new malaria infection and a recrudescence or relapse has resulted in the conventional acceptance of the term prevalence as being synonymous with 'point prevalence' while incidence means always the frequency of cases of malaria over the period, irrespective of whether the disease resulted from a new infection or not. The difference between the two concepts is shown in Fig. 43.

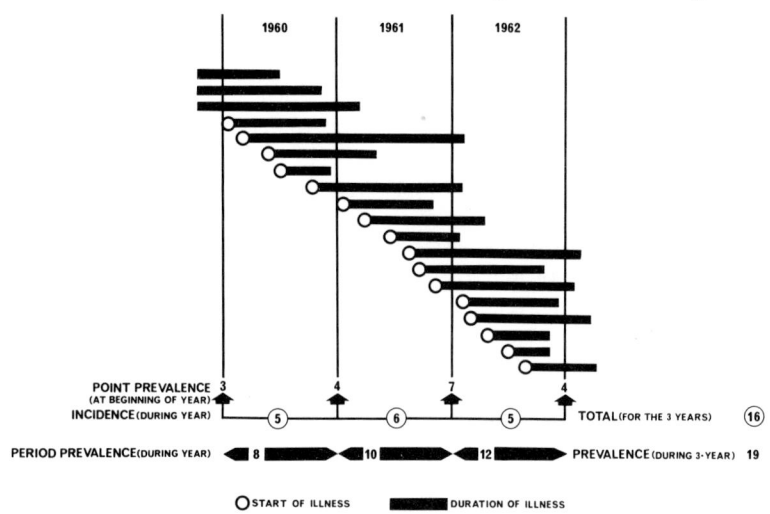

Fig 43 Diagram of epidemiological concepts of prevalence and incidence (WHO, 1966).

The terms *index* and *rate* express the relationships between various frequencies or counts. The word 'rate' usually carries the idea of some simple form of proportion such as percentage. The word 'index' is applied to a measurement of one type of value indicating its relationship to another. Thus the proportion of enlarged spleens is the 'spleen rate' of group but it provides an index of the endemicity of malaria in the relevant population. This semantic difference between the 'index' and 'rate' exists only in the English language. In other languages the term 'rate' is generally expressed as a percentage and only the expression index (or 'indice') is commonly used.

The *morbidity rate* (or morbidity) is the proportion of the number of cases of malaria in a unit time in the population in which they occur. It is closely related if not identical to the incidence of malaria and usually expressed with regard to 1000 or 10 000 population. Except in conditions when the diagnosis and reporting of each case is carried to perfection the morbidity rate is based on recorded admissions or attendances at hospitals and dispensaries. Naturally, in areas of high endemicity with a large proportion of asymptomatic carriers of malaria parasites the morbidity rate refers only to clinical cases and represents only a small proportion of the total amount of malaria.

The true *mortality rate* from malaria is in practice equally if not more difficult to determine than the morbidity rate for similar reasons. The often quoted average mortality rate due to malaria (1%) is not more than an estimate, since the fatality varies considerably in relation to the infecting species of Plasmodium and according to the provision of medical facilities, which depend on socioeconomic conditions of the country or area concerned.

The term *epidemic* may be applied to a sharp rise of the incidence of malaria among a population in which the disease was unknown. Conversely it may refer to a seasonal or other increase of clinical malaria in an area with moderately endemic malaria.

According to Russell (1952) in the genesis of malaria epidemics the following major points should be considered: (1) Increased susceptibility of the human population, often due to introduction of non-immunes into an endemic area; (2) Increased infective reservoir in the population; (3) Increased contact between man and the Anopheles vector; (4) Greater effectiveness of local Anopheles in transmitting the malaria parasite.

The exact causes of an epidemic of malaria are often difficult to determine. The increased susceptibility of the local population may be due to some social or other upheavals such as war or a natural disaster, both of them resulting in poor housing, poor sanitary facilities and malnutrition. However, the relationship between susceptibility to malaria and the state of nutrition is not clear. In areas where malaria is unstable, any previous epidemic would produce a proportion of people partly immune to the infection; but the gradual decline of this immunity would create eventually a large number of people without any immunity. However, the most common factor in the increased susceptibility of a community is the introduction of a large number of non-immunes, as often happens in large scale development projects in the tropics.

The increase of the infective reservoir in the community is most commonly due to the introduction of newcomers from an area with a species or strain of malaria parasite unknown or rare in the main locality. Some carriers of the new infection may be asymptomatic but nevertheless the gametocytes circulating in their blood may be highly infective to local Anopheles. A sudden wave of gametocyte production in a proportion of the population as a cause for an epidemic of malaria has also been postulated. A surge of seasonal relapses of a former infection has been incriminated.

The third and probably most important cause of epidemic outbreaks is due to the sudden increase of the number of vectors and to greater mean longevity of the female Anopheles of the species responsible for transmission. Climatic conditions are usually involved in this phenomenon but often a sharp decrease of animals, in areas where zoophilic Anopheles predominate, compels these mosquitos to seek alternative sources of blood, namely the human population. Other incidental causes such as greater accessibility of vectors to man because of different housing have also been postulated but are less easy to prove. Finally, epidemics have occurred in the past, and will occur in the future as a result of introduction into a potentially or actually malarious area of a new vector species with high susceptibility to plasmodial infection and with marked tendency of feeding on man.

In an epidemic of malaria three periods can be distinguished though they cannot be easily separated from one another. Following on the pre-epidemic increase of transmission due to the higher gametocyte rate and the greater density and infectivity of the Anopheles population, there is a sharp rise in the incidence of the disease. This is the *epidemic wave* which is also accompanied by an increase of mortality, directly due not only to malaria but also to other intercurrent diseases. The severity of an epidemic of malaria cannot be easily related to the increase of transmission which has caused it; even small increases of transmission may produce quite dramatic epidemics. The rise of the epidemic wave is usually faster in *P. vivax* outbreaks than in those due to *P. falciparum*, though the severity of the latter is far greater. During the *post-epidemic* period the incidence of malaria falls to its usual low endemic levels but the spleen rates in the population remain high for some time.

The extent of malaria epidemics varies. Localised epidemics occur in an area where unprotected groups of non-immune workers or soldiers are moved into an endemic zone, especially where human activities have increased the breeding potential of mosquitos, by interference with the environment.

When the incidence of malaria increases sharply over a vast geographical area one refers to *regional epidemics* which are often severe with a high mortality and due to unusual climatic conditions as one of the main factors.

Finally, some epidemics may exceed the natural geographical limits of endemic malaria and are loosely called pandemics. This was the case of the widespread epidemic of malaria in Russia after the First World War.

Malaria epidemics may be seasonal, generally related to climatic factors which increase the breeding activity of Anopheles and their longer survival in summer and early autumn. However, some epidemics may occur in the early spring and are due to relapses of *P. vivax* malaria, from infections received during the previous summer. This was the pattern of seasonal outbreaks of malaria in northern Europe. In some seasonal epidemics where *P. vivax* and *P. falciparum* are both involved the former starts earlier and reaches a peak, to be followed by a second peak of *P. falciparum* infections.

When it comes to dealing with malaria epidemics two aims have the highest priority. The first is to recognise them as soon as possible; the second is to help the population affected and to limit the spread of transmission. Any unusually high admission rate to local hospitals or attendance at health centres should be rapidly reported and investigated. Drug treatment on a large scale is the best method of curbing the amount of transmission with extensive imagicidal measures to follow.

Antilarval operations have no place in these conditions but may be planned for the future.

Endemic malaria

This term is applied to malaria when there is a constant measurable incidence both of cases of the disease and of its natural transmission in an area over a succession of years. Conventionally, if the disease ceased to be transmitted over at least three years one may presume that malaria is no more endemic in the area although the Anopheles vectors responsible for the previous transmission may remain. In these conditions potential endemicity may still exist and if there is a probability of importation of cases of malaria from other parts of the world the *malariogenic potential* is said to be high.

The two factors which determine the level of the malariogenic potential are *receptivity* of the area and its *vulnerability*. The first refers to the number of new cases of malaria that could theoretically originate from one single imported case: the second factor is related to the actual numbers of imported cases entering the area in a unit of time.

Endemic malaria may be present in various degrees and the following classification of it is commonly used.

Hypoendemicity denotes areas where there is little transmission and the effects of malaria on the general population are unimportant.

Mesoendemicity is found typically among small rural communities in the sub-tropical zones with varying intensity of transmission depending on local circumstances.

Hyperendemicity is seen in areas with intense but seasonal transmission where the immunity is insufficient to prevent the effects of malaria on all age-groups.

Holoendemicity denotes a perennial transmission of high degree resulting in a considerable degree of immune response in all age-groups, but particularly in the adults.

This classification is based on epidemiological data obtained in the field usually in the course of a study known as *malaria survey*, described in the following section.

The presence and degree of both the endemic and epidemic malaria depend on a number of factors which can be divided into three groups, namely man, malaria parasite and the mosquito vector. The relationship between these main factors will be the subject of the few following pages. However, a simple qualitative interdependence between the various elements of malaria transmission could be expressed, according to Russell (1952), as a formula:

$$(X\ Y\ Z)\ pibect$$

in which X is the human carrier of the plasmodium, Y the Anopheles vector, Z the human recipient of the infection. The single letters of the acronym 'pibect' refer to **p**–the plasmodium, **i**–immunity, **b**–bionomics (habits – of both the man and of the mosquito), **e**–the environment, **c**–control of malaria in the locality, **t**–treatment.

MALARIA SURVEY

Any attempt at control of malaria in a locality or a larger area should be preceded by an evaluation of the amount and conditions of transmission of the disease. This is called a *malaria survey* and it should extend not only to the area to be protected but also to the contiguous unprotected area. The differences noted between the amount of malaria in the two areas following the application of control measures will indicate their effectiveness. The quantitative methods involved in a malaria survey are often referred to as *malariometry*.

The degree of malaria transmission in any region is determined by a number of interrelated factors. These include:
1) The prevalence of malaria infection in man and its seasonal incidence.
2) The species of Anopheles mosquitos, their relative abundance, feeding and resting habits and infectivity.
3) The presence of susceptible human population.
4) Climatic conditions, such as rainfall, temperature, humidity and environmental features which affect the breeding of Anopheles.

The *malaria survey* proper involves investigations under the following headings:
1. Collection of existing environmental and epidemiological data. 2. Investigations relating to the human host. 3. Investigations relating to the insect vector.

Epidemiology of Malaria

a) For a general knowledge of epidemiological situation information is required regarding malaria morbidity and mortality, vital statistics, meteorological, topographical and other relevant features. This involves the examination of hospital and dispensary returns, records maintained by health services, and interviews with medical officers of health, private practitioners and auxiliary medical personnel.

b) Investigations relating to the human host require:

Spleen examination. The spleen rate is the proportion of enlarged spleens in the indigenous population.

Blood examination. The *parasite rate* is the proportion of blood films showing malaria parasites in the indigenous population.

c) Investigations relating to the Anopheles vectors are based on the collection of four groups of data, as follows:

Estimation of mosquito density in relation to the human population. This is determined by the result of mosquito collections, indicating the number of Anopheles entering dwellings, or feeding on inhabitants.

Estimation of natural infection. The *sporozoite rate* is the percentage incidence of sporozoite infection in the salivary glands of Anopheles. The *oöcyst rate* is the percentage incidence of oöcyst formation on the stomach wall of Anopheles.

Estimation of biting habits. This is determined by the results of the precipitin test of mosquito blood-meals, indicating whether the Anopheles had fed on human or animal blood. It is therefore a means of distinguishing between anthropophilic and zoophilic species.

Estimation of longevity. Various entomological techniques used for this purpose include comparison of the sporozoite rate and total infection rate, comparison of the immediate and delayed sporozoite rate, measurement of the ampulla of the oviduct, and estimation of daily survival rate from the proportion of parous Anopheles females.

Spleen examination

One of the earliest methods used for estimation of the amount of malaria in a given locality is that of determining the proportion of persons with a palpable enlargement of the spleen. This method introduced by Dempster in India in 1848 is still commonly used, although it is admittedly a crude measure.

The object of palpation of the spleen is to determine not only the percentage of individuals with demonstrable enlargement of the organ but also the approximate degree of splenomegaly.

Two techniques of spleen palpation are used: In one the individual is examined lying down, with the examiner seated on the subject's right, so that the right hand can explore the splenic region below the left costal margin. The second method, less cumbersome in the field, has the subject standing, with the examiner sitting on a low stool in front of the examined person. The examiner's right hand gently explores the left side of the abdomen from below the umbilicus towards the costal border. If no spleen is palpable, the subject is requested to breathe deeply, while the exploring hand attempts to feel the tip of the spleen by pressing the abdomen under the costal border (Fig. 44).

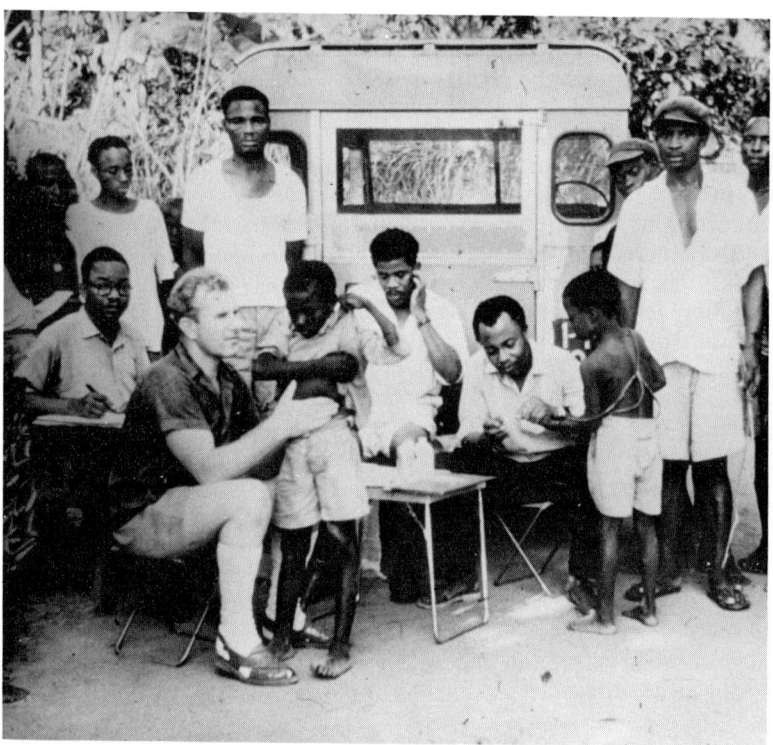

Fig 44 Procedure adopted for malaria surveys in Nigeria. The malariologist palpating the spleen of the child sits on a low stool, which allows him to feel the spleen, even when slightly enlarged. The technician who takes the blood slide and the clerk who keeps the records are in the background.

Palpation of the spleen in children is relatively easy, but in adults with greater muscular development more experience is necessary. The main errors, made usually by non-medical examiners, are to mistake the outer end of the left rib or a hard faecal bolus in the large intestine for the enlarged spleen. On the other hand, very large spleens may be missed if only the upper part of the abdomen is palpated. It should be remembered that occasionally large spleens are due to kala azar (intestinal leishmaniasis) or Manson's schistosomiasis, but generally the proportion of splenomegaly over 10% is due to malaria.

The proportion (expressed as a percentage) of enlarged spleens in a sample of the population is known as the *spleen rate* and is a crude but nevertheless valuable measure of endemic malaria. Usually the spleen rate is determined in children 2–10 years of age; this is because the enlargement of the spleen is greatest when the immune response is building up. However, for a complete picture of the amount of malaria in a locality the proportion of enlarged spleens in adults should also be known.

An important refinement of the method of spleen rate determination is the evaluation of the degree of splenic enlargement. This can be done by classifying the size of the enlarged spleen and determining the proportion of various classes of splenomegaly.

For the determination of the degree of enlarged spleens Hackett's method of arbitrary classification of the size of the palpated spleen is now generally accepted according to criteria given in Table 9 and Fig. 45.

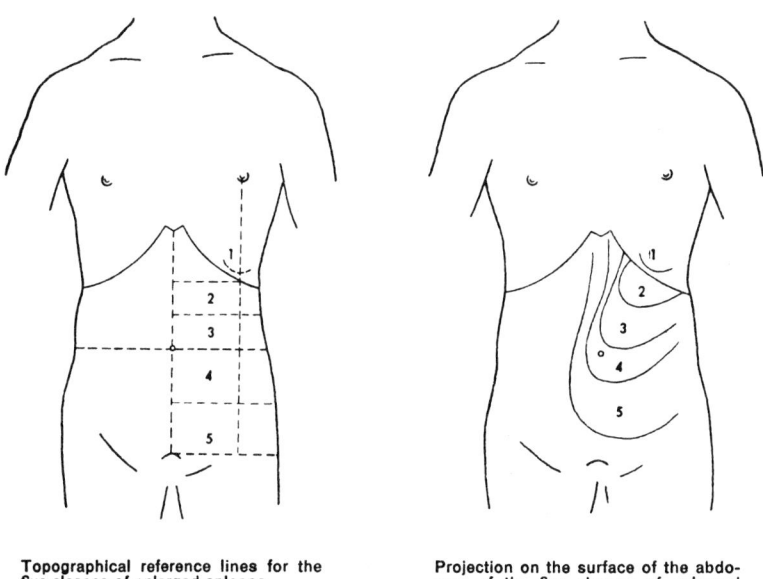

Topographical reference lines for the five classes of enlarged spleens

Projection on the surface of the abdomen of the five classes of enlarged spleens

Fig 45 Classification of spleen sizes according to Hackett's method. (WHO, 1963, Terminology of malaria)

A useful malariometric index is that of *average enlarged spleen* (AES) which can be easily calculated from the frequency distribution of various classes of spleens recorded in the way shown by the following example:

Class of spleen	Age group 2–9 years Numbers of various classes found
0 (not palpable)	14
1	25 ⎫
2	10 ⎪
3	3 ⎬ 41
4	2 ⎪
5	1 ⎭
Total	55

The AES index is calculated by multiplying the number of individuals in each class of enlarged spleen by the class of spleen and dividing this figure by the total number of individuals with splenomegaly. In the table above the spleen rate is 41 out of 55, or 75%. *The average enlarged spleen* will be $25 + 20 + 9 + 8 + 5 = 67/41 = 1.64$.

Table 9

Classification of sizes of the spleen according to Hackett

Class of spleen	Description
0	Normal spleen not palpable even on deep inspiration.
1	Spleen palpable below the costal margin, usually on deep inspiration.
2	Spleen palpable below the costal margin, but not projected beyond a horizontal line half way between the costal margin and the umbilicus, measured along a line dropped vertically from the left nipple.
3	Spleen with lowest palpable point projected more than half way to the umbilicus but not below a line drawn horizontally through it.
4	Spleen with lowest palpable point below the umbilical level but not projected beyond a horizontal line situated half way between the umbilicus and the symphisis pubis.
5	Spleen with lowest point palpable beyond the lower limit of class 4.

Note: This classification obviously does not apply to children with a very distended abdomen or with a pronounced umbilical hernia. The error in classifying the spleen size in these children will be largely eliminated if the child is examined in recumbent position and not standing. The horizontal mid-line in the case of a large umbilical hernia cannot be more than approximate.

Blood examination

The other important measure of the prevalence of malaria in an area is the evaluation of the proportion of persons in a given community who harbour the parasites of malaria in their blood. This epidemiological index is known as *parasite rate*. To be precise the parasite rate must be determined for a relatively narrow range of age-groups from infants, through toddlers, small children, school children, adolescents and adults.

Epidemiology of Malaria

The following age grouping is recommended by the WHO (1963):

Group	Description
0–11 months	Infants, babies
12–23 months	Small children
2–4 years	Toddlers
5–9 years	Juveniles
10–14 years	Adolescents
15 years and over	Adults

The technique of blood examination was indicated in one of the previous sections. The proportion (as a percentage) of the sample of the population showing malaria parasites in the blood is the *parasite rate*, which should be related to one of the age-groups of the population sample as shown above. The infant parasite rate is of special importance as it is a good indicator of a recent transmission of malaria.

It should be remembered that the reliability of results of blood examination depends on the standardised technique of the collection of blood slides and their examination by competent technical staff. For field surveys only the thick film method is normally used. The average microscopist can examine 100 thick film fields in 5 minutes. This represents about 0.1–0.2 mm^3 of blood and some very scanty infections may escape detection.

In some surveys (as indeed in cases of individual infections) it may be useful to know the degree of malarial infection. The term *parasite count* is the number of malaria parasites seen on an average in a number (such as 100) of blood film fields, or in relation to the number (such as 5000 or 10 000) of red blood cells. Usually the parasite count is given in relation to 1 mm^3 of blood, after a suitable conversion. The parasite count may also be calculated in relation to the number (400–500) of white blood cells seen in 100 fields of the blood film when the number of those cells per mm^3 is known.

As in the case of the average enlarged spleen it may be useful to know the average degree of parasitaemia in a sample of a well defined group of the population. Since the range of individual counts per mm^3 of malaria parasites in the blood is very wide, to obtain the *parasite density index* the individual counts are divided into 10 classes as follows:

Class	Parasite count per mm^3 (μl)
1	Less than 100
2	101–200
3	201–400
4	401–800
5	801–1600

Class	Parasite count per mm³ (µl)
6	1601–3200
7	3201–6400
8	6401–12 800
9	12 801–25 600
10	25 601–and over

The *parasite density index* for a given group can be calculated in the same way as the average enlarged spleen. Only the positive slides are included in the denominator.

Example: Out of 120 slides 90 are positive; they are composed of the following classes:

Class	1	2	3	4	5	6	7	8	9	10	Total
Frequency	15	30	13	12	8	6	3	2	0	1	90
	15	60	39	48	40	36	21	16	0	10	285

Parasite rate $\dfrac{90 \times 100}{120} = 75\%$

Parasite density index $\dfrac{285}{90} = 3.17$

In the above calculation of the parasite rate and parasite density index all species of parasites are lumped together and mixed infections are counted as one. This is the *crude parasite rate* or *crude parasite density index*.

If infections with different plasmodia are counted separately one refers to a *species infection rate* or *species parasite density index*.

The determination of the parasite density index is not always necessary but the indication of the frequency of the individual species of malaria parasites is of importance. This can be given either as the *species infection rate viz*. percentage of subjects found with infections of one particular species of plasmodium or as the parasite formula. The latter indicates the relative prevalence of the various species in the total of positive slides. Thus, if in a series of slides from 100 children there are 62 positives (parasite rate 62%) of which 40 show *P. vivax* ($^{40}/_{62}$), 20 *P. falciparum* ($^{20}/_{62}$) and 2 *P. malariae* ($^{2}/_{62}$) the *parasite formula is:* V 64.5, F 32.3, M 3.2. But the *species infection rate* of the examined group will be $^{40}/_{100}$ = 40% for *P. vivax*, 20% for *P. falciparum* and 2% for *P. malariae*.

Classification of endemicity of malaria

The degrees of endemicity of malaria mentioned before have been adopted by the WHO on the basis of spleen rates determined on a statistically significant sample of the population involved. These degrees are as follows:

1 *Hypoendemic malaria:* Spleen rate in children (2–9 years) not exceeding 10%.
2 *Mesoendemic malaria:* Spleen rate in children (2–9 years) between 11% and 50%.
3 *Hyperendemic malaria:* Spleen rate in children (2–9 years) constantly over 50%. Spleen rates in adults also high (over 25%).
4 *Holoendemic malaria:* Spleen rate in children (2–9 years) constantly over 75%, but spleen rates in adults low (Fig. 46).

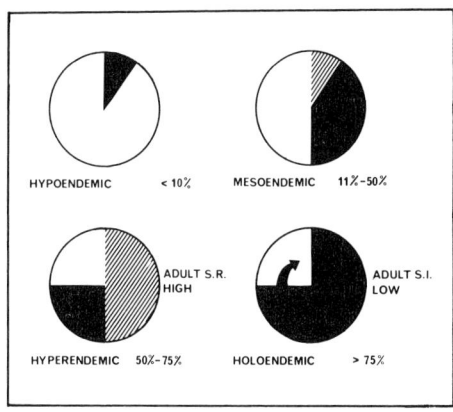

Fig 46 World Health Organization's classification of endemicity of malaria according to the spleen rate.

The reason for the reference to the adult spleen rate in the last two types of endemic malaria is the presence of a considerable immunity acquired in the holoendemic areas, where the population is exposed to an intense and nearly perennial transmission.

An alternative method of classification of endemicity of malaria has been proposed using parasite rates as an indicator of the amount of transmission of malaria.

Recording of data and their statistical significance

For proper recording of data obtained in the course of malariometric surveys the use of standard forms is convenient.

Two such forms are shown in Fig. 47. The first is used in the field while the second is more useful for the consolidation of all results

INDIVIDUAL SPLEEN/BLOOD RECORDS

Place: .... Project: ....

Date: .... Investigator: ....

Serial No. of slide	Name	Age	Sex	Spleen class	Result of blood examination	Remarks

CONSOLIDATED SPLEEN/BLOOD RECORD

Age group	No. of spleens examined	Spleen class						No. of blood films examined	No. of positive blood films	*P. falciparum* trophozoites	*P. falciparum* gametocytes	*P. vivax* or *P. ovale*	*P. malariae*	Mixed infections	Class of parasite count										
		0	1	2	3	4	5								Neg. 0	1	2	3	4	5	6	7	8	9	10

Fig 47 Individual and consolidated spleen/blood records as used for malariometric surveys.

obtained. The number of subjects to be examined within the locality selected on epidemiological grounds is chiefly determined by statistical considerations. The adequacy of a sample size can be determined either in advance of the survey or when reporting on its results. The size of the sample required depends on the general prevalence of the phenomenon that is being investigated. It is obvious that for valid comparisons a smaller sample is sufficient when the spleen or parasite rate is high in the investigated areas; on the other hand a larger sample is needed for the statistical validity of the results.

The range of chance variation of the results that must be considered in relation to the magnitude of the percentage observed in the sample is given in Table 10.

If, for example, in a sample of 100 children parasites are found in 40, then the parasite rate in the total population of chidren of the same age group lies between 30 and 50% and this may be assumed with a 95% probability.

The appraisal of the statistical significance of the difference between

Epidemiology of Malaria

two rates should be done according to the well known methods, in relation to the standard error of the difference. However, the use of a convenient nomogram reproduced in Fig. 48 will dispense with the need of calculation. In this nomogram the left-hand scale, M, refers to the combined numbers of the two samples that are to be tested; and the right-hand scale, P, refers to the combined percentages in the two samples that have a specified characteristic.

The value of M is marked on the left-hand scale, and the value of P on the right-hand scale. A straight-edge is then placed to connect the two points, and the value is read where it intersects the 5% side of the centre scale. If the difference in the two rates exceeds the scale value, then it may be considered to be significant at the 5% probability level. Similarly, significance at the 1% probability level can be found by using the 1% side of the centre scale.

Table 10

Confidence intervals at 95% probability level corresponding to varying sample sizes and sample percentages from 5% to 95%

Sample size	Percentage observed in sample					
	5%	10%	20%	30%	40%	50%
50		3–22	10–34	18–45	26–55	36–64
60	1–14	3–20	11–32	19–43	28–54	37–63
80	1–12	4–19	12–30	20–41	29–51	39–61
100	2–11	5–18	13–29	21–40	30–50	40–60
200	2–9	6–14	16–26	24–38	33–47	43–57
300	3–8	7–14	16–25	25–36	35–46	44–56
400	3–8	7–13	16–24	26–35	35–45	45–55
500	3–7	8–13	17–24	26–34	36–44	46–54
1000	4–7	8–12	18–23	27–33	37–43	47–53
	60%	70%	80%	90%	95%	
50	45–74	55–82	66–90	78–97		
60	46–72	57–81	68–89	80–97	86–99	
80	49–71	59–80	70–88	81–96	88–99	
100	50–70	60–79	71–87	82–95	89–98	
200	53–67	62–76	74–84	86–94	91–98	
300	54–65	64–75	75–84	86–93	92–97	
400	55–65	65–74	76–84	87–93	92–97	
500	56–64	66–74	76–83	87–92	93–97	
1000	57–63	67–73	77–82	88–92	93–96	

QUANTITATIVE EPIDEMIOLOGY OF MALARIA

Many aspects of a malaria survey require some quantitative data, the collection and interpretation of which depends on the use of elementary mathematical principles. In answering the usual epidemiological

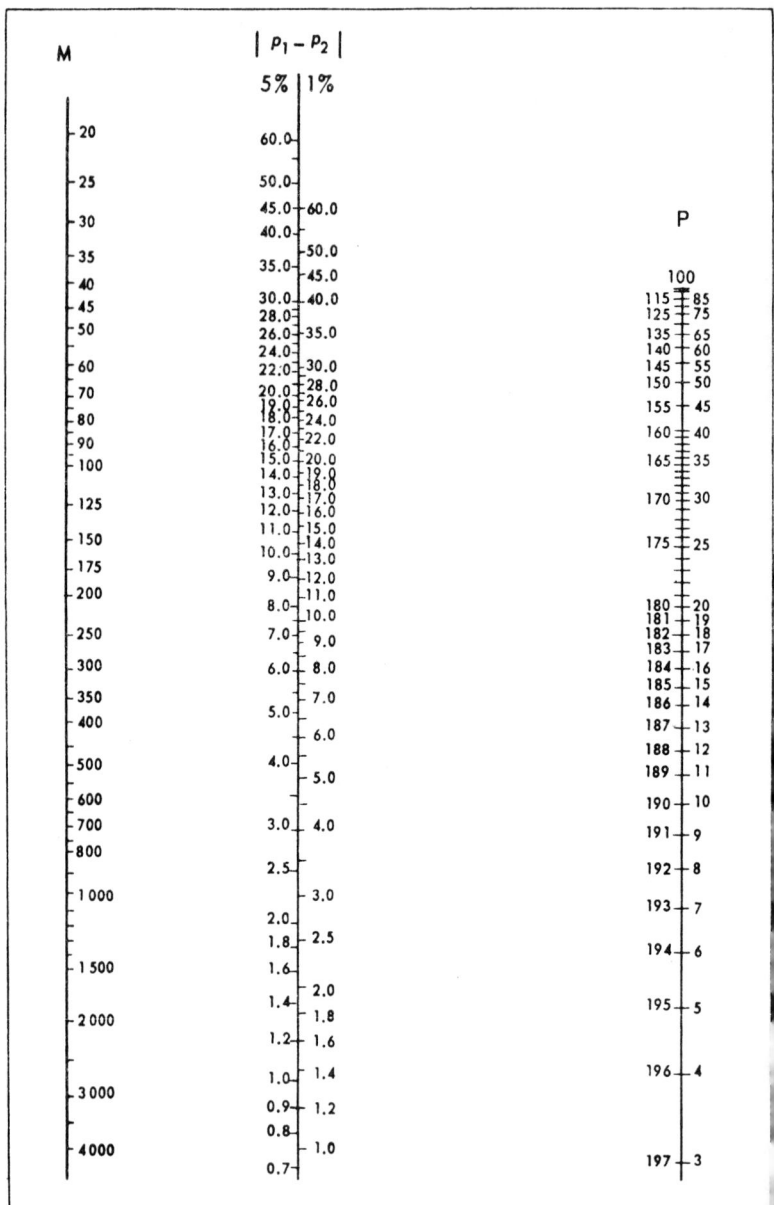

Fig 48 Nomogram for rapid testing of the degree of statistical significance of the difference between two rates. (WHO, 1966)

Epidemiology of Malaria

questions: 'Who? When? Where? Why?' some degree of precision is needed and here the well-known statement of J. J. Thomson should be remembered: 'When you can measure what you are speaking about and express it in numbers, you know something about it, but when you cannot measure it or express it in numbers, your knowledge is of a meagre and unsatisfactory kind.'

It may be worthwhile to quote Ronald Ross's opinion which has been used as the leading maxim of George Macdonald's book, *The epidemiology and control of malaria* (1957).

'To say that a disease depends upon certain factors is not to say much, until we can also form an estimate as to how largely each factor influences the whole result. And the mathematical method is really nothing but the application of careful reasoning to the problems at issue.'

There is no other tropical communicable disease to which mathematical approach has been applied more widely or thoroughly. The first and most inspired attempt at formulating the quantitative laws of epidemiology of malaria and its transmission and control was made by Ronald Ross at the beginning of this century. A number of other studies followed but the interest in this subject died down until the 1950s, when Moshkowsky in the USSR and George Macdonald in Britain revived it in a series of remarkable investigations. The reader interested in this aspect of epidemiology of malaria should study the original works quoted in the list of references.

In the basic outline of the principles of a malaria survey several of the quantitative factors of malaria transmission have already been pointed out. Some of these factors are so obvious that they do not require any additional explanation, others need a few comments.

Anopheles vary greatly in their susceptibility, some being prone to carry malaria while others rarely do so. Certain species have characeristics which exclude them from the role of important vectors, such as a marked preference for animal blood or a very short life. It is therefore possible to put the anopheline vectors into groups of important, less important and unimportant vectors and the grouping is useful so long as the natural flexibility of species is remembered. Very favourable circumstances may convert a usually unimportant vector anopheline into an important one, and the classification is not therefore rigid. In a following section the important vectors in some parts of the world are listed with descriptions of their breeding, biting and resting habits.

Most female Anopheles take a blood feed once in every two to four days, the intervals again depending on temperature. They are by no means invariable feeders on man; some have a marked preference for human blood, choosing it whenever possible; others have a strong preference for animals and rarely feed on man, so that it is very unusual for them to transmit malaria. Between these two extremes there are large groups less set in their habits. The final choice depends to a considerable extent on the availability of blood so that under some circumstances they feed predominantly on man and under others only rarely so. The degree of variation within one species may be wide; in the instance of *A. culicifacies* in India the percentage of human blood feeds may vary between 2% and 80%; this variation in feeding habit may have a great effect on the incidence of disease.

An adult female mosquito acquires malaria parasites by receiving them in a blood feed from a malarious person. She has no prospect of transmitting the disease unless she lives through the time taken for the sporogonic development of the malaria parasite; this is estimated at between 8 and 25 days according to temperature. Even if the Anopheles survives through this time the number of people whom she will bite and so to whom she will transmit the parasite depends on the length of her survival after that time. The length of life of a mosquito in nature is very difficult to measure but some general indication of the range may be helpful. The most robust can survive under ideal conditions for 3 or more months. They rarely meet these ideal conditions in nature, being to a large extent at the mercy of natural enemies and such risks as dry winds which may kill them in a very short time; the best they can hope for seems to be an expectation of about 20 to 25 days, some individuals being more and some less lucky; this corresponds to a daily death rate of 4 or 5%. At the other end of the scale the expectation may be much less than this, as little as 2 or 3 days, but even among these short-livers a sufficient few may live long enough to maintain transmission of malaria. Under such adverse conditions it is clear that only a very small minority of all mosquitos can live long enough to carry the disease from one man to another, and that one mosquito is not likely to infect many people. As a consequence, often large numbers of mosquitos are needed to maintain the disease in a community when these conditions prevail, and if the numbers fall below the requisite figure transmission will become rare and the disease will tend to disappear.

The average number of adult female Anopheles of a defined species, caught sheltering in human habitations or biting exposed individuals indoors or out of doors, is the *anopheles density*. It can be expressed as a relative proportion per room, per person, per day, etc.

The proportion of freshly fed female Anopheles whose midgut (stomach) contains human blood is the *human blood index*. Following the blood feed (on man or on animals) the ovarian development of the female Anopheles begins and ends with egg-laying. This period is known as the *gonotrophic cycle* and averages 2–4 days.

The period necessary for the development of the plasmodium in the mosquito from the fertilisation of the female gamete by the male through the subsequent stages of oökinete, oöcyst and finally sporozoite is known as the *sporogonic cycle*. Its duration depends on the species of the plasmodium and on the environmental temperature.

The percentage of female Anopheles of a defined species caught in nature and showing on dissection oöcysts in the midgut is the *oöcyst rate*. Conversely the percentage of female Anopheles with sporozoites in their salivary glands is the *sporozoite rate*.

The *inoculation rate* or the relative proportion of the human population receiving an *infective* bite in a unit of time, from the average number of female Anopheles found in a room or in a hut may be estimated by multiplying the anopheline density per person per day by the sporozoite rate. Thus if an average of 6 female Anopheles were found every day in a room where 3 persons slept and where the sporozoite rate for the period was 5% then the supposed daily inoculation rate would be:

$$\frac{6 \times 5}{3 \times 100} = \frac{30}{300} = 0.1$$

However, not all female Anopheles found in the room would have fed on that night. Assuming that the gonotrophic cycle is 48 hours or 2 days, only half of Anopheles would be involved. In view of this the previous figure of 0.1 must be halved and the postulated figure would be 0.05. Thus every person in this room would receive one infective bite every 20 days. This reasoning is arbitrary as it leaves out many variables such as the actual infectivity of Anopheles with sporozoites in salivary glands or the value of the assessment of anopheline density based on collection of mosquitos in rooms. The latter index is particularly uncertain when it is taken to represent the mosquito/man contact.

The mosquito/man contact can be defined as *man biting rate* viz. the average incidence of anopheline bites per day per person. It may be expressed as ma where m is the relative density of female Anopheles to man; a is the *man biting habit* or the probability that a mosquito will feed on man during a day. The incidence of bites per day of an individual female mosquito on the human population is composed of the feeding frequency per mosquito per day (24 hours) multiplied by the proportion of such bites on man. This is the *human blood index* obtained from the results of precipitin tests.

The *inoculation rate* of malaria by the Anopheles depends on the man biting rate multiplied by the infective sporozoite rate. However, since the actually infective bites of Anopheles cannot be determined in the field, only an estimate of this factor is possible from entomological data. A different approach has been used by Macdonald (1957) who calculated the inoculation rate in a community from the known parasite rate of infants. Details of this investigation are beyond the scope of this book but it may be pointed out that generally the inoculation rate estimated by this method is 20 to 100 times less than the inoculation rate derived from entomological data. This discrepancy is pronounced when the endemicity of malaria is high and indicates the effect of immunity transmitted by the mother as well as other intervening factors.

The key factor in the mathematical analysis of transmission of malaria is the *longevity of the vector*. The duration of the sporogonic period of the development is at least about 9 days for *P. vivax* and 12 days for *P. falciparum* at 26°C. Obviously any mosquito that lives less than this period will not be able to transmit the infection through sporozoites.

The direct estimation of the average age of mosquitos may be obtained if we know the mean duration of each gonotrophic cycle (from blood meal to oviposition) and the mean number of such cycles in female Anopheles. Such a direct estimation of physiological age of mosquitos is possible by methods developed by Soviet entomologists. This is technically difficult and cumbersome and various indirect methods are easier and more widely applicable. One such method of estimating the mean age of the anopheline population is based on calculating the proportion of Anopheles females that had laid at least one batch of eggs (*parous* females) in relation to the total number of female Anopheles of the same species collected. From this proportion the probability of survival through one day can be derived and from that the calculation of the *mean expectation of life* of the vector population is simple enough.

Finally the expectation of life of Anopheles surviving long enough to become infective to man, after having fed previously on blood containing gametocytes, presents no great difficulty.

The *expectation of infective life* of a vector population can be defined as their mean number of days of life in the infective condition. It is a function of the daily survival rate of the female mosquito and of the sporogonic period of a given species of the malaria parasite. This is the most important factor in the transmission of malaria and any decrease of it is the key to malaria control by use of insecticides.

During the past decade much attention has been given by various authors and especially by Macdonald (1957) to a quantitative approach to epidemiology of malaria. This requires a precise measurement of the various factors involved in the transmission of the infection in order to elucidate their respective relationship.

The most important factors of the complex epidemiological picture resulting from the vectorial capacity of an anopheline population are as follows: The man biting rate; the man biting habit; the probability of vector's survival through the sporogonic period of the parasite species; the expectation of life of the female Anopheles vector; the vectorial capacity of the vector population and, finally the basic reproduction rate, which is the estimated number of secondary malaria infections potentially transmitted within a susceptible population from a single non-immune individual.

The mathematical relationship and derivation of these factors from a series of quantitative indices was presented by Black (1968) and shown in Table 11.

Although the basic reproduction rate is an important cumulative epidemiological factor it represents the theoretical estimate of the intensity of transmission. In practice the *net reproduction rate* is much closer to real conditions. The *net reproduction rate*, viz. the actual number of secondary infections, is always much lower than the basic reproduction rate and can be estimated from the equation

$$\frac{p^n}{p^n - s}$$

where p^n is the probability of survival of Anopheles through n days of the duration of sporogonic period and s is the sporozoite rate.

Another valuable epidemiological factor is the *index of stability* of transmission of malaria. It depends on the man biting habit of the main vector *(a)* and its probability of survival through 1 day *(p)* and can be derived from the expression

$$\frac{a}{-\log_e p}$$

This brief account of the modern principles of quantitative epidemiology of malaria gives only a rudimentary idea of the complexity of theoretical and practical field work connected with it. For those who are interested in this approach the sources quoted in the list of references will be of value for future reading.

Synopsis of quantitative approach to the transmission of malaria and to its control

In the development of quantitative epidemiology the study of malaria occupies an important place from the beginning of this century when Ronald Ross defined the basic approach to the 'theory of happenings' relevant to the transmission of this infection. Malaria has not only the usual numerical features applicable to morbidity or mortality of human groups exposed to a specific disease. Infection of an individual and of the population has also the quantitative characteristics of the incubation period, proportion and size of enlarged spleens, rate,

Table 11

Factors composing the vectorial capacity of a mosquito population and the basic reproduction rate of malaria (after Black, 1968)

Factor	Definition of index	Common name of index	Method of obtaining the index	Macdonald's (1957) expressions
1	Bites *per man* per night by vector population	Man-biting rate	Night-biting captures on human baits (e.g. 10 bites per man)	ma
2	Bites *per mosquito* per night	Man-biting habit	Composed of (i) the feeding frequency based on the observed gonotrophic cycle in nature (e.g. 0.4 where the female oviposits and feeds once in 2.5 days on average); and (ii) the human blood index, assessed by the precipitin test applied to daytime resting samples (e.g. 0.5): $a = 0.4 \times 0.5 = 0.2$	a
3	Proportion of bites on man ('Human blood index')			
4	Probability of vector's survival through sporogonic period of parasite	Expectation of infective life of the vector population	Based on age-grading or proportion parous and knowledge of gonotrophic cycle duration (e.g. 0.60 days (see footnote*)	p^n
5	Expectation of life of female vectors			$\dfrac{1}{-\log_e p}$
6	Expected inoculations of man per infective case per day	Vectorial capacity of vector population	Multiplication of factors $1 \times 2 \times 3 \times 4 \times 5$. (e.g. $10 \times 0.2 \times 0.6 = 1.2$). (When this value descends below 0.01, basic reproduction rate 1 for *P. falciparum*)	$\dfrac{ma^2 p^n}{-\log_e p}$

To obtain the basic reproduction rate:

7	Proportion of vector females developing parasite normally following ingestion of gametes	Mosquito's receptivity (susceptibility) to infection	Only assessable by infections of captive samples on malaria cases (e.g. 0.9)	b
8	Days of infectivity per case (i.e. reciprocal of proportion of cases recovering in one day)	Reciprocal of recovery rate	Longitudinal observation of local cases of malaria in the absence of transmission (e.g. 100 days)	$\dfrac{1}{r}$
8	Expected new infections per case in the absence of immunity	Basic reproduction rate of parasite	Multiplication of factors 6 × 7 × 8 (e.g. 1.2 × 0.9 × 100 = 108).	$\dfrac{ma^2\,bp^n}{-r(\log_e p)}$

* To compute the factors from the proportion parous it is necessary to know also the mean difference in age between the nulliparous and the youngest parous females in the sample, and the sporogonic period of the parasite. Graphs are available to enable the field worker, who has observed these parameters, to read off from his data the proportion surviving one day, the expectation of infective life and the expectation of life.

Note: e is the base of natural logarithms (2.718)

count and density of parasite, gametocyte rate, duration of infection and the frequency of relapses, to mention only the main elements.

The infection is carried by mosquitos which have the characteristics of relative numbers, range of flight, proportion and frequency of female Anopheles feeding on man, their oviposition interval and mean duration of life. In the host/parasite relationship there are the factors of ambient temperature relevant to the duration of sporogony, proportion of infective Anopheles and numbers of their oöcysts and sporozoites. There is no other disease in which the various elements of transmission of the infection lend themselves to more accurate measurement, and no one in which they are so fascinatingly interconnected.

In the series of factors of the epidemiology of malaria some of the most important relate to the vector. The proportion of the population of mosquitos which live long enough for the development of malaria parasites in them depends on the mortality to which they are exposed. Next comes the question of how long the mosquitos may be expected to survive before they transmit the infection to another person.

The curve of the longevity of an Anopheles population decreases exponentially in relation to their daily mortality and this has an important bearing on the probability of transmission. The concept of the mean expectation of life of mosquitos which depends on the environmental conditions, runs like a red thread through the weave of the pattern of epidemiology of malaria.

The keystone to the understanding of the dynamics of transmission of the infection is the *basic reproduction rate* or the number of secondary infections that would originate from a single primary case of malaria if there had been no suppressive effect of the immune response of the human host enhanced by the possibility of superinfection.

The probability of survival of a proportion of the anopheline vector population through one day and through the extrinsic period of the development of the parasite forms an important element in the expression of the reproduction rate. Other factors related to the behaviour pattern of the mosquito are also of significance since they govern the degree of contact between the human host and the vector.

The mean daily number of infective bites inflicted on the human victim is the inoculation rate which has been usually estimated from the entomological data. An alternative method of assessing this index 'a posteriori' from the infant parasite rate shows the difference between the results obtained by the two methods and is due to the effect of immunity which rises with the increasing exposure to infection.

The antiparasitic and antitoxic effects of immunity protecting the individual received much attention but another manifestation, namely the restriction of the gametocyte output (thus lessening the infectivity of man to the mosquito) has a protective effect on the community. This is one of the facets of the biological system by means of which the transmission in an endemic area may be stabilised at a tenable level.

Together with the behaviour characteristics of the vector the expectation of life of the Anopheles population enters into the components of the index of stability of the disease and determines why malaria should be in some places apparently static and in others almost unpredictably epidemic. It explains the dependence of the chain of transmission on the environmental conditions and defines quantitatively the features of the environment which influence the pathogen and the two types of host. It also denotes the amenability of the control of transmission through the decrease of the reproduction rate so that each successive number of cases will be progressively smaller until the disease eventually fades out.

The aim of malaria eradication is to reduce the reproduction rate below one and to maintain it consistently below this critical level. The attack on the vector using residual insecticides has normally a rapid effect on transmission because it drastically reduces the probability of anopheline survival. The degree of this impact can be estimated by various entomological methods. Its overall effect on the vector can now be assessed by measuring the 'vectorial capacity' – a term that expresses the mean number of probable inoculations transmitted from one case of malaria in a unit time. The periodic regional epidemics of malaria have often revealed the constant menace of this disease. Such events are due either to the sudden increase of the density of the vector and its enhanced longevity, or to the change of the behavior pattern of the vector or to the introduction of the new sources of infection into the receptive area.

EPIDEMIOLOGICAL CHARACTERISTICS OF MALARIA IN SOME SELECTED AREAS

In Northern and Central Europe, where malaria slowly disappeared during the nineteenth century thanks to improved agriculture and draining of marshy areas, the brackish water breeding *A. atroparvus* was the main vector of indigenous malaria in coastal areas. *A. messeae*, the fresh water breeding member of the *A. maculipennis* complex, was responsible for outbreaks of malaria in exceptional circumstances when its numbers were very high and there was a shortage of domestic animals, on which this mosquito usually fed.

The Mediterranean area and the Middle East. Throughout much of this area malaria has been effectively controlled, but in some parts of it a considerable degree of endemic malaria still persists. The disease was seasonal throughout the whole of the area and severe regional epidemics were well known in countries on both shores of the Mediterranean. Several vectors are involved. The two most widespread are *A. labran-*

chiae in the western parts and *A. sacharovi* in the eastern. Both of them are preferentially grassy pool breeders, and hence malaria was specially associated with swamp formation. One notorious vector prevalent in the eastern parts, *A. superpictus*, bred in clear sunlit water, usually without vegetation, and typically in shingly streams, a fact which made many river valleys extremely unhealthy. There were also other vectors of local significance, such as *A. claviger* which was notorious as a result of its habit of breeding in domestic water cisterns in the Middle East, and *A. sergenti* which from time to time caused severe epidemics often in the neighbourhood of springs and irrigation systems of date palm groves.

Much of this has, however, gone and there is no indigenous malaria in Mediterranean countries of southern Europe, while in those of northern Africa the amount of malaria has greatly decreased. The same applies to some countries of the eastern Mediterranean. There have been some setbacks to malaria eradication or control in Asian Turkey, Afghanistan, Iran and Iraq where anopheline resistance to insecticides has occurred.

North-East India, Assam, Northern Bengal. Formerly malaria was seasonal and highly endemic and large areas of this part of the subcontinent were uninhabited on account of their insalubrity. *A. minimus* is by far the most important carrier in these areas. It seems to be more dependent on man for its food than any other species, and is long-lived and susceptible to infection. It bites mainly in the second half of the night, shelters in houses and cattle sheds, and breeds in cool water. This preference for relatively cool water determines the type of breeding place which varies with the season. In winter larvae are found along the grassy banks of major rivers, in grassy pools and other places; in the summer breeding becomes confined, occurring particularly in running water and in exposed subsoil water, as in primitive wells and seepages. Larvae can only persist in the presence of some vegetation such as grass along the edge, but they do not occur where the overhanging vegetation is dense; therefore the typical breeding place is an exposed sunlit drain or stream with grassy banks. This mosquito is the commonest vector in this part of the world.

A. leucosphyrus is now known to be of great importance in limited areas where it occurs. It is much attracted to man but rests in houses for only a short period after feeding; in consequence it is rarely found in day-time catches. It breeds in small pools in the forest, and since it does not seem to fly far, it is important only in the neighbourhood of heavily overgrown land.

Other mosquitos may be of local importance. Thus *A. annularis* has been incriminated, and *A. maculatus* is apparently a vector in the hills near Shillong. *A. philippinensis* is not a carrier in Assam, but is important in parts of Bengal; the dividing line is not exactly drawn. *A. sundaicus* is a coastal mosquito which breeds exclusively in brackish water, and might be important in some coastal areas.

The plains of India and of Pakistan. Malaria throughout the plains is seasonal and shows a marked tendency to epidemics over large areas, particularly in the Punjab and Sind, and in some coastal areas of Tamil Nadu and Kerala.

A. culicifacies is by far the most important vector; it prefers feeding on cattle rather than on man and its life is relatively short. Malaria is maintained by force of numbers of the vector and where they are insufficient to keep the disease going, one may find quite healthy areas. Where, however, they are numerous the malaria they carry may be severe and subject to extreme fluctuations in amount from year to year. *A. culicifacies* is a pool breeder, occurring in natural and artificial pools exposed to the sun and often in those without vegetation, rarely in permanent swamps. Roadside pools, borrow-pits and such like are much favoured, as are also rock-pools and sand-pools in the beds of dry rivers. This last preference explains why malaria in some places, particularly in the extreme south, is closely linked with dry weather; failure of the rains is more likely to precipitate epidemics than excess rain. Excess irrigation which raises the subsoil water and makes pooling common is a frequent cause of high endemicity. In the Punjab pools of these types are rare; most breeding occurs during the monsoon, an excess of rain causing epidemics (Fig. 34).

A. stephensi is a vector of malaria in Bombay, Delhi, and in Karachi as also in other towns where larvae are found in wells, cisterns and any type of water containers around houses; in the country it is a pool breeder. When they are able to, the adult Anopheles have a strong preference for feeding on cattle rather than man; in consequence, malaria transmission becomes possible either in the absence of cattle or when the mosquitos are abundant.

There are other vectors of local importance. *A. annularis* is important in some parts of Orissa and Bengal; it breeds in pools, swamps and rice fields. *A. varuna* is a local vector of considerable importance. *A. philippinensis* is the common carrier in the plains of Bengal; it breeds in ponds and tanks with much surface vegetation. *A. sundaicus* is a carrier in the coastal areas of Bengal and Orissa and perhaps in a part of Andhra Pradesh; it breeds in brackish water only, and occurs near the sea.

The Western Ghats and hills of Peninsular India. These hills were notorious for the severity of malaria and there were many areas which were not populated for this reason. Control was first achieved by the application of the knowledge of the habits of *A. fluviatilis*, largely in the form of training and flushing streams. Later the full efficacy of the residual insecticides has been realised. Malaria is now greatly reduced in these areas.

A. fluviatilis, which is a close relative of *A. minimus*, is the principal vector. Much attracted to man and feeding very largely on him, it rests in houses and breeds in places similar to those favoured by *A. minimus*, except that it does not demand the presence of vegetation, occurring in rocky streams in which *A. minimus* could not maintain itself. It also occurs in rice fields fed by seepage water, from any part of which the total output may be insignificant, though the gross output from the entire area may be much more than enough to keep malaria transmission going.

Sri Lanka (Ceylon). There are very great variations in the incidence of malaria in different parts of the island, depending on the climate. Generally speaking it is absent at heights over 1000 m and in areas where the annual rainfall is heavy, but highly endemic in those where it is low. As a result of the monsoon distribution the disease was very prevalent in the north and east, extending in its severity round a part of the south coast. In the south-west corner, where the south-west monsoon occurs in full force, it was absent. Between these two areas is an intermediate one extending from Chilaw to Kurunegala in the north and then along the lower parts of the hills to the south where the incidence of malaria varied very greatly from year to year; periodic epidemics of disastrous severity occurred.

The sole vector of importance is *A. culicifacies*, an account of which has been given above in describing malaria of the plains of central and north India and Pakistan. The type of pool preferred as a breeding place is much associated with slight rain rather than continuous downpours, a fact which causes the spatial and seasonal distribution of malaria. In the areas of highest malaria incidence breeding may be found in almost any type of pool, but in the epidemic areas it occurs more particularly in the pool of river beds during the dry season. Monsoon failure is therefore related to epidemics.

The history of control included long and energetic efforts at prevention of breeding, with local success which did not amount to general control. Residual insecticides were brought into use soon after the war, their application became general, and in 1947 a campaign throughout malarious areas of the entire country was started. Soon malaria as a serious public health problem ceased to exist. In 1960 a further expansion was made and the objective has been changed, from control to eradication of the disease. However, since 1967 adverse climatic conditions and a certain slackening of the rigorous search for remaining cases have caused a considerable increase of malaria incidence amounting to an epidemic of vivax malaria.

Epidemiology of Malaria

South-East Asia and the Philippines. Malaya (West Malaysia) had a history of disastrous outbreaks of malaria. This phase came to an end, largely as the result of the introduction of rational methods of control; there was a marked exacerbation during the war but since then there has been a marked reduction in general incidence. It seems that the main anopheline carrier, *A. maculatus*, is attracted more to cattle than to man, and may not always be an important vector. Development of the country provided favourable conditions for it through the multiplication of breeding places by estate clearance, the introduction of non-immune labourers, and the growth of groups of people without domestic animals. These three factors working together caused the epidemics and as each of them is now coming to an end the incidence of malaria is correspondingly in decline. Extensive clearing or the aggregation of new labour forces could, however, easily precipitate a recurrence of past conditions.

The chief vector is *A. maculatus*. Also important, but in much more restricted areas, are *A. sundaicus* and *A. letifer*. *A. campestris* has been incriminated as a vector in the lowlands near the coast. *A. umbrosus*, which breeds in stagnant pools of peaty water in well-shaded jungle swamps, may occasionally carry human malaria near its breeding places, but it is chiefly a vector of monkey malaria.

A. maculatus occurs in streams, rock pools, and seepages, but only when they are exposed to broad daylight. Clearance of forests can expose such places and make them highly dangerous or can be selective and do no harm. *A. sundaicus* is a strictly coastal mosquito as it breeds in saline water, usually between high neap tide level and spring tide level. Its control was for long based exclusively on the construction of embankments with controlled internal drainage which prevented the access of saline water to this area and removed fresh water from it. *A. letifer* breeds in brown peaty water pools and stagnant agricultural drains, with and without vegetation, in the low country. *A. campestris* (formerly known as the dark-winged *A. barbirostris*), breeds in ricefields and in pools, often containing decaying vegetation, in the lowlands near the coast (Fig. 35).

In Viet-Nam and the Khmer Republic where *A. minimus* and *A. sundaicus* are the main endophilic vectors both responded well to the residual insecticide spraying but the exophilic *A. balabacensis* which does not commonly feed in human habitations has not been affected. The same is largely true in Thailand, where the increase of human activities in forested areas exposed the population to these Anopheles. In the Philippines the main vectors are *A. minimus flavirostris*, which breeds in clear, slow-flowing streams; two other vectors, *A. mangyanus* and *A. litoralis*, a brackish water breeder, are of local importance. In most of these countries problems of resistance of malaria vectors and of *P. falciparum* have impeded the success of control methods.

Indonesia and Borneo (Kalimantan). Conditions in Indonesia resemble those in Malaya, both in past history and in the nature of the common carriers, the chief of which are *A. maculatus* and *A. sundaicus*. A number of other mosquitos have, however, been incriminated in different places. Two of these, *A. hyrcanus* and *A. aconitus*, breed in extensive exposed sheets of water such as rice fields during some part of the cultivation cycle. *A. aconitus* has been successfully discouraged by ensuring that all rice fields in one locality were in the same stage of cultivation, so that a common off-season occurred when no suitable harbourage presented itself. However, the association of these species with agriculture, and that of *A. sundaicus* with the fish industry, made control very difficult until the arrival of the new residual insecticides. Extensive schemes of control have been initiated with the objective of general control throughout the country. These schemes are in progress, covering large areas in Java and Bali. Full success has not been achieved partly because of resistance to both DDT and dieldrin in *A. sundaicus* and *A. aconitus* in some areas.

Malaria is widely distributed in Borneo, and commonly of the low epidemic potential type. The most important vector is *A. leucosphyrus*, a mosquito with the habit of resting for only a short time in houses after having fed in them. It breeds in the forest, in seepages and pools often under tangled undergrowth surrounded by swampy areas, in places which are inaccessible for any routine weekly antilarval measures. The shade afforded by the forest is apparently essential to the survival of larvae in the water. *A. leucosphyrus* is not a strong flier; it carries malaria only within a short range of dense bush. Other carriers of local importance are *A. sundaicus* and *A. umbrosus*.

Australasia and the South Pacific. The South Pacific includes a very large area which is free from malaria; the disease does not extend east of 170°E or south of 20°S. In continental Australia malaria had in the past a restricted distribution in the more extreme north, chiefly in coastal areas in the east to north-western Australia.

Very high incidences occur in New Guinea, particularly in coastal areas, and in the neighbouring islands. Incidence is also high in the Solomon Islands and in the New Hebrides, though these two are of progressively lower grades than New Guinea, typically with seasonal epidemic malaria. Experience of the war showed that extremely serious outbreaks may be expected in any imported human groups.

The carriers are all of the *A. punctulatus* complex, which bites man readily but can be diverted by cattle, on which they often feed by preference. They are pool breeders, with larvae occurring in sunlit water of the most diverse types, including such sites as wheel ruts in roads. One of the varieties of this species may breed in sea-water pools. They enter houses to feed, but tend to shelter out of doors in the nearby bush; relatively poor fliers, they do not move far from their breeding places.

Tropical Africa. Throughout most of Africa south of the Sahara malaria shows a high endemicity, but has a low epidemic potential. Exceptions to this last statement are to be found on the slopes of mountains in Kenya, at the periphery of the distribution of malaria in Zimbabwe-Rhodesia and the Republic of South Africa, and formerly in Mauritius, in all of which places epidemics were well known. In the centre of the continental area transmission is nearly perennial, though there are seasonal exacerbations, and very high endemicities are common in the coastlands and other places at a low altitude. Endemicity is reduced, though still high, on the plateau of East Africa which is at an average altitude of 1400 m; the disease occurs up to a height of 2300 m on some mountains, though more as occasional outbreaks than a continuous endemicity. Epidemics in the lowlands of the central region are rare unless precipitated by obvious causes such as the importation of labour from non-malarious places or construction work producing many new breeding places.

There are three vectors which are important wherever they occur in this region, *A. gambiae*, *A. melas* and *A. funestus*, and a number of other carriers which may be of local importance but are not of general significance.

A. gambiae complex is the most important vector. It is very widely distributed and feeds predominantly on man; it is normally robust and long-lived, readily susceptible to infection, and often numerous. Though this is not an invariable habit, it commonly rests in houses, but is easily driven out of doors. In the warmer parts of Africa it bites at night in the house; in the cooler parts it may bite in the open. It seems to disappear or nearly so from the limits of its distribution during the cold season.

The larvae are commonly found in pools, usually exposed to the sun, and though they occur in all types of such pools they are more common in temporary ones than in those of long standing. Breeding in rice fields and in swamps may occur. Owing to the nature of the breeding places, this species tends to be more numerous in the rainy season than in dry weather.

A. melas is a close relative of *A. gambiae*, distinguished from the latter by preference for brackish water for its breeding places. It is therefore confined to coastal districts, where it may be of great importance, and is responsible for most of the malaria of many parts of the West African coast. In its other general characteristics it resembles

A. gambiae. Owing to the nature of its breeding places the control of this species requires special methods.

A. funestus is a very widely distributed carrier, second in importance only to *A. gambiae*. It feeds predominantly on man, is robust and long-lived, shelters almost exclusively in houses, and is readily susceptible to infection.

The larvae are commonly found in streams, and particularly under shade; swamps, seepages, fallow rice fields, and the grassy edges of rivers may be important breeding places. Owing to the nature of its breeding places its season is often different from that of *A. gambiae* and in many places the one species takes over from the other as chief vector when the season changes. It has a long flight range, but has not demonstrated the invasive tendency shown by *A. gambiae*. Moreover, it responds more readily to residual insecticides.

Some anophelines in equatorial Africa which are important in limited localities include:

A. moucheti in the Congo and Cameroun, probably an important carrier in large riverine forest tracts.

A. nili in coastal West Africa may be an important secondary carrier in some places; it breeds in streams.

A. pharoensis. A common carrier in Egypt; it may play a minor role in the drier parts of West Africa, the Sudan, Uganda and Kenya.

The Caribbean Area. In this area eradication programmes have made great progress (except for Haïti). Formerly the general incidence of malaria on the islands of the Caribbean was much less than in most of the areas already described, though there were localities with high prevalence. Throughout the area the disease was of the high epidemic potential type, liable to marked fluctuations from time to time and from place to place.

The Bahamas are free from malaria, though they have experienced it and could do so again. All the other islands were to some extent malarious, the disease having a very patchy distribution. Malaria eradication has been achieved in Jamaica, Dominica, Grenada and Carriacou, Barbados, Trinidad and Tobago, Puerto Rico and Cuba. In the Greater Antilles (Cuba, Jamaica, Puerto Rico and Hispaniola) the chief carrier is *A. albimanus*, a mosquito of the plains, very prevalent in irrigated areas where it breeds in cane fields, rice fields and other similar stagnant water. It is a relatively poor carrier, possibly being normally short-lived, and is important only by reason of large numbers.

In the Lesser Antilles, notably in Trinidad and neighbouring islands, *A. aquasalis* is the common carrier. It is always coastal in its distribution, but as the islands are mostly small this is little restriction. It breeds

Epidemiology of Malaria

in brackish water, in drainage channels, slow streams, mangrove swamps, borrow-pits, and a great variety of waters within five or six miles of the coast. It feeds on cattle in strong preference to man, and is very short-lived, characteristics which would have made it a very poor carrier if it had not often been present in enormous numbers. It is apparently diverted by cattle and the amount of malaria may be in inverse proportion to their numbers in some places.

Another carrier in Trinidad is *A. bellator*, an unusual vector. It breeds high above the ground in bromeliads, parasitic plants growing on trees and common trees in cacao plantations. It bites mainly out of doors and in the hours of daylight. The disease it carries is therefore often an occupational one of plantation workers. Nevertheless it has proved susceptible to control by the use of residual insecticides in houses. The additional method used is destruction of the bromeliad by spraying with copper solutions, or the cutting down of the parent trees.

South America. On the mainland, there are areas in which *A. aquasalis* is the vector, but the most important is *A. darlingi*, which breeds profusely in the irrigation channels, irrigated fields, and swamps which between them constitute the economy of the inhabited lowlands. It is strongly attracted to man, shelters exclusively in houses, and may be rather short-lived. It is a fairly potent carrier, and its ubiquity has made severe malaria a feature of several countries. The first large-scale control by residual insecticides was started in Venezuela and Guyana, and resulted in the actual elimination of the mosquito from the main coastal belt.

A. darlingi is also the vector in the hills of the interior, where it is not universally distributed but can readily establish itself near human settlements. Fortunately its susceptibility to control is likely to be as marked as in the lowlands.

Other vectors of malaria in South America include *A. punctimacula* (in Peru and Colombia), *A. aquasalis*, *A. pseudopunctipennis*, *A. albitarsis* (in Brasil), *A. albimanus* in coastal lowlands. Special attention has been given recently to *A. nuñez-tovari*, a forest dwelling mosquito with elusive habits, which maintains a degree of transmission in the border areas of Venezuela and Colombia.

In parts of Brazil *A. cruzi*, with peculiar breeding habitats in water-containing bromeliad plants, deserves mention.

In Central America the list of vectors include, *A. darlingi*, *A. aquasalis*, *A. punctimacula* but the most important of all is *A. albimanus*, which breeds in pools, puddles, ponds, marshes and artificial containers and has gained much notoriety because it has become resistant to nearly every insecticide available at present.

In the USA *A. quadrimaculatus* was the major if not the only vector of malaria in the past, though in some localities *A. freeborni* was incriminated. Today there is no more transmission of endemic malaria in that country, even though isolated cases of infection from imported carriers may occur. In the southern part of North America *A. albimanus* is the main vector in the lowlands adjacent to the Pacific Ocean.

Chapter 8

Chemotherapy and Chemoprophylaxis

Antimalarial drugs have a selective action on the different phases of the parasite life cycle and may be divided generally into *causal prophylactic* drugs which prevent the establishment of the parasite in the liver and *schizontocidal* drugs which attack the parasite in the red blood cell, preventing or terminating the clinical attack.

When the term *schizontocidal drug* is used alone it refers to its action on blood schizonts; the term *tissue schizontocide* refers to compounds acting on exo-erythrocytic forms. The *gametocytocidal* drugs destroy the sexual forms of the parasite; some of these drugs have a pronounced anti-relapse effect and are extensively used for radical treatment of malaria. Finally, *sporontocidal* drugs inhibit the development of the oöcysts on the stomach wall of the mosquito feeding on the carrier of gametocytes so that no sporozoites are produced and the mosquito cannot transmit the infection. This relationship between the phase of the development and the action of the drug is shown diagrammatically in Fig. 49.

Certain drugs bring about rapid cure of falciparum malaria but for complete and permanent cure of vivax, ovale and quartan malaria other drugs are necessary.

In addition to these clearly definable differences between the action of drugs on the four species of malaria parasites there are differences between strains of the same species, so that generalisations which are

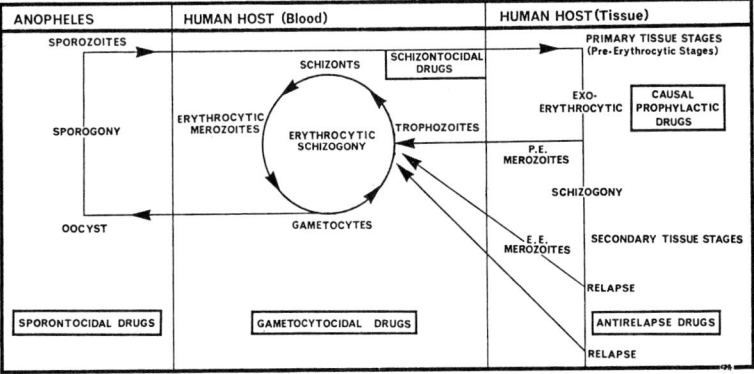

Fig 49 Diagram of action of antimalarial compounds in relation to the stage of development of the malaria parasite in Anopheles and in the human host.

true about malaria in one part of the world may appear to be quite incorrect in other parts.

The state of immunity has a bearing on the use of drugs, since persons who have, by prolonged exposure to the infection, acquired a degree of immunity can be cured or protected much more easily than those who have not. Evidence obtained from treatment or prevention of the partially immune groups cannot be applied to non-immunes or to other groups whose immunity may be less, and much confusion has resulted from efforts to do so.

Although it might appear that the availability of a wide range of antimalarials should satisfy all the requirements of individual treatment, prevention of infection and other needs of malaria eradication programmes, the truth is that most of the known drugs have a relatively short and incomplete action when given in a single dose and must be administered regularly over a number of days to have the desired effect. This is difficult in underdeveloped countries where the rural health services are inadequate. Hence the often expressed but still unfulfilled hope that one day a drug will be developed which will combine prolonged action with full effectiveness against all stages of malaria parasites.

USES OF ANTIMALARIAL DRUGS

A drug may be put to several uses, in each of which its utility may be affected by several factors, such as the species of malaria parasite concerned, its response to the relevant compound, the presence of partial immunity in the human host, the risks of toxic effects, as well as by other simpler ones such as availability, preference, and cost. The main uses of antimalarials are:

Protective (prophylactic) use; *Curative (therapeutic)* use, and *Use to prevent transmission* (Table 12).

1. *Protective (prophylactic) use.* This implies that the drugs are used before infection occurs or before it becomes obvious, with the aim of preventing either the occurrence of the infection or any of its symptoms.

Absolute prevention of infection implies destruction of sporozoites soon after they have been inoculated by the bite of an infected Anopheles. There is no drug that can achieve this.

On the other hand there are drugs that act on the early stages of the parasite, while it is still confined to the liver tissue, and destroy these stages before merozoites are liberated into the blood stream. In such a case one defines the relevant drug as *causal (or true) prophylactic*. When the drug is unable to achieve this effect within a short time and yet, if given over a longer time (exceeding the normal duration of the incubation period), it keeps the number of malaria parasites in the blood at such low level that they will not cause any clinical symptoms, then it acts as a *suppressive* (or *clinical prophylactic*) drug, as long as the subject continues to take it at adequate dosage. In practice it means that when the drug administration is discontinued the parasites remaining in the body may start multiplying once again and this may lead to a renewed attack of the disease.

All blood schizontocides are clinical prophylactic drugs or suppressants and it is obvious that if they are administered for a long time they may eventually eliminate the malaria infection simply by exhaustion of the supply of parasites.

Such an objective known as *suppressive cure* can be attained in the case of falciparum malaria, the common tropical infection.

2. *Curative (therapeutic) use.* Therapeutic use of drugs refers to the action on the established infection and comprises the treatment of the acute attack, and radical treatment.

Treatment of the acute attack implies drug administration against the erythrocytic stages of the parasite using schizontocidal drugs. The result of the treatment may be either a temporary cure with a transient relief of symptoms or a permanent cure.

In infections with species of malaria parasites that produce relapses, permanent cure can be achieved by *radical treatment*. This requires the use of anti-relapse drugs that will act not only on the erythrocytic parasites but also on the secondary tissue stages of plasmodia.

3. *Use of drugs to prevent transmission.* This refers to the prevention of infection of mosquitos and implies an action on gametocytes in the peripheral blood of the human host or interruption of the development of the sporogonic phase in the mosquito, when the latter feeds on the blood of an infected person who has been given the appropriate compound.

In malaria control the operational use of drugs distinguishes several aims. When antimalarial compounds are used by individuals for prevention of the infection or of the disease one refers to *individual protection* or *individual prophylaxis*. When such drugs are used by the whole community or by a well defined portion of it one talks about *collective drug protection*.

In malaria control programmes the main types of drug administration are: presumptive treatment, radical treatment and mass drug administration.

Presumptive treatment means generally treatment given to a presumptive malaria case at the time when a blood sample is taken for confirmation of the malaria infection. It usually consists of a single dose of a schizontocide (at times combined with a sporontocide) and its aim is to relieve symptoms, possibly due to malaria, and to prevent the spread of the infection by mosquitos. Presumptive treatment is thus a precautionary measure limited to selected individuals.

Table 12

Action of commonly used drugs on the cycle of development of malaria parasites

Drug	Sporozoites	Primary tissue phase (during the incubation period)	Erythrocytic phase Asexual parasites	Erythrocytic phase Sexual forms (gametocytes)	Secondary tissue phase (responsible for relapses)	Development of gametocytes in the mosquito (sporontocidal action)	Chemical class of the relevant antimalarial compound	Remarks
Quinine	No action	No action	Fast action	Active against *P. vivax* and *P. malariae*. No direct action on *P. falciparum*	No action	No action	Cinchona alcaloid	Used for emergency treatment
Mepacrine	No action	No action	Fast action	As quinine	No action	No action	9-amino-acridine	Obsolete drug
Chloroquine Amodiaquine	No action	No action	Fast action	As quinine	No action	No action	4-amino-quinolines	Most reliable drugs unless resistant *P. falciparum* present
Primaquine	No action	Active but not used for prophylaxis	Active but only in toxic doses	Direct and fast action on all species but particularly *P. falciparum*	Highly active	Highly active	8-amino-quinoline	Used for radical cure

Drug							Chemical class	Remarks
Proguanil	No action	No action	Active particularly on P. falciparum	Active but relatively slow	No direct action	No action	Active	Biguanide	Essentially a prophylactic drug
Pyrimethamine	No action	No action	As proguanil	As proguanil	No evidence of direct action	Some action on P. vivax	Highly active	Diaminopyrimidine	As proguanil
Sulphones	No action	No action	Possible action, but no evidence	Incomplete action when given alone. Less effective on P. vivax	As pyrimethamine	No evidence	Little evidence	Sulphones comprise several short-acting compounds	Used mainly in association with pyrimethamine or other antifolates
Sulphonamides	No action	No action	Possible action, but no evidence	Incomplete action when given alone. Less effective on P. vivax	As pyrimethamine	No evidence	Little evidence	Sulphonamides of value are long acting compounds more effective in P. falciparum than in P. vivax	As above for treatment of P. falciparum resistant to chloroquine
Mefloquine	No evidence	No evidence	No evidence	Active esp. on P. falciparum	No evidence of direct action	No evidence	No evidence	Quinoline-methanols	As above. Used often after a previous treatment with quinine

Radical treatment has been explained before. Its purpose in malaria control is to eliminate all remaining or imported relapsing infections and to prevent the spread of the disease.

Mass drug administration means that in areas where the disease is highly endemic every person must receive regularly the prescribed dose of the drug. The frequency of distribution depends on the purpose of the programme, the nature of the drug and other conditions. Practical difficulties of this method are often considerable. One of the methods of mass drug administration is by the use of medicated salt.

AVAILABLE ANTIMALARIAL DRUGS; THEIR STRUCTURE AND RELATIONSHIP

There are several chemical groups of antimalarial compounds in general use. For practical purposes, the drugs belonging to the eight most important groups are given here under their international non-proprietary names: (1) Quinine; (2) Mepacrine; (3) Chloroquine, Amodiaquine; :4) Proguanil and Chlorproguanil; (5) Pyrimethamine; (6) Primaquine; (7) Sulphones and Sulphonamides; (8) Quinoline-methanols.

Some knowledge of the chemistry of these compounds will be useful for understanding their antimalarial action (Fig. 50).

Quinine is one of the four main alkaloids extracted from the Cinchona tree bark. It has a complex molecule one part of which is the quinoline nucleus.

Mepacrine belongs to the group of 9-amino-acridines; the quinoline ring in it is broadened to form the acridine ring.

Chloroquine and amodiaquine both have a quinoline ring in which the active side chain (as in chloroquine) or a substituted anilino group (as in amodiaquine) are linked with the ring in the position 4 of the carbon of the quinoline ring. Both compounds belong therefore to the 4-aminoquinoline class of antimalarials.

In the case of *primaquine* the quinoline ring has an alkylamino chain attached in the position 8 and this compound, together with other similar ones (pamaquine, quinocide), belongs to the 8-amino-quinolines.

Proguanil (known as chlorguanide in USA) represents the biguanide class of antimalarials. It is characterised by having a biguanide chain attached at one end to a chlorophenyl ring. The metabolic product of proguanil is chemically very close to the structure of pyrimethamine. *Pyrimethamine* has a pyrimidine ring with two diamino- groups attached to it; it belongs to the diaminopyrimidine class of antimalarial compounds.

The two latter compounds destroy the malaria parasite by interfering with its biochemical processes through binding an essential

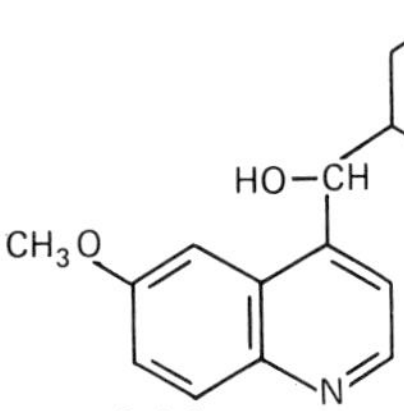

Quinine
6-methoxy-α-(5-vinyl-2-quinuclidinyl)-4-quinolinemethanol

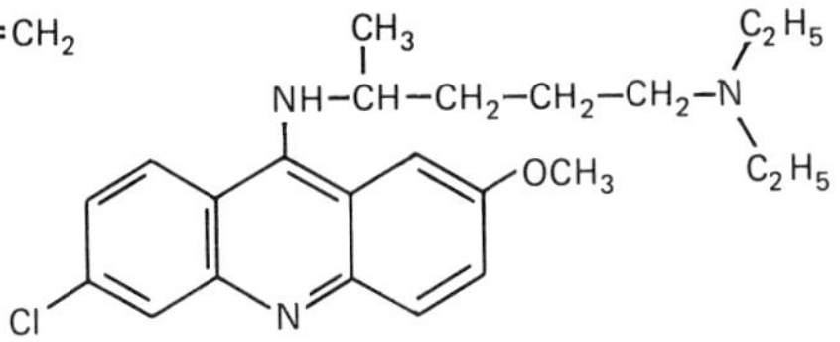

Mepacrine
2-methoxy-6-chloro-9-(4'-diethylamino-1'-methylbutylamino)-acridine

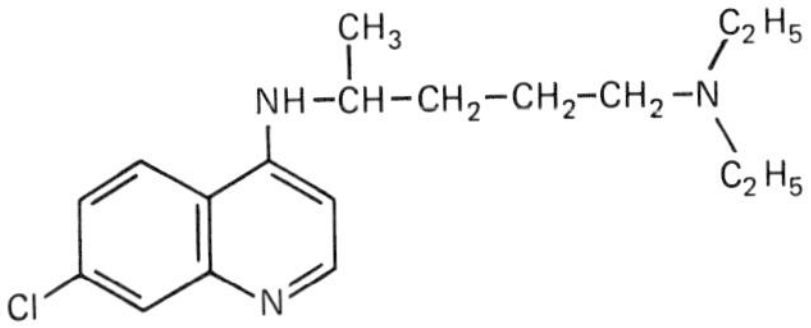

Chloroquine
7-chloro-4-(4'-diethylamino-1'-methylbutylamino)quinoline

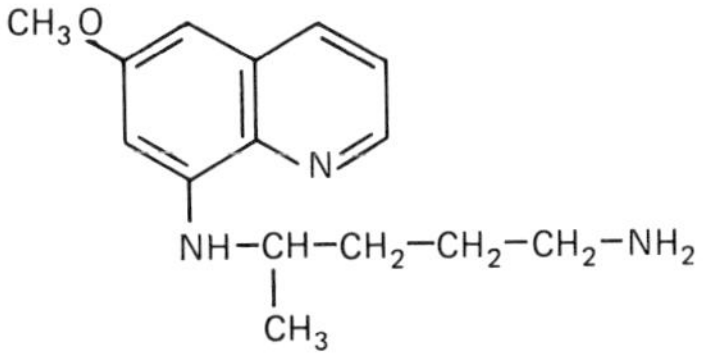

Primaquine
6-methoxy-8-(4'-amino-1'-methylbutylamino)quinoline

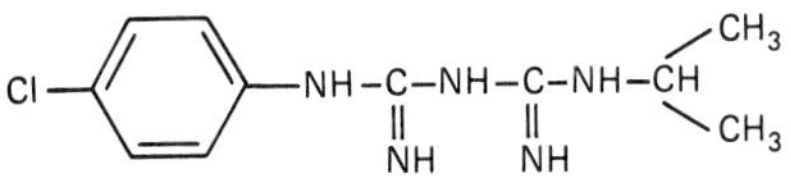

Proguanil
N^1-(p-chlorophenyl)-N^5-isopropyldiguanide

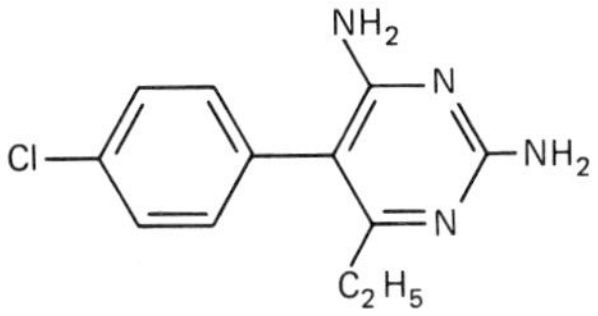

Pyrimethamine
2,4-diamino-5-p-chlorophenyl-6-ethylpyrimidine

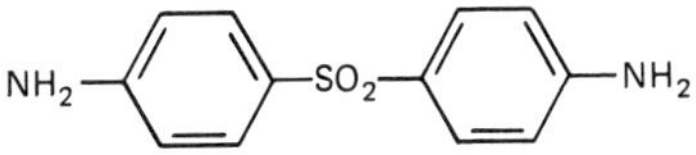

Diaphenylsulfone (Dapsone)
4,4'-diaminodiphenylsulfone

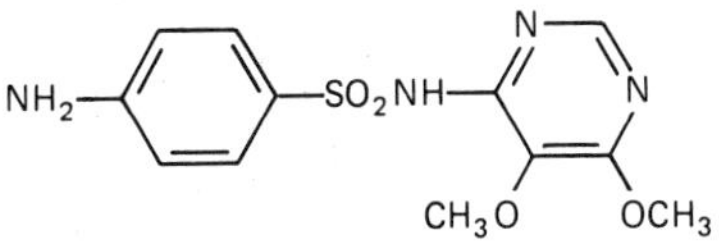

Sulformetoxine (Sulfadoxine)
5,6-dimethoxy-4-sulfanil-amidopyrimidine

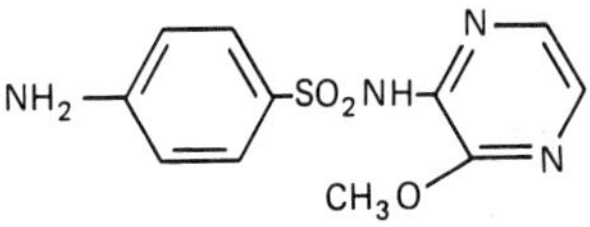

Sulfalene
3-methoxy-2-sulfanilamido-pyrazine

Fig 50 Chemical formulae of commonly used antimalarial drugs.

enzyme: dihydrofolate reductase. The two compounds are frequently called dihydrofolate reductase inhibitors or antifolates (also known as 'antifols').

Another compound with the same properties as pyrimethamine is *trimethoprim*; it is less effective than pyrimethamine in binding the enzyme of the parasite.

Sulphones and sulphonamides, which in the 1930s proved to be excellent anti-bacterial drugs, were tested for their antimalarial properties but in spite of some action appeared to be disappointing in comparison with other compounds. Their mode of action is due to the fact that when ingested they compete with the para-aminobenzoic acid for the enzyme which transforms it into the next essential product of metabolism of the plasmodial cell.

Sulphones are represented by the diamino-diphenyl sulphone known as DDS or dapsone. There are large numbers of derivatives of *sulphonamides* of which sulphadiazine is one of the earliest used for treatment of malaria; some newer sulphonamides (sulphamethoxypyridazine, sulphadimethoxine, sulphadoxine, sulphamethoxazole) are bound with the protein of blood plasma and act for a considerable time after a single administration.

The first three groups (quinine, mepacrine, chloroquine and amodiaquine) are essentially therapeutic drugs; primaquine is a radically curative drug as it has a specific action against the tissue forms of malaria parasites responsible for relapses of tertian and quartan malaria. Proguanil and pyrimethamine are mainly protective (prophylactic) compounds, although they have also a useful action on the parasite developing in the mosquito. Sulphones and sulphonamides have an action on the blood forms of malaria parasites similar to the first three groups, but this action is relatively slow; a combination with pyrimethamine increases very greatly the therapeutic action of these compounds.

Quinolinemethanols represent a new series of valuable compounds studied during the past decade by the US Army Research and Development Command and evaluated on experimental animals and then on clinical trials in man. Several promising compounds of this group are still under study, but one of them now known under the generic name of *mefloquine* appears to be a very effective drug for treatment of malaria due to drug resistant *P. falciparum* in some parts of the world. Unfortunately mefloquine is not yet available for general use. Another related compound of the series of phenanthrenemethanols is also being evaluated at the present time.

The main properties of the drugs generally used are classified according to their effects in Table 12.

Clinical uses of common antimalarial compounds

Quinine. For more than three centuries cinchona and its alkaloids, especially quinine, were the only effective drugs available for the relief of malaria. Within recent times, however, the new substances described below have been synthesised and these have proved not only superior to quinine but also less toxic. Today quinine is recommended mainly for emergency treatment of falciparum malaria but also, and increasingly so, if no other drug is fully active on some resistant strains of malaria parasites.

Quinine is particularly useful for emergency treatment of severe malaria and in such cases it must be administered by injection, preferably by slow intravenous infusion in a suitable diluent in single adult doses not exceeding 650 mg (10 grains) or, if repeated dose is necessary, not more than 2000 mg (about 30 grains) in 24 hours. Administered over 10–14 days at the dose of 650 mg (10 grains) 3 times daily quinine will effect a radical cure of falciparum malaria but given alone it has no prospect of doing so in cases of vivax or quartan malaria. Resistance by malaria parasites to quinine is very rare.

As a preventive drug, quinine has proved inferior to other drugs and there is no excuse for its continued use for this purpose. Its prolonged administration is sometimes connected with the onset of blackwater fever. It produces some side effects, such as noise in the ears, and when given in very large doses it may cause a restriction of the visual field.

Mepacrine. Mepacrine would seem to be just as generally useful as the more modern drugs but has many disadvantages. It accumulates slowly in the body to reach an effective concentration and may be slow in action unless it is first given in high doses. Given at a dose of 1 g on the first day, followed by 300 mg daily during the next week, it has a pronounced schizontocidal action on all types of malaria but has little effect against strains of *P. falciparum* showing resistance to the 4-amino-quinolines. Given in adequate doses (that is, 0.1 g or 100 mg once every day) it is a good suppressant of malaria, but it has the marked disadvantage of being deposited in the skin so that those who take it become a bright yellow colour. It can also cause skin eruptions and mental disturbance when given in high doses.

The toxic characteristics of mepacrine are sufficient to command much caution in its use. Intramuscular injection of mepacrine is dangerous in children as it may produce fatal collapse or brain damage.

Mepacrine is not recommended for routine use and is now considered as an obsolete drug. It is mentioned here because large supplies of it may still be found in some countries and could be used if no other drugs are available.

Chloroquine. This is an excellent preventive and curative drug with a wider range of useful qualities than any other drug. It is a highly effective and rapid blood schizontocide. It destroys gametocytes of *P. vivax, P. malariae* and *P. ovale* but has no immediate action on 'crescents' of *P. falciparum*. For curative purposes the regimen advised for an adult is an initial dose of 0.6 g (600 mg) of chloroquine base[1] followed by an additional dose of 0.3 g (300 mg) six to eight hours later, followed by a single dose of 300 mg on each of the following two to four days. In certain areas it may be advisable to continue treatment with a once weekly administration of smaller doses of chloroquine (300–600 mg of base) for 4–8 weeks to prevent recrudescence of falciparum malaria. Chloroquine is the most effective drug available for the speedy control of any malarial fever in a person who is able to swallow tablets. Indeed in a person who is partially immune to malaria an attack can be controlled by a single dose of 600 mg of chloroquine. Patients with severe malaria who cannot take drugs by mouth should receive the initial treatment by injection. Chloroquine in single doses up to 300 mg of base (for an adult) may be given by intramuscular or intravenous injection and this dose may be repeated twice or even three times in the first 24 hours. Chloroquine by injection should not be given to young children but if this is necessary, great caution is advised. Divided doses in several injections are a good safety measure and the total dose in the first 24 hour period must not exceed 5 mg per kg of child's body weight. As soon as possible the treatment should revert to the oral route.

Chloroquine may be considered a dual-purpose drug in that it is efficient for the control of the attack of malaria and in the light of experience has proved to be a reliable suppressant. When used for relatively long periods after leaving the malarious area chloroquine may eliminate the infection with falciparum malaria.

Malaria can usually be suppressed by taking chloroquine at an adult dose of 300 mg of base per week. In some parts of the world where malaria is intense a weekly dose of 600 mg of base is taken by non-immunes. In areas where resistant strains of *P. falciparum* are present, a 'breakthrough' with acute attacks may occur either during or soon after the cessation of suppression. In persons exposed to *P. vivax* or other relapsing infections attacks of malaria are liable to occur when the suppressive regimen is terminated.

---

[1] All antimalarial drugs in common use are organic bases and form salts with acids. With the exception of pyrimethamine (and some preparations of amodiaquine) antimalarial drugs are employed in the form of salts. Because only the base components are therapeutically active, and as there are considerable differences in the content of base in various salts, doses of antimalarial drugs should be expressed in terms of base content. Nevertheless, some drugs such as quinine and proguanil are commonly prescribed in terms of the salt content.

Chloroquine does not produce any significant side effects in the dosages normally advised for antimalarial purposes but pruritus, some blurring of vision and headache have been reported in some individuals, especially when high doses were used.

Chloroquine is occasionally given in combination with other drugs such as pyrimethamine or primaquine; this has the effect of making the individual non-infective to mosquitos for some time. This effect is particularly valuable in malaria eradication campaigns.

Amodiaquine. Chloroquine and amodiaquine belong to the same group of 4-aminoquinolines and have many pharmacological and clinical aspects in common. Thus what has been said of the former applies very largely to the latter.

There is a slight difference in the dosage of these drugs mainly because amodiaquine is often formulated in tablets of 200 mg base each. A new type of tablet containing pure amodiaquine base (Basoquin) has no bitter taste and may be easier swallowed by children. There is no injectable amodiaquine preparation but an alternative compound, amopyroquine (Propoquine), is available.

Amodiaquine has the same properties as regards resistance by *P. falciparum* as has chloroquine; parasites resistant to the latter are generally resistant to amodiaquine, though some strains are more susceptible to the action of this drug.

Primaquine. This drug succeeded pamaquine which was one of the early synthetic antimalarials but was found to be too toxic for general use. The most important property of primaquine and some closely related compounds of the series of 8-aminoquinolines is that they prevent relapses of malaria, through destruction of the forms which persist in the liver. They are also active against gametocytes but not on other forms of malaria parasites circulating in the blood. Because they are poor schizontocides 8-aminoquinolines should not be used alone for treatment or prevention of malaria.

For radical cure of *P. vivax, P. malariae* or *P. ovale* infections primaquine is given following the standard treatment with chloroquine, amodiaquine or quinine. However, if medication is started in a latent interval between relapses it may be given alone. It may be used in this latter way to cure residual infection with vivax malaria in people leaving countries where the infection is widely prevalent.

Once weekly administration of 45 mg primaquine together with 300 mg of chloroquine base has been used as a prophylactic regimen in some areas because primaquine has an effect on persisting tissue forms of *P. vivax*. However, the usual dosage of primaquine is 15 mg base daily for 14 days.

In some individuals affected with the glucose-6-phosphate dehydrogenase deficiency whose red blood cells are unduly sensitive to primaquine and undergo haemolysis, an alternative regimen of 30–45 mg of primaquine once a week for 8 weeks has been found useful and without undue harmful effects. Some strains of *P. vivax* are less sensitive to this dosage of primaquine. On the other hand any attempt to shorten the treatment by giving primaquine for 5 days instead of 14 is bound to increase the chance of relapses. Treatment with primaquine should be given under medical supervision as this drug may cause a number of side effects that may be dangerous in some individuals.

Proguanil. The great advantage of this drug is safety, in which it excels all other drugs. When given in proper doses it causes no ill-effects, whether immediate or remote. This drug has a slow schizontocidal action on erythrocytic forms of malaria parasites but is effective against the primary tissue phase of *P. falciparum* and has a sporontocidal effect on this species. It is less active against *P. vivax*.

Proguanil (chlorguanide) was first used for treatment of malaria (at two doses daily of 300 mg for 10 days). Though it was successful in a proportion of cases, there were many failures, and it is now not recommended for this purpose.

It is, however, very valuable as a preventive drug, at the adult dose of one tablet of 100 mg (0.1 g) every day but in areas with highly endemic malaria a daily dose of 2 tablets could be used for a limited time. Such daily doses are advantageous because daily medication is easy to remember. Once- or twice-weekly doses do not give adequate protection to non-immunes, but they have in some places been used for the protection of semi-immune populations.

Proguanil is rapidly absorbed and excreted, and is not accumulated in the tissues. Since its main action is on the early stages of the parasites which develop in the liver, while parasites which have entered the blood stream are much less sensitive to the drug and may not be affected by continuous administration of it, this may account for some failures of prevention by this compound.

In some localities where proguanil was at first effective its value has decreased due to the development by the malaria parasites of resistance to it. This has happened in some areas in Malaysia, New Guinea and East Africa, but is not sufficiently widespread to contra-indicate the use of the drug in general. Responsible local advice should always therefore be sought on its suitability. Subject to this qualification, proguanil is the best preventive for self-medication by people who remember to take the daily dose.

A compound closely related to proguanil is *chlorproguanil* with very similar properties. As it persists in the blood for a longer time, it may be used once a week, at 20 mg in a single dose.

Pyrimethamine. This compound has some characteristics in common with proguanil, the chief practical difference being that it is effective in much smaller doses. For preventive purposes once weekly administration is adequate as this drug is rapidly absorbed and slowly excreted. It has, like proguanil, the great advantage of freedom from side-effects; it is safe when taken in proper doses, it is tasteless and therefore well suited for medication of infants and young children.

Like proguanil, pyrimethamine has slow blood schizontocidal activity but considerable activity on the primary tissue forms of *P. falciparum* and, to a lesser extent, of *P. vivax*; on the other hand it has a pronounced sporontocidal effect so that an individual with gametocytes in the blood is non-infectious to mosquitos.

Pyrimethamine alone is not recommended for the treatment of attacks of malaria; it is normally reserved for preventive purposes. The usual adult dose is 25 mg once a week. At this dosage it effectively prevents infections with falciparum malaria, and suppresses vivax malaria, exactly as does proguanil, though it is subject to the same qualifications about resistance.

Resistance has appeared in several localities, in which pyrimethamine automatically becomes less effective. These are usually limited areas, not amounting to country-wide distribution in parts of East Africa, West Africa, and the Far East. Responsible local advice should therefore be sought to confirm the appropriateness of the drug before full reliance is placed on it. Moreover, since there is a connection between resistance to proguanil and that to pyrimethamine it is not advisable to change from one to another in the case of resistance developing when resort should be made to chloroquine. In view of the possibility of stimulating resistance, pyrimethamine alone should not be used for mass drug administration.

Though very safe in normal dosage, as detailed above, pyrimethamine can cause serious and even fatal effects if taken in excessive quantities by children. Parents should never give this drug daily when a weekly regimen has been recommended.

In malaria eradication programmes aiming at the prevention of malaria, a single adult dose of 50 mg has a sporontocidal effect for as long as 3 or 4 weeks, though it may not eliminate the parasites or cure the clinical effects. It is occasionally given in combination with chloroquine; the latter for its clinical value, pyrimethamine for its sterilising effect.

Sulphones and sulphonamides. The activity of diamino-diaphenyl-sulphone (DDS or dapsone) against malaria parasites has been known since the 1940s, but the interest in this and other compounds increased during the past decade because of the appearance of resistance in *P. falciparum*. The early clinical trials confirmed the schizontocidal effect of dapsone especially against *P. falciparum* but the drug was much slower in action than chloroquine. This late action is evident in both chloroquine-sensitive and chloroquine-resistant strains and dapsone was used for prevention of malaria, as a suppressive rather than therapeutic drug. Several derivatives of dapsone were subsequently introduced and among these is the diformyl diphenylsulphone which is more slowly excreted and perhaps more useful as a repository compound for prolonged action. Dapsone may produce side-effects in susceptible subjects and this has limited its usefulness. At the present time it is mainly used at a dosage of 100 mg once a week in combination with pyrimethamine, although at a daily dose of 25 mg it may be occasionally added for short term treatment together with schizontocidal compounds.

Sulphonamides, like sulphones were occasionally used for treatment of malaria some 40 years ago, but with uneven results, due to a different response of various strains of *P. vivax* and *P. falciparum*. Moreover, their short carry-over effect and need for high doses coupled with toxic effects were sufficient to justify the reluctance to use them as antimalarials.

However, the introduction during the past decade of long acting sulphonamides for antibacterial treatment has revived the interest in these compounds, particularly for treatment of *P. falciparum* infections resistant to chloroquine. Three of the long-acting sulphonamide compounds were found to be of particular value as antimalarials although their wider acceptance was due to the potentiating effect of antifolate drugs (pyrimethamine, trimethoprim) given in association

Results of experimental chemotherapy on human malaria transmitted to Aotus monkeys indicated that when delivered in combination the action of a sulphonamide (such as sulphadiazine) and pyrimethamine was mutually enhanced by 30 times for pyrimethamine and by 50–100 times for sulphadiazine when the infection was due to strains non-resistant to either of the two drugs.

Sulphadimethoxine has a relatively short half-life of 30–40 hours in human blood. At an average daily dose of 250 mg it has a substantial but shortlived schizontocidal effect. This drug is of value as a component of a synergistic drug combination.

Sulphalene also known as *sulphamethoxypyridazine* has a plasma half-life of 65 hours. It is a good schizontocide and suppressive in chloroquine resistant malaria but some strains of *P. falciparum* respond less quickly to it. At a single dose of 1.0 to 1.5 g together with an antifolate compound this is a valuable therapeutic antimalarial combination in areas of drug resistant malaria. Among the antifolate compounds used, trimethoprim or pyrimethamine are most common. The combination of sulphamethoxypyridazine with pyrimethanine is known as 'Metakelfin'.

Sulphadoxine also known as *sulphorthomidine* (Fanasil) is of particular importance as it is rapidly absorbed from the gastro-intestinal tract and has a remarkably long half-life of 150–200 hours in human plasma. Thus effective drug levels can be maintained by a single or once weekly oral administration. This compound is less effective against *P. vivax* than against *P. falciparum*. Single doses of 1.0–1.5 g are sufficient and overdosage should be avoided. The real value of sulphadoxine lies in the synergistic combination with antifolate compounds such as pyrimethamine. This combination at a ratio of 20:1 has gained a wide acceptance. The reason for it is a reciprocal potentiation between the two components due to a sequential action on two enzymes which are needed in the consecutive stages for the biosynthesis of folinic acid in malaria parasites.

The evaluation of the long-term effect of sulphones and sulphonamides is still incomplete. One of the potential problems is the possibility of producing sulphonamide resistant strains not only of malaria parasites but also of various bacteria including those responsible for cerebrospinal meningitis. The other problem is related to the possible though admittedly rare side effect on some individuals. For this reason these drugs should be reserved for conditions when *P. falciparum* are resistant to chloroquine. Long acting sulphonamides must not be given indiscriminately and only for short periods.

Repository antimalarial drugs

Some progress has been made in the developing of long-acting injectable prophylactic antimalarials. Repository preparations such as cycloguanil embonate[1] and an injectable derivative of diacetylsulphone[2] given at the single dose of 5 to 10 mg per kg of body weight has given considerable protection for several months against malaria infections with susceptible strains of plasmodia. Field trials have shown the advantages of this method and also some limitations, since 10–15% of persons given intramuscular injections of these drugs have local reaction at the site of the injection and occasionally sterile abscesses.

New antimalarials

Among several promising groups of new antimalarial compounds developed during the past decade in the USA (4-quinoline methanols,

---

Cycloguanil embonate is a derivative of the dihydrotriazine metabolite of proguanil. The proprietary name of this injectable drug is Camolar.
The diacetyl derivative of dapsone (acedapsone) for injection as a repository antimalarial is known under the name of Hansolar. The mixture of this drug and of Camolar has been used under the name of Dapolar. They are still undergoing clinical trials and are not available commercially.

9-phenanthrenemethanols, 2–4 diamino-quinazolines, and 2–4 diaminotriazines) the first group represents the most successful advance. One of the compounds of this group known under the code name WR 142490 has now received its generic name of mefloquine. Extended trials of this compound have confirmed its value for treatment of falciparum malaria resistant to other drugs. Although mefloquine is not yet available for general use its discovery is a good augury for future progress of chemotherapy of malaria. In fact two other compounds of this group may be even more active than the first. It appears that a short course of quinine followed by a single dose of 1.5 g of mefloquine is a very effective treatment of malaria due to *P. falciparum* resistant to 4-aminoquinolines.

Many antibiotic drugs have been tested for antimalarial activity. When aureomycin, chloromycetin, fumagillin and terramycin were used experimentally on malaria of birds or rodents some action was found but its practical importance was limited. More recently tetracycline and its derivatives, (doxycycline, lincomycin) alone or in combination with quinine were used on cases of human malaria and found to be of some promise. However, the present consensus of medical opinion is that these highly active antibiotics have several side-effects, especially on the kidneys and on the intestine; colitis has been frequently caused by lincomycin and clindamycin. Thus antibiotics should be used only in cases where their specific antibacterial action is needed.

PHARMACOLOGICAL CONSIDERATIONS OF MALARIA CHEMOTHERAPY

As a general rule, the action of a drug depends on the presence of an adequate concentration of the active compound in the fluids bathing the tissues and on the susceptibility of the cells to it. The concentration attained by the drug in contact with the cells on which it acts depends on absorption, distribution and clearance.

A drug may have to pass through a succession of cellular membranes to reach its site of action in the body. The gastro-intestinal tract, the tubules of the kidney, the sinusoids of the liver and the brain are surrounded by layers of cells controlling the uptake of substances into these organs. These membranes are essentially a double layer of oriented lipid molecules, between two polypeptide layers. Drugs and nutrients pass across these membranes by various transfer mechanisms, such as diffusion through the lipid phase, filtration through pores or active transfer by ionised carrier mechanism.

The absorption from the gastro-intestinal tract depends on the function of this organ, which can be influenced by such factors as fever. The rate of absorption from an injection varies in relation to the type of the drug, its solubility and physical characteristics of the preparation.

The distribution of the drug in the body is related not only to the type of the compound but also to specific functions of internal organs. Many drugs are bound to plasma proteins, particularly to the albumin fraction; this binding is reversible and there is a dynamic equilibrium between the bound and unbound form of the compound. The bound drug can be regarded as a storage depot since only the free form is active. This is of great practical importance in the use of some sulphonamides.

It is obvious that for the effective treatment of an acute attack of malaria one should aim at an adequate plasma concentration of the drug such as quinine or chloroquine, to affect the parasite in the red blood cells. However, the concentration of the drug in these cells need not be more than a fraction of the concentration in plasma.

Clearance of drugs from the body occurs in two ways; some are excreted unaltered but most of them are first metabolised and then excreted; however, some compounds are unaltered and fixed by specific tissues. While the liver is the most important organ concerned with the metabolism of drugs, the main organs of excretion are the kidneys. The biochemical changes which drugs undergo in the body may lead to pharmacological activation or inactivation. Inactivation can occur through processes of oxidation, reduction, and hydrolysis. The rate of inactivation has an important bearing on the duration of its effect. Drugs can be inactivated by conjugation reactions which are synthetic processes, involving adenosine triphosphate, glucuronic acid, acetylation etc. Drugs can also be transformed into active compounds; thus proguanil is oxidised to an active antiplasmodial substance. Many drugs are metabolised by enzymes located in the intracellular microsomes of liver cells. The rate of clearance of antimalarial drugs varies enormously; the range is from less than an hour to well over a week. However, most of the drugs are cleared in an exponential manner so that when a single dose of drug is given, the amount of it removed in a unit time is a constant fraction of the amount still present. This implies that in practice it is impossible to produce a prolonged action by giving a massive dose of a drug that is rapidly excreted. Prolonged action of such compounds can be obtained by delayed absorption or frequent dosages (e.g. quinine treatment of acute malaria). Cumulation results when the intake of a drug exceeds its clearance from the body. If a drug that is cleared in an exponential manner is given at regular intervals and if a constant fraction of the drug present in the body is cleared in the interval, then it is easy to calculate the extent to which the drug will cumulate. Certain therapeutic agents have exceptional powers of slowly cumulating in some tissues; this is the case of mepacrine, the concentration of which in the skin produces staining and may have an irritant effect on parts of the central nervous system.

The wide variations that occur in the fate of drugs in the human body indicate the reasons why the frequency of drug administration varies greatly. With most of the drugs that have important therapeutic action it is necessary to produce an effective concentration in the blood as quickly as possible and to maintain this concentration for an adequate time. This is achieved by the principle of an initial 'loading dose' followed by lower maintenance doses. Intravenous injection is often the only available method of rapid and intensive action; when a steady and more prolonged action is needed the intramuscular route provides a suitable method of administration, providing that the drug will be tolerated by the site of the injection. However, when it comes to a uniform concentration of the drug in the body fluids, the oral administration is still preferable even if influenced by the bio-availability of the effective compound related to its pharmaceutical formulation.

DOSAGE OF ANTIMALARIAL DRUGS

Usually all the doses of antimalarials quoted without special explanation are meant to be administered to adults of approximately 70 kg (154 lb) body-weight. Naturally, they should be adjusted, so that people of very light or very heavy build may be given up to 20–25% of the drug less or more, as the case might be.

In the past, the dosage of quinine was normally expressed in grains, one grain being equivalent to 65 mg. Thus 10 grains is equivalent to 650 mg. Nowadays, dosages of all drugs are given either in milligram (e.g. 100, 150, 1500 mg) or when it comes to amounts exceeding 1000 mg they may be expressed in grams with appropriate decimal fraction (e.g. 1.5 g).

Synthetic antimalarials are usually prepared as salts of basic compounds, but the dosage should always be expressed in terms of base e.g. tablets of chloroquine diphosphate 250 mg contain 150 mg of chloroquine base. The labels of available drug preparations refer normally to the content of base, but this should be checked to avoid confusion of dosage. In fact, the need to distinguish between the content of tablets in salt or in base applies only to chloroquine, amodiaquine and primaquine. Proguanil and pyrimethamine are prepared only as base and confusion is not likely. The dosage of quinine is always reckoned in terms of salt.

Dosage for children can be calculated according to Young's formula as follows:

$$\text{Child's dose} = \text{Adult dose} \times \frac{\text{Age of child (in years)}}{\text{Age of child} + 12}$$

Chemotherapy and Chemoprophylaxis

Another rough and ready reckoning of dosages for children is based on the following table:

Age of child	Fraction of adult dose	
Infants up to 2 years	⅛ – ¼	Allowance should be made for size and weight of child so that a heavier child may receive the upper limit of the relevant range
Children 2–6 years	¼ – ½	
Children 6–12 years	½ – ¾	
Over 12 years	¾ – 1	

NOMENCLATURE OF ANTIMALARIAL DRUGS

Most antimalarial drugs are known under a variety of names and this is responsible for much confusion. During their experimental development by research laboratories the tested compounds are known under a code number. If considered suitable for general use they are then put on the market under a manufacturer's trade name which takes the place of the code number. Under certain conditions, which amount to an official approval of value (not necessarily a greater value than others), they are admitted to the official pharmacopoeias such as the British, French, the US and the International Pharmacopoeias. Since the name under which they are already known is a trade name, viz. the property of one manufacturer, they are then given a non-proprietary name which anyone can use and it becomes the permanently accepted name in the country recognising the pharmacopoeia concerned.

However, in addition to various proprietary or trade names the same drug may be known in different countries under different non-proprietary names. As an example, the drug commonly known as paludrine was originally known under the code number *M 4888*; it was then issued to the public under the trade name *Paludrine*, which is the property of Imperial Chemical Industries; it is entered in the British Pharmacopoeia under the name *proguanil* which anyone can use. This is now the correct generic name of this substance within the United Kingdom and those other countries which recognise the British Pharmacopoeia, and should be used to describe it.

However, in the USA the non-proprietary name of proguanil is *chlorguanide*, and in the USSR, *bigumal*. There are at least a dozen different trade names of this compound. The use of trade names should be avoided unless products of specific manufacturing firms are intended; when it is necessary to use them they are normally written with an initial capital letter (e.g. Paludrine). In the USA the protected status of such names is indicated by an addition of a sign ® indicating that this is a trademark. Non-proprietary names are spelled with a small letter (e.g. proguanil). The World Health Organization keeps an up to date list of international non-proprietary names of compounds on which there is an international agreement.

Table 13a

(1) Antimalarial drugs in common use

Non-proprietary name	Formulation	Some proprietary names	Dose for prevention (adult)	Dose for treatment (adult)	Remarks with regard to usage
Quinine (dihydrochloride or sulphate)	Tablets at 650 mg (10 grains)	No proprietary names (excepting certain formulations)	Not used	2–3 tablets daily for 10–14 days	Mainly when malaria parasites are resistant to chloroquine and amodiaquine. In severe cases the drug to be given by injection and additional drugs and other measures are needed.
Quinine (dihydrochloride or sulphate)	Solution for i.v. injection 60 mg per ml	—	—	650 mg repeated 2 or 3 times (max) in 24 hrs.	*Very slow* i.v. injection preferably as i.v. drip. Oral medication as soon as possible.
Chloroquine (phosphate or sulphate)	Tablets at 100 mg 150 mg and 300 mg of *base*	Aralen Avloclor Resochin, Nivaquine and other names	300 mg or 600 mg-over the week	600 mg at once, followed 6 hours later by 300 mg. Then 300 mg daily for the next 2–4 days.	*For prevention*: Either 1 tablet (100 mg) every day (French pattern) or 1 tablet (150 mg) twice a week or 2 tablets (300 mg) once a week.
Chloroquine (phosphate or sulphate)	Solution for i.m. or i.v. injection, 5% equivqalent to 40 mg base per ml	As above	—	200–300 mg i.m. repeated in 6 hours if necessary. Or i.v. drip 300–400 mg in 500 ml saline	Intramuscular or intravenous injections may be dangerous in small children. If necessary, to be given in divided small doses. Correct dosage related to the weight of child important.

Drug	Formulation	Trade names	Dose	Notes
Amodiaquine (hydrochloride or base)	Tablets at 200 mg or 150 mg of base	Camoquine Flavoquine Basoquine, etc.	400–600 mg over the week	*For prevention*: usually 2 tablets (300 or 400 mg) once a week, but also 1 tablet (150–200 mg) twice a week. No parenteral formulation of amodiaquine, but injection of amopyroquine is an alternative.
Primaquine (diphosphate)	Tablets at 5 mg and 7.5 mg of base	Neo-Quipenyl, etc.	Not used	Only as antirelapse treatment: 3 (at 5 mg) or 2 (at 7.5 mg) tablets daily for 14 days	Following the usual treatment by quinine, amodiaquine or chloroquine. The dosage not be exceeded and preferably under medical supervision, especially in dark-skinned subjects.
Proguanil (hydrochloride)	Tablets at 100 mg	Paludrine, Chlorguanid Bigumal etc.	1–2 tablets daily	Not used	In some areas parasites are resistant to this drug and cross-resistant to pyrimethamine.
Chlorproguanil	Tablets at 20 mg	Lapudrine	1 tablet once a week	Not used	As above.
Pyrimethamine	Tablets at 25 mg	Daraprim Malocide, etc.	1 tablet once a week	Only when combined with other drugs	In some areas parasites are resistant to this drug and cross-resistant to proguanil.
Cycloguanil emboate	Oily suspension 140 mg per ml	Camolar	2–2.5 ml deep intramuscular injection	Not used	Protection for about 3 months. May give rise to local reaction. Detailed recommendations for the technique of injection must be followed. Possible breakthrough in areas with resistance to proguanil and pyrimethamine.

Note: The adult doses quoted in this table refer to persons 70 kg (154 lb) body weight. These doses should be adjusted to the usual rules for weight and age of children.

i.v. – intravenous; i.m. – intramuscular.

Table 13b

(2) Combinations of antimalarial compounds

Non-proprietary name	Formulation	Some proprietary names	Dose for prevention (adult)	Dose for treatment (adult)	Remarks
Pyrimethamine and chloroquine sulphate	25 mg + 150 mg (base)	Daraclor	1 or 2 tablets once a week. Children under 6 years of age ½ the tablet	4 tablets the first day, 2 tablets on each of the next 2 days	Mainly for single-dose treatment (presumptive treatment) of cases suspected of malaria infection prior to confirmation of the diagnosis. Used in malaria eradication programmes.
Amodiaquine and Primaquine	150 mg (base) + 15 mg (base)	Camoprim	2 tablets once a week for limited periods	2 tablets the first day, 1 tablet on the next 2 days, then 2 tablets once a week for 4–6 weeks	Mainly for limited mass drug administration programmes. To be used with caution in dark-skinned individuals. Also available as Camoprim Infatab at half the dosage of amodiaquine. For limited paediatric use.
Pyrimethamine and Dapsone	12.5 mg + 100 mg	Maloprim	One tablet once a week	Not generally used	To be used for individual protection. Not for children or pregnant women. May be used in areas with resistance of *P. falciparum* to other drugs.
Chloroquine and Chlorproguanil	150 mg + 20 mg	Lapaquin	One tablet a week	Not normally used	Mainly for individual prevention of malaria but occasionally used for limited mass drug administration.

Pyrimethamine and Sulphadoxine	Tablets at 25 mg + 500 mg Ampoules for i.m. injection 20 mg + 400 mg.	Fansidar	Limited use 2 tablets every 2 weeks or preferably 1 tablet every week	2–3 tablets as a single dose. Also available in ampoules	For treatment of falciparum malaria resistant to chloroquine and other drugs. When used for prevention, the duration of its use to be limited to a few months. In pregnancy under medical supervision and much caution advised.
Sulphalene and Trimethoprim	750 mg + 500 mg	Metakelfin	As above	2–3 tablets as a single dose	As above

Naturally, all non-proprietary compounds have also their own chemical names which indicate their fundamental chemical structure. While each different compound has a different and usually very complicated chemical name there are series of drugs of similar general structure and these 'generic' compounds are often given under the name of their chemical group. Thus for instance chloroquine and amodiaquine belong to the group of 4-aminoquinolines, while primaquine is a drug of the 8-aminoquinoline series.

A list of common antimalarial compounds together with their usual formulations and other characteristics is shown in Table 13a and b.

TREATMENT OF ACUTE MALARIA

The initial treatment of acute malaria is the same irrespective of the species of the parasite, except for some special circumstances such as severe infection with falciparum malaria in children or non-immune subjects. It is in the additional 'follow-up' therapy that the chemotherapy of relapsing malaria is different.

For acute malaria the most active drugs are chloroquine and amodiaquine; quinine is still of value in some circumstances, such as resistance of parasites to other drugs, and for parenteral administration in very severe infections. The generally advocated oral treatment of moderately severe malaria in adults of average weight (70 kg) is as follows:

	Chloroquine	**Amodiaquine**	**Quinine**
Day 1 followed six hours later by:	600 mg 300 mg	600 mg —	650 mg 650 mg and eight hours later again the same dose
Day 2	300 mg	400 mg	650 mg three times a day
Day 3	300 mg	400 mg	650 mg twice a day
Day 4	300 mg (if necessary)	400 mg (if necessary)	650 mg twice a day
Days 5 to 7	300 mg (if necessary)	400 mg (if necessary)	650 mg twice a day
Total dose	1500 to 1800 mg of chloroquine base (more if indicated)	1400 to 1800 mg of amodiaquine base (more if indicated)	10 500 to 14 300 mg over 7–10 days

Freedom from recrudescences of falciparum infection can be assured by a 'follow-up' treatment of 300 mg of chloroquine or amodiaquine, taken once week for one month.

Relapsing malaria. A radical cure for relapsing malaria (such as due to *P. vivax*) can be obtained when the usual treatment by chloroquine or amodiaquine is followed by administration of primaquine at the adult dosage of 15 mg of base every day for 14 days, or 30–45 mg once a week for 8 weeks. Daily treatment may occasionally produce cyanosis, abdominal pain and other symptoms in some individuals. This explains why a degree of medical supervision is necessary when primaquine treatment is given.

All these drugs are very bitter and must be given with a generous drink of milk, fruit juice or other flavoured fluid. Care must be taken to make certain that the patient swallows the tablets and does not later vomit. Proper nursing and relief of general symptoms are important in the treatment of malaria. Some variation of the dosage of antimalarials is needed according to the weight of the patients and their condition.

Treatment of severe falciparum malaria. Treatment of patients with complications of *P. falciparum* malaria such as involvement of the central nervous system, anaemia, very high fever, dehydration, cardiovascular, gastro-intestinal, renal and liver symptoms, etc., must be instituted rapidly.

In such cases antimalarial drugs should be administered by intramuscular or intravenous injection.

Quinine and chloroquine are the best drugs for this purpose. Intravenous injection acts somewhat more rapidly than intramuscular injection but presents a relatively greater risk in some patients. For intravenous injection both quinine and chloroquine are almost equally acceptable. The first acts rather more quickly but (unless given very slowly) may cause a rapid fall in blood pressure and cardiac arrhythmia or other symptoms. For this and other reasons, treatment of severe malaria requires strict medical supervision.

Intravenous quinine or chloroquine must be given with caution and in high dilution. Quinine dihydrochloride solution may be given at the adult dose of 500 to 650 mg (8 to 10 mg per kg of body weight) diluted in 20 ml of isotonic saline with 5% glucose or in plasma. It should be injected very slowly (at least 20 minutes), or preferably, given as a slow (2–4 hours) intravenous drip in 500 ml of plasma or isotonic saline with glucose. This may be repeated, if necessary, after 6 to 8 hours. The dose of 2000 mg over 24 hours should not be exceeded.

Intravenous injections of chloroquine diphosphate or other salts of this compound can be given at a single dose of 200 mg base (4 ml of 5% solution) with the same precautions as with quinine. Higher doses, but not exceeding 400 mg of base, may be given, but it is preferable to give such a dose by i.v. drip in 500 ml of dextrose saline or plasma over a period of not less than 1–2 hours. This can be repeated, if necessary, after eight hours but the dose of 800 mg of chloroquine base over 24 hours should not be exceeded.

As with many other drugs, faulty technique of intravenous injection of concentrated quinine or chloroquine solutions may produce a local necrosis of surrounding tissues; this risk is greater with quinine than with chloroquine.

Intravenous injections of any antimalarial drugs in children below seven years of age may be dangerous and should be avoided if possible. Intramuscular injections should be given only when really necessary viz. in severe infections requiring rapid treatment, and the dosage of the drug must be based on the weight of the child. It is safer to give the drug in divided doses separated by an interval of 1–2 hours. Oral treatment of all cases of malaria in children should be preferred whenever possible. Should there be any suspicion that the patient was infected in an area where chloroquine resistant *P. falciparum* is present, quinine should be employed for emergency treatment.

Naturally, in addition to specific treatment by antimalarials supporting treatment is of equal importance. Severe anaemia calls for blood transfusion. An hourly temperature, pulse, respiratory rate and blood pressure chart should be kept since hyperpyrexia, cardiovascular collapse and respiratory depression can occur. Hyperpyrexia is treated in the same way as a heat stroke by sponging the body with water and aiding evaporation under a fan. When the temperature reaches 38°C the cooling of the patient must be stopped. Chlorpromazine (25–50 mg) may be given by injection to promote peripheral vasodilatation.

Blood urea and electrolyte estimation should be monitored, to give an idea of renal impairment or other disturbances. If sterile condition can be assured an indwelling catheter should be passed for collection and examination of urine. The volume of urine and vomit should be measured to assess the degree of hydration of the patient. When renal failure occurs haemodialysis or, failing this, peritoneal dialysis may have to be undertaken. The development of acute pulmonary oedema calls for the administration of oxygen. When any of these conditions, and especially cerebral oedema or sudden intravascular haemolysis occur then large doses of corticosteroids (such as dexamethasone or prednisolone phosphate 40–60 mg or more) by intramuscular injection, may be beneficial. Diazepam (Valium) at 5–10 mg or chlorpromazine (25–50 mg) is useful to sedate the patient if convulsions are present. Signs of shock with cardiovascular collapse require parenteral fluids. Heparin has been advocated to prevent intravascular sludging but the value of this treatment is doubtful. In every case the best possible nursing services should be provided.

DRUG RESISTANCE

It is not surprising that the malaria parasite, in response to an increasing use of antimalarial drugs, has found its defence in the development of resistance. It had been already observed that there were considerable variations in the susceptibility of some parasites to quinine, but these proved to be no more than normal differences displayed by various species or strains of plasmodia. The term *resistance* means the ability of a strain of a parasite to survive and to multiply in spite of the administration of an active drug given in usual or higher than usual doses.

The observation of resistance to proguanil and pyrimethamine some 20 years ago was of limited importance since these drugs are not normally used for treatment of acute malaria. Whenever there is sufficient evidence that these two drugs fail to give the protective viz. prophylactic effect, chloroquine or amodiaquine can be used. However, the reports on resistance of *P. falciparum* parasites to 4-aminoquinolines (chloroquine and amodiaquine), first observed in 1960–61 in Colombia and in Brazil, were of greater consequence since together with quinine these are the most valuable drugs for treatment of acute malaria. Further reports on drug resistance came from Thailand, Malaysia, Cambodia, Philippines, Indonesia, Viet-Nam, Laos, Burma and other areas of south-east Asia. In each of these countries the actual foci of resistance may not cover the whole area, parasites in many localities being still normally susceptible to the drug. The occurrence of resistance even in small areas, is, nevertheless, disturbing because occasionally it has been found that cross-resistance extended to all the other known synthetic antimalarial drugs and in exceptional conditions apparently also to quinine. If this resistance were to become common it would result in a dramatic depletion of our range of drugs for prevention and treatment of malaria.

In practice, drug resistance is suspected when acute cases of malaria (*P. falciparum*) do not fully and rapidly respond to proper treatment with drugs or when recrudescence of symptoms and parasites in the blood is seen soon after their temporary disappearance after such treatment. Recrudescence of the infection may be due to a number of causes. One should remember, however, that there are strains of plasmodia that require somewhat larger doses of certain drugs to be given over a longer period. Moreover, there may be differences between individual patients in the way they absorb and utilise drugs.

Wherever resistance of *P. falciparum* to chloroquine is confirmed alternative drugs such as quinine, sulphonamides with antifolic compounds and mefloquine are used for treatment of individual patients. The question of the best prophylactic here is difficult to answer at present. Proguanil or pyrimethamine give a good protection but cannot be relied on if resistance to these drugs occurs. It is likely that in such a situation a sulphone or sulphonamide with pyrimethamine may be indicated for individual protection for a limited time of 6 months to a year. The value of other drugs is being assessed. Fortunately there is no evidence of any widespread resistance to chloroquine on the continent of Africa although recently a few cases were apparently seen in the eastern part of that continent. Thus at the present time there is no justification for shunning the use of chloroquine and amodiaquine in Africa. It has become 'fashionable' to employ sulphonamide compounds for treatment of malaria in Africa and to regard chloroquine as an obsolete drug. This trend should be deplored as it undermines confidence in the value of 4-aminoquinolines which are still our most dependable and least toxic antimalarial compounds.

How malaria parasites become resistant to chloroquine is still not fully known. Two explanations have been proposed: one suggests that such parasites are deficient in chloroquine binding sites which normally concentrate the drug in the blood. The other hypothesis is that such resistant plasmodia have different biochemical pathways of amino-acid synthesis. There is a distant but not confirmed possibility that the widespread use of chloroquine as a suppressant may be partly responsible for the emergence of resistance to the drug in some parts of the world. It is therefore suggested that wherever there is no resistance of malaria parasites to pyrimethamine and proguanil, one of these two drugs should be used preferentially for prophylaxis of malaria in individuals and in small groups of people.

Any reports of apparent resistance of malaria parasites to chloroquine should be based on a careful investigation of each case to exclude the possibility that the drug has not been taken by the patient or that it has been vomited. Attention must be paid to the quality of the drug, and the dose should be adjusted to the weight of the patient. Accuracy of the blood examination following the administration of the drug is essential.

Criteria for recognition of suspected resistance of malaria parasites to 4-aminoquinolines have been proposed and a standard procedure for determining the response of malaria parasites to chloroquine in the field has been recommended by the WHO (Fig. 51).

Previous methods of assessing the sensitivity of *P. falciparum* to chloroquine and other drugs were based on observing changes in the level of parasitaemia after a standard treatment of infected individuals. Major advance in this method took place a few years ago, when infections with human malaria parasites were successfully established

Chemotherapy and Chemoprophylaxis

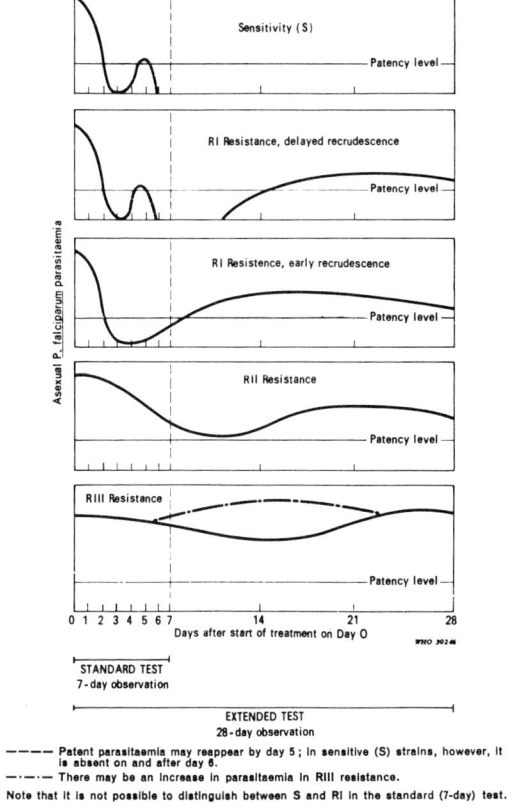

Fig 51 WHO field test for response of malaria parasites to chloroquine. Diagram shows degrees of response ranging from sensitivity to high resistance. Chloroquine administered by mouth at the dose of 25mg/kg. (WHO, 1973)

and maintained in the owl-monkey (*Aotus trivirgatus*). Since then another method was proposed because of the acute shortage of Aotus monkeys and also because it offers greater possibility of standardisation. The method, introduced by Rieckmann, consists of cultivating a sample of the infected blood *in vitro* and observing the effect of the tested drugs on the development of asexual parasites. The simplest and most widely used technique involves the mixing of blood containing parasites of *P. falciparum* with nanogram or microgram quantities of the tested drug, in flat bottomed screw-capped glass vials, in the presence of a glucose solution. The contents of the vials with known amounts of the drug and adequate controls are incubated for 24 hours; after that the contents are diluted with plasma, thick films are made and stained in the usual way. The extent to which the normal maturation of trophozoites to schizonts is inhibited by the drug indicates the degree of drug resistance.

This new method presents considerable advantages; its results assessed in the field correspond to the results obtained on Aotus monkeys or evaluated in human cases. In some conditions this method may be the only means of determining the drug resistance of malaria parasites.

Lately Rieckmann's method was improved still further by introducing a technique which is based on collection of capillary blood samples from a fingerprick, for titration on standard microplates. This enhances the value of the method for wider field use. Final confirmation of drug resistance can be obtained from the study of malaria infections on human volunteers in a special reference centre.

Should the drugs of the 4-aminoquinoline group given at the adequate dosage fail to produce the desired therapeutic effect, quinine is still one of the most reliable alternative drugs. However, there is evidence that the administration of sulphones or sulphonamides combined with antifolates is justified when the condition of the patient does not respond to chloroquine (or other 4-aminoquinolines) and one of the following drug combinations has been proposed.

(1) Sulphadoxine (Fanasil)   1000–1500 mg   To be given
     Pyrimethamine   50–75 mg   as a single dose (2–3 tablets)

(This drug combination is available under the trade name of Fansidar in tablets containing 500 mg of sulphadoxine and 25 mg of pyrimethamine. An injectable preparation is also available containing 400 mg and 20 mg of respective compounds in a 2 ml ampoule. Some authors advocate 1–2 injections of quinine followed by oral Fansidar.)

(2) Sulphalene (sulphamethoxypyrazine)   1000 mg   Single dose
     Pyrimethamine   50 mg
(3) Sulphalene (sulphamethoxypyrazine)   750 mg   Single dose
     Trimethoprim   500 mg
(4) Following a standard quinine treatment an additional administration of:
     Pyrimethamine   50 mg daily for 2–3 days and
     Dapsone (diamino diphenyl sulphone)   25 mg daily for 3–4 weeks

It should be stressed that the last of the proposed types of treatment is still not generally used and no firm recommendations on its value can be given at present.

Wherever Fansidar or other similar proprietary drug combinations are not available, various other therapeutic drug regimens for treatment of chloroquine-resistant *P. falciparum* malaria have been recently proposed. Most of them start with the administration of quinine (650 mg three times daily for 3 days) together with sulphadiazine (2 g daily for five days) and pyrimethamine (50 mg daily for 3 days) or as an alternative to the last two drugs, the proprietary combinations of sulpha-methoxazole with trimethoprim or pyrimethamine. The value of these treatments has not been assessed and caution is advocated before adopting them.

Lately, cases of resistance of *P. falciparum* to the combination of sulphonamides with pyrimethamine have been reported from Indonesia.

Finally, although mefloquine is not yet generally available, its therapeutic dosage is 15 mg per kg of body weight as a single oral administration, preceded or not by quinine injection.

TOXIC EFFECTS OF ANTIMALARIAL DRUGS

Side-effects of conventional antimalarial drugs taken by mouth are few provided that their dosage is appropriate to the weight and the condition of the subject. *Proguanil* and *pyrimethamine* are usually better tolerated than any other drugs. However, many cases of accidental fatal poisoning of children have occurred after they had swallowed as few as 5–10 tasteless pyrimethamine tablets. Thus this drug must not be left on the table or anywhere within the reach of children. A new method of packaging the tablets in plastic strips prevents these tragic accidents. Large doses of this compound given over a long time may have a depressive effect on the bone marrow and should not be given to pregnant women.

Mepacrine taken over a long period produces a yellow discoloration of the skin, dark patches under the nails and on mucous membranes and occasionally various skin lesions; given in large doses it may be responsible for transient mental disturbances or for more serious effects in children.

Quinine may cause buzzing in the ears, tremor and ocular symptoms; injections of quinine can produce a sudden and dangerous fall of blood pressure unless administered very slowly. *Chloroquine* and *amodiaquine* given on an empty stomach may cause abdominal discomfort and vomiting; the practical importance of such mild side-effects must not be under-estimated as they could adversely influence the acceptance of this drug in mass drug administration. While there is no evidence that the taking of the usual prophylactic dose of chloroquine produces any adverse effect, high doses given daily for 5–10 years may affect the eye. Chloroquine when used for the treatment of rheumatoid arthritis and some other conditions is given in very large daily doses over a prolonged period and in a number of cases retinopathies have been described. On the other hand there is no evidence that chloroquine (or amodiaquine) given at the usual weekly dose of 300–400 mg for up to 3–4 year of continuous chemoprophylaxis has a deleterious effect on the eye.

Table 14
Protective value of antimalarials

Drug	Action	Side-effects	Acquired drug resistance by parasites	Remarks
Quinine	Fair suppressive	Very rare	Absent	Daily regimen in non-immunes. Association with blackwater fever. Bitter taste, unless coated tablets.
Mepacrine	Good suppressive	Frequent	No evidence	Daily regimen in non-immunes. Not recommended for children. Bitter taste. Toxic effects. Staining of skin. Obsolete drug.
Chloroquine	Very good suppressive. Suppressive cure of *P. falciparum*	Rare	May appear though limited to some areas	Twice weekly or once weekly regimen in non-immunes. Bitter taste.
Amodiaquine	As chloroquine	Rare	As chloroquine	Once weekly regimen in non-immunes, otherwise like chloroquine. Basoquine – no bitter taste.
Proguanil	Good suppressive. Causal prophylactic of *P. falciparum*	Very rare	May appear	Daily regimen in non-immunes. Wide margin of safety. Slightly bitter taste.
Pyrimethamine	Good suppressive. Causal prophylactic of *P. falciparum* and occasionally *P. vivax*	Very rare at standard doses	May appear	Once weekly regimen in non-immunes. No bitter taste. Attention: accidental poisoning of children.
Pyrimethamine with dapsone	Good suppressive	Rare at standard doses	May appear	Once weekly regimen in non-immunes. Not for pregnant women and infants. Caution in G6PD deficiency.
Pyrimethamine with sulphadoxine or with sulphalene	Good suppressive	Rare at standard doses	May appear though infrequent	Once weekly or once a fortnight (for non-immunes). Once monthly (for immunes). Not for pregnant women and infants. To be used for a limited time only.

Attention has already been drawn to the danger of intramuscular injection of chloroquine (and mepacrine) particularly in small children. The dosage of these drugs in children must be adjusted to their weight and general condition; when an appropriate and relatively large dose of these drugs must be given, it is preferable to divide it into two or three smaller ones adequately spaced. *Primaquine* and other *8-aminoquinolines* may cause abdominal pain, nausea, vomiting, cyanosis and other symptoms, especially in some dark-skinned people. Slight cyanosis may be tolerated but serious and even fatal haemolytic effects on the blood and bone-marrow may occur in individuals with sensitivity to this group of compounds.

Although sulphones and sulphonamides may induce haemolysis in some persons with inherited blood enzyme deficiencies it appears that both in normal persons and in otherwise healthy carriers of G6PD deficiency, administration of standard doses of these drugs such as those found effective for treatment or suppression of infections with chloroquine-resistant *Plasmodium falciparum* does not often produce marked haemolysis; if it does, such symptoms disappear when the drug is withdrawn. The combination of long-acting sulphonamides with pyrimethamine is not recommended for treatment or prophylaxis of women during pregnancy and is contraindicated for infants. In other persons it is preferable to limit the use of these drugs as suppressives to 6–9 months. Overdosage of these drugs is dangerous.

INDIVIDUAL DRUG PROTECTION

Any individual wishing to visit or to live in a malarious country without the risk of sickness due to malaria may be protected by taking drugs that will either prevent the infection from becoming established or that will suppress the clinical symptoms of the disease. The first type of action is called *causal prophylaxis*, the second goes by the name of *suppression*. However, the distinction between the two terms is not rigid in practice, as suppression may be so complete that it leads to successful elimination of the parasite; thus, as far as the protected person is concerned, it may be tantamount to true prophylaxis. Thus the term 'prophylaxis', 'prophylactic drugs' is often used in the general sense to embrace the protective action of any antimalarial compound. Causal prophylaxis may be easily attained in falciparum malaria since the parasite has only the primary tissue phase and does not produce relapses. Other malaria parasites have the secondary tissue phase, responsible for long term relapses, and causal prophylaxis is more difficult to achieve.

Proguanil and pyrimethamine are essentially prophylactic drugs which eliminate malaria infection at its source in the liver cells by acting on

Table 15

Dosage of antimalarials for individual protection

Drug	Frequency	Infants	1–3yr	4–6yr	7–10yr	11–16yr	Adults
Proguanil[1]	Daily	25	50	50	75	100	100–200
Pyrimethamine	Once weekly (on Sundays)	–	6	12	18	25	25
Chloroquine (base)[2]	Once weekly*	35	75	100	150	225	300
Amodiaquine (base)	Once weekly[1]	50	100	100	200	300	300–400
Pyrimethamine and dapsone (Maloprim)	Once weekly	Not recommended	Not recommended	¼ tablet	½ tablet	As adults	12.5 mg + 100 mg. 1 Tablet
Sulphadoxine and pyrimethamine (Fansidar)[3]	Once weekly or once every two weeks	Not recommended	Not recommended	½ tablet 1 tablet	¾ tablet 1½ tablets	As adults As adults	500 mg + 25 mg. 1 tablet (weekly)

*2 tablets once a week or 1 tablet twice a week

Notes: [1] In some parts of the world where malaria is intense the dosage of proguanil may be doubled (viz. 2 tablets = 200 mg daily) for limited periods.
[2] In French-speaking parts of tropical Africa the usual regimen of chloroquine prophylaxis for adults is 100 mg either daily or for 6 days a week.
[3] For limited periods only in areas where plasmodial resistance to conventional drugs has been confirmed.

the pre-erythrocytic forms of parasite which evolve from the sporozoites inoculated by the mosquito. These two drugs are safe and highly effective, especially against *P. falciparum*, failing only with strains resistant to these compounds. They are less effective against *P. vivax*; primaquine is more effective against this species of malaria parasite, but is rarely used for this purpose because of its toxic effects (Table 14).

All therapeutic (e.g. schizontocidal) drugs are good suppressive drugs as they eliminate the parasites present in the red blood cells or keep the number of plasmodia at a very low level. Drugs such as chloroquine suppress the symptoms of the disease when the administration of small doses of these compounds is regular and prolonged. When taken for a prolonged period they are likely to cure falciparum malaria (*suppressive cure*) but they do not necessarily eliminate the vivax infection, for which anti-relapse drugs (primaquine) must be given.

Quinine is now not used for suppression as its long-term administration may cause blackwater fever. Chloroquine and amodiaquine are powerful suppressants and relatively non-toxic. Various combinations of dapsone or sulphonamides with pyrimethamine are being promoted or tested in the field; it appears that they are of value in areas where resistance to other drugs is confirmed. The use of prophylactic or suppressive drugs may fail in parts of the world where resistance to one or another group of compounds exists. It is necessary to check by local inquiry that the drug used is effective in that area. The highest transmission rates of *P. falciparum* are today in Tropical Africa where the malaria parasites are still sensitive to 4-aminoquinolines.

Visitors or short time residents in malarious areas should start their drug prophylaxis either on arrival or preferably a few days before departure simply to get used to the new habit. On their return from the tropics it is most important that the taking of antimalarials should continue at least for one month to eliminate the parasites that may remain in small numbers in the internal organs and may cause recrudescence of the infection.

The state of immunity affects the use of drugs: anyone who by prolonged exposure to the disease acquired partial immunity can be protected or cured by smaller doses of drugs than those given to non-immunes. However, persons born and raised in endemic tropical areas, who have resided for several years in non-malarious countries may have lost some of their acquired immunity. On their return to the tropics they should be protected for about a year by the same dosage of drugs as applied to non-immunes.

The dosage of drugs for general protection is given in Table 15. Taking protective antimalarial drugs every day (e.g. proguanil) presents an advantage because of the development of a regular habit (e.g. at breakfast) and thus gives a wider margin of safety.

COLLECTIVE DRUG PROTECTION

The application of collective drug protection is justified only when more permanent methods are either disappointing or impracticable. Nevertheless general protection of groups of people residing in malarious areas and of populations living there permanently can be achieved temporarily by collective chemotherapeutic measures.

This method has been used with success in army units, organised labour forces or similar communities. The rapid excretion of all existing drugs means that they must be administered frequently and regularly to every man, woman and child. This obviously poses formidable problems of organisation, distribution and above all, persuasion. Mass-chemotherapy for malaria protection can be of use in exceptional circumstances and in relatively small numbers.

Nevertheless it should be remembered that this is the quickest method of bringing a malaria epidemic under temporary control. Drugs may also be used in the initial phases of the eradication campaign if the action of insecticides proves too slow or where conditions interfere with their full application.

Collective drug protection brings into play not only the protection of each individual but also the gradual reduction of the infective seed-bed with the decrease of the transmission in the mosquito.

Prevention of infection by the elimination of parasites from the organism before they start multiplying in the blood is possible with proguanil given at an adult dose of not less than 100 mg daily, or with pyrimethamine at not less than 25 mg once a week. These two drugs are safe and efficient prophylactics of *P. falciparum* unless the relevant strains of this species have become resistant to either drug or both drugs. They are less effective for prophylaxis of *P. vivax*.

Given to indigenous inhabitants of malarious areas, usually infected from their early childhood, these drugs have a slow and incomplete effect on the infection even if they may initially prevent its spread by their action on gametocytes developing in the mosquito. However, both drugs have a tendency to produce resistant strains and it is likely that after some time their effect will greatly decrease and that the transmission of the infection will be resumed. As a short term measure for temporary protection these drugs and especially pyrimethamine may be given to small semi-immune groups providing that there is a regular assessment of the degree of protection thus provided. Any cases of malaria occurring in individuals covered by this measure must be treated by 4-aminoquinolines. Resistance is much less likely with regard to chloroquine and amodiaquine which are excellent suppressants and will achieve a radical cure of infections caused by *P. falciparum* susceptible to these drugs.

Chemotherapy and Chemoprophylaxis

The following points should be considered whenever any collective drug distribution is undertaken.

1. Value of such a method as a public health measure.
2. Indication for limitation of such a method of malaria control to a specific group of the population.
3. Possibility of undesirable long-term effects on the community.
4. Selection of appropriate drug and dosage.
5. Method of distribution, its timing, regularity, frequency, means of supervision.

1. The question whether a collective drug distribution is of immediate benefit to the indigenous population living in a malarious area can be answered in the positive. It has been shown in Africa that regular drug distribution decreases the total amount of sickness due to all causes, that it somewhat reduces absenteeism in schools and that in other groups it may be followed by a modest but definite gain of weight and increase of haemoglobin levels.
2. It is not less obvious that wherever any collective drug distribution is proposed, this must be adapted to the epidemiological conditions of the area. In areas with moderate endemicity and seasonal transmission it is conceivable that all the groups of the population would benefit from drug distribution (adjusted to the start of the transmission period) while in highly endemic areas the near-perennial protection of young, more vulnerable age groups is preferable.
3. The possible undesirable long-term effects of a distribution of an antimalarial drug should be considered from two angles: toxic action of the drug and possible interference in highly endemic areas with the acquired tolerance of the infection. As far as the first point is concerned, it seems that with the exception of mepacrine, and some 8-aminoquinolines, harmful effects of most of the well-known drugs are very few, particularly when assessed in the light of the benefits that the drugs confer. When it comes to the possible interference of regular drug distribution with the degree of acquired immunity to malaria, it must be confessed that definite information on this point is lacking, probably because in all field trials the absolute regularity of drug distribution has never been achieved and any reinfection, even of short duration, has been sufficient to maintain a degree of immunity. Recent studies in Nigeria compared two groups of children, one protected and the other unprotected from malaria transmission. The results followed by serological tests showed that the antibody levels were only slightly lower in the protected children.
4. With regard to the selection of an appropriate drug for collective protection, the general principles outlined previously are important. A good schizontocide, if given at an adequate dosage, acts on all the four

species of human plasmodia in their asexual stage of the erythrocytic cycle and has slow general effect by attrition on the gametocyte reservoir. For this purpose, the 4-aminoquinolines are unsurpassed and there is little to choose between amodiaquine and chloroquine.

Proguanil and pyrimethamine have a causal prophylactic effect and also a direct sporontocidal action on the gametocyte reservoir. Their large-scale use is not justified in conditions of continuous and high level transmission because of the probability of the selection of resistant strains in a population already infected. Their use in small well supervised groups alone or in combined form with a 4-aminoquinoline is much less open to objections although some observations on the resistance to pyrimethamine developing even when the drug is given together with chloroquine cannot be dismissed.

5. The frequency of administration is related not only to the dosage of the drug but also to the convenience of its distribution. Generally once weekly administrations of chloroquine or amodiaquine are most appropriate to assure regularity, though fortnightly distribution may be adequate. The frequency of drug administration depends on many local conditions and a reasonably strict observance of weekly or fortnightly routines is not too difficult. In schools this regimen is certainly the most suitable to minimise the effect of one or two defaults in the weekly drug distribution. It is obvious that in areas of high endemicity the risk of reinfection is the greater when the treatments are more widely spread. Interruptions of this drug distribution in schools due to holidays are unavoidable.

6. When it comes to the method of distribution there is little doubt that two groups of the population must be given the highest priority: (a) pregnant and nursing women and (b) infants and children. The distribution of drugs to these two groups is not difficult through the normal health services and schools but there will always be a proportion of women and children missed since the total drug coverage is almost impossible to achieve in rural areas.

It is obvious that the drug protection from malaria should be the responsibility of the national health services and that the cost must be met mainly by the government, though various forms of overseas aid may provide a substantial assistance to the organisation and expenditure involved.

Table 16 shows the dosage of the main drugs that could be given for collective drug protection in relatively small groups with little immunity or in semi-immune communities living in an endemic area.

For the control of epidemic malaria in rural communities these doses may be inadequate and a double dosage of fully active schizontocidal drugs (chloroquine or amodiaquine) is recommended.

At the appropriate dosage none of these drugs taken for general protection has any serious side-effects.

Table 16

Dosage of drugs for collective protection

Drug	Groups with little immunity (adult dosage)	Semi-immune communities in endemic malarious areas (adult dosage)	
Proguanil	100–200 mg daily	300 mg once a week	With the proviso of regular assessment of effect
Pyrimethamine	25–50 mg once a week	25 mg once a week	
Chloroquine	300–600 mg base once a week	150–300 mg base once a week or once a fortnight	
Amodiaquine	As chloroquine	300–400 mg base once a week or once a fortnight	

Special responsibility lies with the distributors of the drug; they must ensure that the drug is really swallowed and not spat out or vomited and that the whole population benefits from this measure.

Drug distribution should continue for one month after the confirmed end of the epidemic. The possibility of relapsing vivax and malariae infection some weeks or months after the cessation of the drug distribution should be taken into account.

Various drug combinations (chloroquine with pyrimethamine; chloroquine with chlorproguanil; amodiaquine with primaquine; pyrimethamine with dapsone; sulphadoxine with pyrimethamine) have been used for protection of relatively small groups of semi-immune people with varying results related to the regularity and completeness of the 'total coverage' of the relevant population and reflects the degree of acceptance of the drug. It is still too early to give any definite recommendations as to the best drug and its dosage.

MASS DRUG ADMINISTRATION THROUGH DISTRIBUTION OF MEDICATED SALT

Mass drug administration can be achieved either by direct and supervised distribution of tablets or by incorporation of the drug into common salt used for normal daily preparation of food. The latter form of indirect drug distribution is often referred to as Pinotti's method, from the name of the Brazilian doctor who introduced it in the 1950s.

A number of difficulties have been met in using this method in the field. A community may draw its salt from a wide variety of sources; thus there may be considerable problems in trying to canalise the supply of salt through one point where the antimalarial compound is added to it. It is difficult to ensure the even distribution of the active drug through salt in bulk since in damp conditions chloroquine may tend to concentrate ('leach out') in one part of the container. The individual consumption of salt differs considerably and hence the range of dosage with the antimalarial varies. Some people consume little or no salt and therefore escape the action of the drug; this applies particularly to infants and they are therefore the group most at risk. These difficulties have bedevilled the application of what at first sight seemed to be a simple and effective method. In consequence, the utility of medicated salt distribution is likely to be confined to very special circumstances. This method proved to be very successful in Guyana, Iran and Surinam, and it may be applicable in other areas where a single source of salt can be identified and controlled. The procedure involves the purchase of a chloroquine or amodiaquine salt concentrate which is mixed locally with the bulk of salt consumed. This is done by machinery (e.g. in a concrete mixer) and involves a limited capital expenditure. Nevertheless, the whole process demands a fair degree of management, which is only possible to governments or large industrial concerns.

The antimalarial compounds suitable for use with medicated salt are chloroquine and amodiaquine. When pyrimethamine was used for this purpose in the early field trials, rapid development of resistance to this drug invariably followed. Chloroquine has been most commonly used for medicated drug distribution, though amodiaquine base (less bitter than chloroquine) was employed with success in Surinam.

The general requirements for Pinotti's method are as follows:
1. The salt supply of the population must be such as to ensure that only the medicated salt will be consumed. This may require some legislative action and much public health education.
2. The salt intake must be regular and well known to calculate the concentration of the compound in relation to the average daily consumption of the inhabitants.
3. The final concentration of the drug must be adjusted so that the intended weekly dosage of chloroquine or amodiaquine should be 300–400 mg of base.
4. The concentration of chloroquine in salt must not exceed 0.4% as beyond this limit the medicated common salt becomes bitter.
5. Mixing and bagging procedure must be such as to prevent irregular drug concentration and 'leaching-out' on storage.
6. A regular follow up of results is necessary to detect any technical, operational or human problems that may occur.

Chapter 9

Rationale and Technique of Malaria Control

Before considering in detail the concept and methods of malaria control, it may be useful to stress the great differences that exist between various epidemiological types of malaria. It is obvious that they have an important bearing on the selection of control methods and especially those that aim principally at the vectors of the infection.

EPIDEMIOLOGICAL TYPES OF MALARIA

The differences in the features of these types produce different pictures of the disease as it affects the community as a whole; the disease may be endemic or epidemic. Endemic malaria is constantly present in considerable degree and without great fluctuations in quantity; epidemic malaria shows great fluctuation in quantity and severity from time to time.

Apart from the endemic and epidemic types in some parts of the world a minor change in conditions may precipitate a great epidemic whilst in others the disease tends to be stable in its incidence and unexplained epidemics are rare. There is a high epidemic potential over very large parts of India, Sri Lanka, south-east Asia, north-west Africa and some countries in South America, and a low epidemic potential in much of equatorial Africa. In these areas of high epidemic potential disastrous outbreaks are easily precipitated although control can be readily established. The explanation of this potential has been the subject of much study and controversy but can be rationally proved on a basis of the factors which influence the prevalence of the disease.

Endemic malaria of low epidemic potential

This type of malaria occurs over the greater part of equatorial Africa, in the hills and foothills of India, the plains of Assam and in other places. It is due to transmission by anophelines which preferentially bite man and which commonly have a relatively long life, in places where the temperature is high for long periods. Malaria tends to be highly endemic, a fact often obscured by the development of some degree of immunity by the local peoples, but made manifest in children and in immigrants who suffer severely. Epidemics in the indigenous population are almost unknown except following a major increase in the numbers of mosquito breeding places. The disease can be maintained by relatively small numbers of mosquitos; entirely non-malarious parts are rare. Thus control measures which operate by reduction of mosquito numbers must be very nearly perfect to secure visible results, minor measures having little effect. Control by residual insecticides, which operates by reduction of expectation of life rather than by reduction of mosquito numbers, can be effective if it produces a sufficiently high Anopheles mortality, such as is attainable by the energetic use of the most effective insecticides, but which may not be reached when there is any degree of slackness in application.

Endemic malaria of high epidemic potential

This occurs over much of the plains of South America, India and Sri Lanka, and in south-east Asia. It is due to transmission by anophelines which tend to bite animals in preference to man or which normally are relatively short-lived. Its character is accentuated in areas where both these conditions apply. There are great variations in endemicity. In some places a high incidence is normal and the indigenous population may acquire some degree of immunity with results comparable to those in the type previously described. Some non-malarious localities may be found, and all gradations between these extremes occur. Considerable fluctuations in the amount of malaria from year to year are common and there may be severe periodic epidemics in previously non-malarious parts.

The precipitating causes of these epidemics are difficult to explain as they may be quite minor in character; when they are major, epidemics such as those of 1934–35 or 1967–68 in Sri Lanka may occur. As a minor manifestation of this instability the disease may appear without apparent explanation in previously healthy places; it may disappear from them again with as little obvious cause.

The number of anophelines needed to maintain transmission is relatively high and control by reduction of breeding, though perhaps not easy, is at least readily feasible. Control by residual insecticides is effective provided that a daily mosquito mortality of about 25% is kept up. This is within the range of effect produced by the routine application of active insecticides.

Hill malaria

The greatest altitude at which malaria occurs differs very much from place to place in the tropics, from nearly 2500 m in Kenya to under 1000 m in Sri Lanka. Near the upper limit of its altitude range the disease is almost always unstable with a tendency to epidemic manifestations, which are likely to occur following unusually rainy weather.

Control is relatively easy, when the method used is the application of residual insecticides.

Sub-tropical seasonal malaria

In those places where the temperature sinks below the minimum at which malaria is carried for most of the year, sharply defined summer epidemics occur. There may be three waves of the disease. In some places there is a spring epidemic occurring before transmission starts, due to relapses from the previous year and cases in which the incubation period has been prolonged by cold weather to several months. The second wave consists of fresh cases, chiefly due to vivax malaria which may rapidly reach its peak. The third wave comes in the late summer or autumn and is characterised by the greater prevalence of falciparum malaria. These seasonal epidemic waves are annual; when the epidemic potential is high there may be great differences between the sizes of epidemic waves in consecutive years; when it is low a more or less uniform type is likely to occur. A high potential with great variations is to be seen in the sub-tropical parts of north-west India and Pakistan, the Punjab and Sind. To a lesser extent it can be seen in parts of the Middle East and in North Africa.

Malaria of labour forces

The assembly of a labour force in any part of the world always increases the epidemic potential of the locality, and for a number of reasons. Bringing people together, often from a considerable distance, always involves the introduction of some who have no tolerance to malaria as it is found locally. Not only do they suffer themselves but, by providing a focus from which infection spreads, they also increase the load on others and start epidemics amongst them. Their activities often include the clearing of land, exposure of streams and seepages, digging of borrow-pits, and other works which increase the collection of surface waters and provide more facilities for mosquito breeding. In the early stages of development a labour force does not own cattle, so that mosquitos which might feed on cattle are driven to feed exclusively on man. Where the local vector prefers to feed on man, as it does over most of equatorial Africa, this will make little difference; where it chooses cattle in preference, if it can find them, the result of the change may be marked.

Whatever the cause, epidemic malaria is extremely common in labour forces and particularly in those places where the epidemic potential amongst the local inhabitants is high. Disastrous outbreaks have occurred on many occasions. Not only for the benefit of the workmen but also for the success of the enterprise concerned, labour forces must have a degree of protection greater than the local population.

THE PRINCIPLES OF MALARIA PREVENTION AND CONTROL

The control of malaria may be an individual matter, for the protection of one man or one house, or a community. It may have to be undertaken at short notice in the middle of an epidemic, or may be planned and arranged during the off-season; it may be necessary for a short period only, or for a long season throughout most of the year. In each of these cases different tactics are necessary.

Generally speaking the measures for prevention of malaria in individuals and for larger scale control of the disease can be divided according to the classification proposed by Russell (1952).
1. Measures designed to prevent mosquitos from feeding on man.
2. Measures designed to prevent or reduce the breeding of mosquitos by eliminating the collections of water or by altering the environment.
3. Measures designed to destroy the larvae of mosquitos.
4. Measures designed to destroy adult mosquitos.
5. Measures designed to eliminate the malaria parasites in the human host.

Protecting the people from bites of Anopheles, or curing the person from whom the mosquito gets its infection, is sound in theory, and as much as possible should be done to this end in practice. However experience has shown that, despite high hopes once rested in the latter method, it can never be relied on to give complete control of the infection in a community. In the endemic types of malaria many people are free from symptoms and are not discovered or treated. Protection from mosquito bites should always be put into practice, and may be expected to yield valuable results particularly in the presence of acute epidemic malaria, but which rarely can be relied on exclusively.

PROTECTION AGAINST THE BITES OF MOSQUITOS

Nets. The use of bed-nets as a protection from mosquito bites during the night has been practised from very early times. They still remain the most important of all measures of personal protection. The size of the mesh is determined not only by the number of holes to the square unit of the material, but also by the thickness and the type of thread of which the netting is made. In woven cotton nets the mesh is stated in terms of the sum of the number of holes counted along a line of the warp and a line of the bobbin falling within an area of one square inch (6.5cm^2), the hole at the corner of the square where the two lines meet being counted twice. A netting suitable for protection against most vector Anopheles is one of 25/26 mesh, woven of 30/s cotton. The number of holes to the square inch (6.5 cm^2) would be about 150

Nowadays, mosquito nets are made of nylon or other synthetic material, which is lighter and easy to wash. The mean size of holes of nylon nets is 1.2–1.5 mm; there should be 6–8 holes to 1 cm.

The material should be white to allow for easy detection of mosquitos. The best pattern is the rectangular net with a reinforced lower end; there should be no tears and no openings in the side for the purpose of entering the net. When in use it should be hung inside the poles and tucked all round under the mattress. It should be let down before dark in the evening, and when going to bed a thorough search should be made for any mosquitos which may be inside it, preferably using an electric torch. A useful precaution is to spray the outside of the net with an aerosol dispenser or a hand-sprayer using an appropriate insecticide preparation (Fig. 52).

Protective clothing. 'Mosquito boots' made of soft leather or canvas are useful to protect the ankles in the evening. Alternatively, a pair of thick socks may be pulled up outside the bottoms of the trousers. Sleeves should be rolled down and trousers substituted for shorts or skirts after

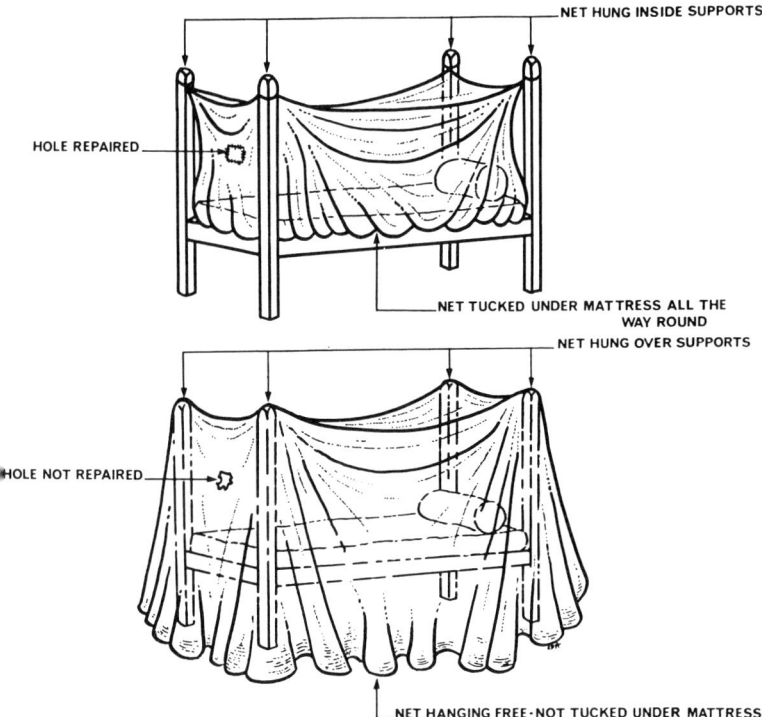

Fig 52   The right way (above) and the wrong way (below) of using the bed-net

sunset. Veils and gloves are sometimes used to protect men on guard at night.

Repellents. These are substances applied to the skin, clothing or bed-nets to repel mosquitos and prevent them from biting. In the past, citronella- or eucalyptus oil were used on the skin but its effect is very short, not exceeding 15–20 minutes. More recently a number of synthetic repellents have been developed, with a duration of protection of 2–4 hours. The most useful of those developed are indalone, Rutgers 612, dimethyl phthalate (DMP), dibutyl phthalate (DBP) and a mixture known as 6-2-2. The most effective against Anopheles is DBP (average protection 4 hours) and DMP (average protection 3 hours). Several new compounds are now available and among these diethyltoluamide (DET) shows much promise as the best repellent. A new group of mosquito repellents has been recently studied; these are dihydroacetone monoesters of carboxylic compounds. Their activity while promising, did not exceed that of diethyltoluamide but the combination of the two appears to prolong their action. Whatever preparation is used it should be applied liberally, especially about the neck, ankles and wrists. Eyelids and other sensitive skin surfaces or mucous membranes are irritated by these substances and should be avoided. Generally repellents are applied at dusk or dawn when Anopheles are most active. Synthetic repellents are plastic solvents and when spilled over or carelessly spread they may damage rayon stockings, fingernail polish, plastic pens, varnish and similar objects. For added protection repellents may be applied to clothing (especially socks) or to bed-nets; in the latter case mosquito nets sprayed with dimethylphthalate will retain repellent action for a few days and may be particularly welcome for protection against midges which can pass through ordinary nets. Special wide-mesh netting impregnated with repellents for use as head nets etc. has been widely used in the USSR. Mosquito-coils or joss sticks containing pyrethrum can be considered as a type of repellent. Their value varies greatly, since it depends on the amount of the active substance that the smoke emits when the coil smoulders.

However, a new type of the mosquito-coil principle has been recently developed and released commercially. It consists of a small semi porous mat, similar to a miniature beer-mat, impregnated with a synthetic pyrethroid compound, with the addition of perfume and a blue dye. When inserted in a small electrical heater, the mat slowly releases the insecticide and perfume by vaporisation. The amount of insecticide released is sufficient for several hours to prevent mosquito from entering the room and biting. Once spent the mat changes colour from blue to white and must be replaced.

Screening. The use of wire gauze in dwellings, especially where electricity is also available for light and fans, has made a great difference to the health and comfort in the tropics.

The building to be screened must be well-built and in good repair. Door frames should be made of seasoned wood with metal brackets at the corners and should not sag on their hinges. They should open outwards and be made to fit against a batten all round; they should have a strong spring to ensure tight closing. It is an advantage to have double doors, with a porch at least 2 metres in length between them. Every aperture in the building must be screened. Outside privies should also be made mosquito-proof.

The size of aperture in the screening material will vary with the diameter of the wire used. As there are several different gauges in use it is best to specify sizes of wire. It was found that 14–16 mesh (14–16 holes along the linear inch or 2.5 cm) and 28–30 Standard Wire Gauge or S.W.G. (aperture 1.2–1.5 mm) is the optimum for general use.

Many materials have been used for screening, zinc-coated steel, brass or aluminium being the most common. A salt-laden atmosphere is very destructive to screening and under such conditions it is an economy in the end to install the most resistant screen available. Certain plastic screens are of good quality and quite durable. Frequent inspection is necessary for the detection of rents in the screen and defects in the wooden framework, the latter being especially likely to develop where there is extreme variation in humidity between the dry and wet seasons.

Site selection. Selection of a suitable site for new housing, temporary or permanent, may avoid much subsequent difficulty. The principles are simply to place the housing upwind from the nearest water source and so that there is the minimum possible breeding of mosquitos within a half-mile (0.8 km) radius and only a little within a mile (1.6 km); local specialist advice may enlarge on or modify these general points.

It may be less expensive to pump water some distance from the pond or river than to site the buildings near the water and then incur the heavy expense on some special methods of mosquito control. At one time such site selection was literally vital to the success of many concerns, and it still considerably affects their prospects though the availability of better methods of control makes it nowadays less important. Systematic malaria control measures should be practised in any villages which may exist within one mile from the periphery of the camp.

Site selection should be kept in mind whether the site is to be occupied for a night only or if it is to be permanent.

MOSQUITO CONTROL

The control of mosquitos is undoubtedly the best method of protecting a community against the disease. Original development early in this century was by 'source reduction', namely the prevention of breeding, the only means then available. The pioneer work was carried out in Malaysia. In that country there was a rational assessment of the nature of the problem, of the species of vectors, the type of water in which they bred, and then a programme of work directed at that type of water only. This method, known as 'species sanitation', made economic practice possible in all those places where the necessary skilled supervision could be provided, a limitation which prevented its extension to many rural areas. This rational approach was not attempted in many other countries, and in some it was found less useful, because the majority of water types were dangerous.

Insecticides directed against the adult mosquitos (imagicides) were first used on a large scale about 1935. Pyrethrum was the first, and good results were achieved with it in southern Africa and in parts of India, but the new insecticides such as DDT, known as residual compounds, replaced it after the Second World War. They have had brilliant success, incomparably greater than many of the older methods which they soon almost entirely replaced throughout most of the world. Despite their general adoption, it would be wrong to conclude that prevention of breeding has now outlived its usefulness. Each of the two main methods of mosquito control has its place, according to epidemiological conditions of the area and other factors.

In places where malaria is of high endemicity control by prevention of breeding cannot be effective unless it is very near perfect, the smallest observable density of adult anophelines being enough to keep the disease going on a substantial scale. Perfection, or near perfection, may be attainable where the breeding places are limited and of a distinct, easily recognisable type; it is not attainable where the breeding places are diffuse and various. High epidemic potential in areas of low endemicity offers conditions for easier control of malaria and the same perfection of technique is less important. It can therefore be particularly successful where breeding places are distinct.

The pattern of amenability to control by residual insecticides is the same in principle but very different in degree. The object is not to kill all Anopheles at once, but to prevent a large proportion of them surviving for 12 or 14 days; even with the most potent vectors this can be achieved if the daily mortality inflicted on them is of the order of 40 or 50%. This is about the upper range of efficiency of insecticide applied by present techniques, but it can always be exceeded by a more thoughtful and generous application, which secures absolute control in most of the highly malarious places. In those places described as of low endemicity and high epidemic potential malaria is very sensitive to changes in the factors controlling it. A daily mosquito mortality of perhaps 20 to 25% will achieve the objective and this is well within the range of purely routine applications. Insecticides directed against the adult mosquito can therefore be prescribed to control the epidemic degrees of malaria, and routine applications by standard techniques will easily control the transmission of infection.

Another consideration is strictly economic. Prevention of breeding demands attention to a large area of ground around inhabited places, and varies little with the number of people in the area. It is therefore more costly per person in sparsely populated areas. On the other hand, insecticides against the adult mosquitos are applied in the house, at a cost per house which varies only a little with the density of population. They are therefore very much preferable in rural areas but may lose some of their advantages in thickly populated places.

The techniques of larval control require real skill and discrimination on the part of the worker. Those involving insecticidal spraying against the adult mosquito require skill, but of another sort which can be acquired by routine drill and which does not demand the same degree of understanding or discrimination. They can therefore be taught to large numbers of persons in a short time; this is probably the most important element in their success, in contrast to larvicidal techniques.

As a general principle the residual insecticides are faster in their effect than methods of prevention of breeding and should be considered in the first instance. There are, however, exceptions to their superiority, particularly in towns and thickly populated areas, or where the breeding places are of a limited and easily discernible form; in such places anti-larval measures are preferable.

ANTILARVAL MEASURES OF CONTROL

The application of antilarval measures for control of malaria has been neglected during the period when residual spraying aiming at the destruction of adult Anopheles seemed to offer the best solution. However, more recently the importance of measures directed against the aquatic stages of malaria vectors has been reassessed and is gaining greater popularity. The extent to which larval control operations are capable of a substantial degree of malaria is governed by technical, operational and economic considerations.

Technical considerations demand the assessment of effects of antilarval measures in comparison with residual spraying or distribution of antimalarial drugs. Thus the presence of exophilic species of Anopheles may warrant the selection of antilarval measures.

The technical reliability and effectiveness of larvicide measures have been fully demonstrated in the field, since the beginning of this century. Some problems, such as maintaining effective coverage of water surfaces at reasonable cost, have now been greatly reduced thanks to the introduction of newer compounds and better formulations. Larviciding is the most valuable and economical malaria control measure where the mosquito breeding areas are clearly defined so that they can be dealt with on a time schedule according to the life cycle of the species of the Anopheles vector. The selection of appropriate larvicide and of the method of its application varies greatly in relation to the type of the breeding place. Special conditions of wells, garden pools, rice fields, swamps, irrigation ditches etc. may require special measures.

Operational reasons refer to situations where the breeding areas of Anopheles vectors are limited and well known; obviously the advantages of antilarval measures are far greater than those of any other method. This is particularly true in urban areas.

Economic reasons are related to operational conditions. Generally operational convenience is also more economical. Permanent antilarval measures while more expensive at first may be much more economical in the long run, especially when repetitive maintenance and supervision are not required, as in the case of filling in of ponds or marshes.

One of the first principles true in both the urban and the rural areas is to avoid the creation of conditions in which the breeding of mosquitos does occur or can do so during the rainy season. Man-made malaria is a curse of the tropics, and much of it can be avoided. The breeding places may be created by digging large holes in the ground to obtain earth for road making; by faults in irrigation systems; by leaking taps in water pipes; by engineering works which interfere with the natural lines of land drainage. The correction of all these errors is usually much more difficult and costly than their avoidance (Fig. 53).

Control of existing breeding places may be by the use of chemicals by drainage, or by biological modification of the water to make it unsuitable as a breeding place. It must be carried out within the radius of flight of the local vector, commonly a mile (1.6 km), and throughout the entire transmission season which usually starts a month or so before the first clinical cases occur. It must be based on a knowledge of the local vector and particularly of its breeding habits, and depends on a detailed survey of the area showing all water surfaces of the potentially dangerous type within the radius prescribed. The collection of this information demands knowledge, the execution of a local survey and the use of skilled labour; all of these may be available or possible in advanced communities or in highly organised industrial undertakings but they are not features of the general rural conditions.

All antilarval operations of any but the small size projects should be based on technical requirements and on the assessment of the administrative and financial feasibility of the proposed method. Major items

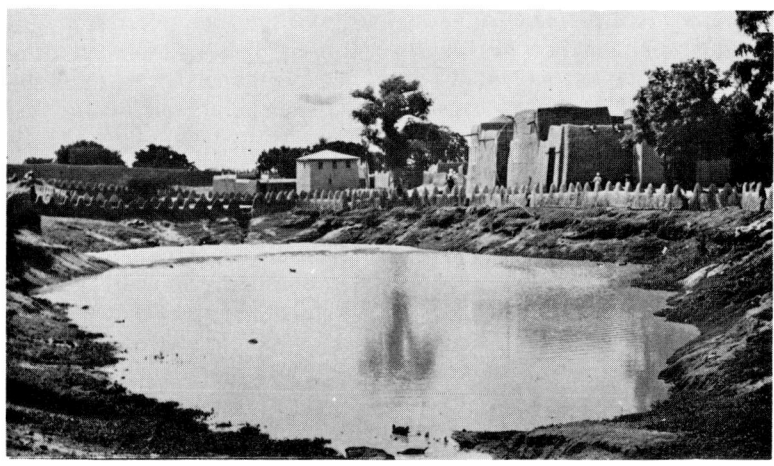

Fig 53 Man-made malaria. A typical borrow-pit at the periphery of a village in northern Nigeria. These pits, dug for the purpose of getting the mud (adobe) for building, collect rain water and are often used as source of domestic water supply. They usually breed large numbers of mosquitos including Anopheles. If no piped water supply is available it is not easy to deal with such borrow-pits by filling in or oiling. Paris green or newer insecticides (such as temephos granules) will control the breeding of larvae, but the treatment must be regular in order to decrease the amount of local transmission. (Wellcome Museum of Medical Science)

that should be considered are: personnel (permanent and temporary), equipment, chemical compounds, transport; supervision of field staff is of importance as also their training. Entomological evaluation of the effectiveness of the method used is indispensable. Among various ways of evaluating the results of antilarval control methods the use of *capture stations* is most advisable. These are selected shelters suitable as resting places for Anopheles mosquitos located in various quarters of the area to be protected. They are visited regularly and the mosquito collector sprays them with pyrethrum insecticide and picks up the killed mosquitos from a sheet previously placed on the floor. This is a valuable means of testing the efficacy of control measures; the presence of adult mosquitos is the most reliable test of antilarval work, and often leads to the detection of breeding places which would otherwise be overlooked. Anti-larval operations can be classified into: source reduction, biological methods, and chemical methods.

Source reduction

This category of anti-larval operations includes filling of unnecessary depressions in which water collects, regulation and improvement of natural water courses, drainage activities, weed control, intermittent drying etc.

Filling is a permanent measure of mosquito control resulting in complete elimination of waterlogged areas. It is a simple operation which can be carried out by unskilled personnel and with simple equipment. However, it can be greatly speeded up when motorised earth-moving machinery can be utilised.

Filling on a minor scale is a simple operation consisting of levelling a host of excavations such as water holes, borrow-pits etc. Filling on a large scale makes use of the spoil from such operations as harbour dredging, demolition, mining etc. Access to such material is extremely valuable since whole swamps and vast mosquito breeding areas can be converted into dry land. A special type of filling is that of 'sand pumping' in which sand mixed with water is pumped from estuaries, lagoons and creeks into the coastal swamp, which is gradually filled and converted into valuable land.

Drainage results in a reduction of water and speeding up of its flow. If the project is large and the area involved includes much flat land surveys are essential, so that the lines of drainage may be laid off accurately on the map. Where the drainage scheme is small the eye alone may be sufficient to establish the drainage line suitable for the existing fall (Fig. 54).

Small drainage projects can be carried out by unskilled personnel under the direction of a technician given special training in simple methods of ditching, which do not require any complicated equipment.

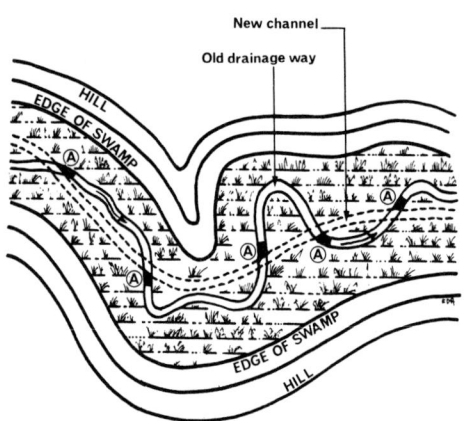

Fig 54 Lay out drains as straight as possible, but the drain should follow the low land, so that deep drains will not be needed. When a new channel cuts across the old, winding watercourse, an earth dam should be built to prevent water from flowing into the old channel.

Rationale and Technique of Malaria Control 221

Several types of drainage can be adapted to the existing topographical conditions of the area involved (Figs. 55a b).

Open drains. As a general rule these should be narrow and deep rather than broad and shallow; their banks should be kept clear of vegetation and sloped to an angle of about 45 degrees; tributaries should enter at an acute angle, and not at right angles in order to lessen the deposit of

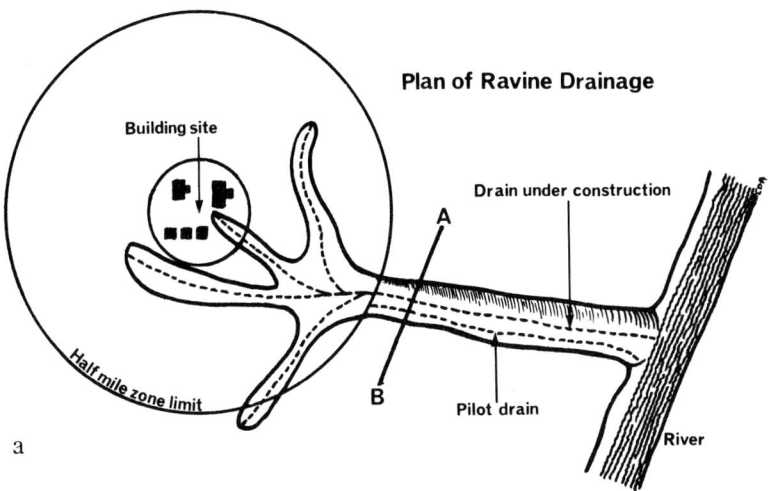

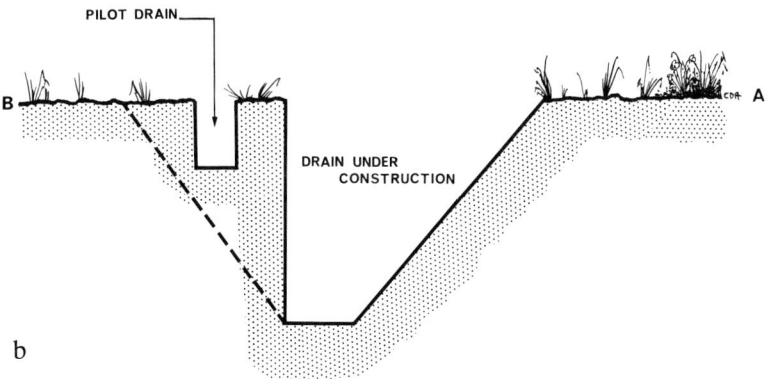

Fig 55a b Plan of drainage of a deep narrow gorge near a building site. Note in Fig 55b the method of construction of the main drain, following the digging of a temporary pilot drain.

ANTI MALARIAL DRAINS

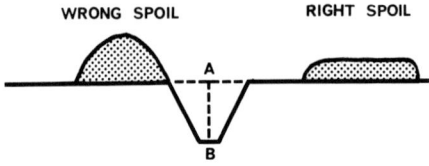

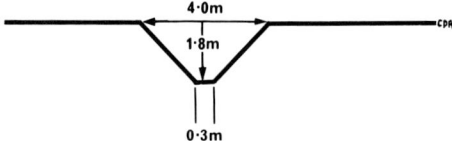

MEASUREMENTS FROM GROUND LEVEL IN METRES

Fig 56 Characteristics of earth drains in relation to the type of soil and the disposal of spoil.

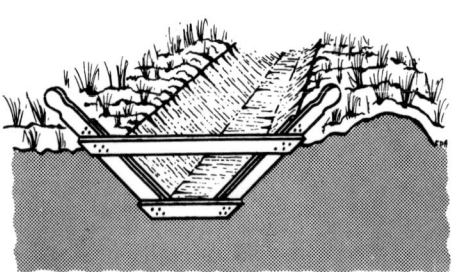

Fig 57 The use of a wooden template facilitates the completion of a uniformly shaped slope of an earth drain.

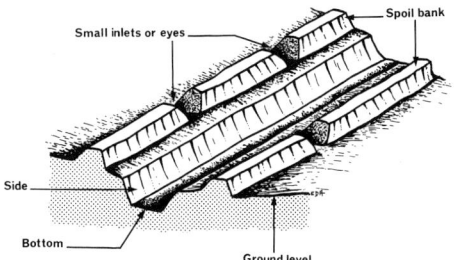

Fig 58 When a drain is dug the removed 'spoil' is used to fill low spots near the drain or is spread or piled up evenly on each side at least 1–2 metres from the edge of the drain; such piles must be separated by small inlets to let the water run into the drain. If the drain crosses a sloping ground the spoil should be piled up on the low side.

silt and debris at the point of junction. The bottom of a narrow drain should be rounded and not V-shaped, but in broad drains a shallow V is preferable to a flat bottom. A few simple precepts concerning the uniform shape of drains and the disposal of spoil are indicated in Figs 56, 57 and 58.

In the case of hill-foot seepages, the best method is to construct a system of contour drains at right angles to the direction of flow, to intercept the seepage at the point at which it arises.

Drains should be as few and short as possible, and their gradient should be carefully considered before starting work. The excavation for drainage should start at the outfall end. Sharp bends should be avoided wherever possible. The main drain should be constructed first and the tributaries afterwards (Fig. 59).

It is obvious that the drainage channels should be so sited that the land can be thoroughly drained. A number of different systems are in use. The herring bone drainage system consists of a main drain with a series of parallel laterals set at an angle to the main drain. This system while suitable for draining of flat land is often erroneously employed for swampy valleys. There, water running from the surrounding higher contours collects between the lateral drains and creates new breeding places for mosquitos. The alternative system of gridiron design intercepts most of the water from the surface and undergound. The use of the gridiron system avoids the multiplicity of junctions at which blockage may take place: moreover its advantage lies in the possibility of using each drain at the outer end as a contour drain aiding in the removal of seepage water (Figs. 60, 61).

Open drains may be either lined with concrete, brick, stone, etc., or they may be open earth drains. A lined drain should never be con-

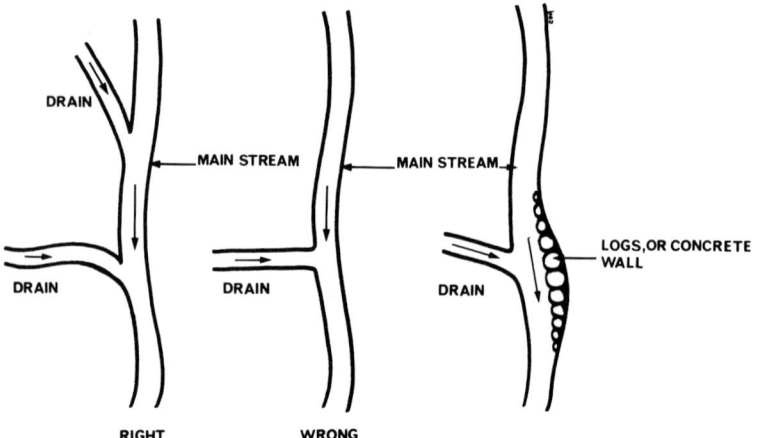

Fig 59 Where two drains or a drain and a stream join, the smaller drain should enter the main stream at an angle of about 30° in the direction of the flow. When a drain must enter the main stream straight into it, the bank opposite the flow should be reinforced with stone, logs or concrete.

structed without first making an earth drain to determine the requisite depth of the drain, and to see whether the flow is satisfactory. Concrete drains may be constructed by connecting a series of precast concave sections in the bottom of an earth ditch.

Lined drains should be made with a central deeper channel, (cunette) to take the water along quickly when its level is low. At the

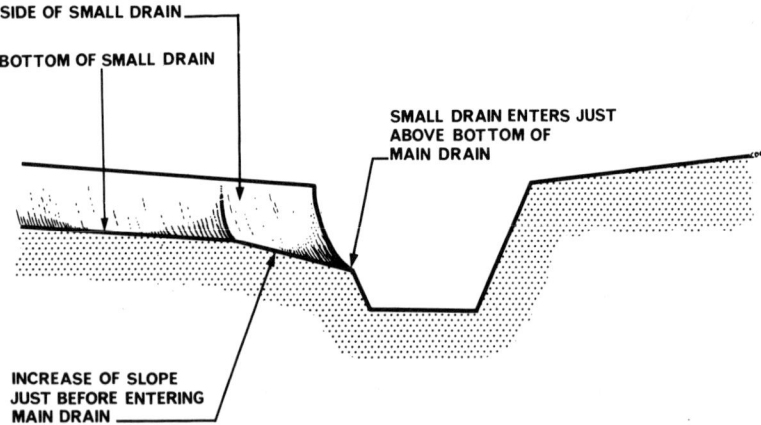

Fig 60 Where two drains join, the grade of the smaller drain should be increased just before it enters the main drain and it should enter just above the bottom of the main drain.

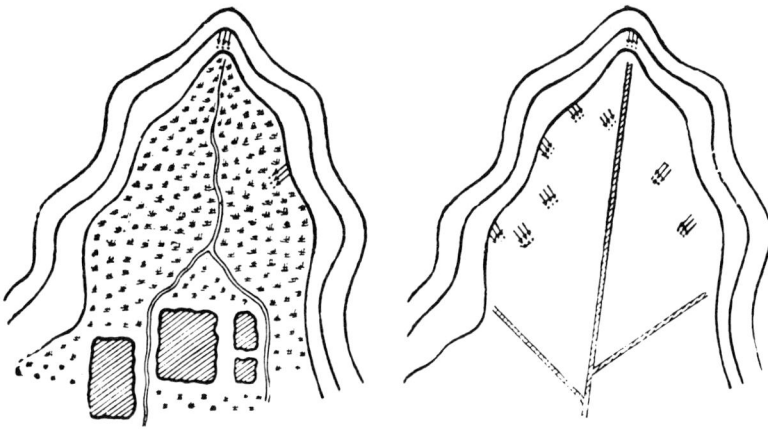

Fig 61 Stages in a scheme of anti-mosquito drainage for a swampy ravine. (From Scharff, 1935)
1. Ravine and swamp due to the obstruction of natural drainage. 2. Removal of obstruction, provision of one central and two herringbone earth drains. Seepages from the higher contours continue and create Anopheles breeding places. 3. Addition of intercepting contour drains with an outflow to the previous drainage system provides an answer to the problem. These drains may be simple earth drains or subsoil drains. The central drain may now be concreted to decrease the amount of maintenance.

point of junction with a side channel, the opposite side of the drain should be strengthened and raised to prevent overflow. Weep-holes should be made in the sides of the drain so that the subsoil water may get into it; these should slope downwards towards the bottom of the drain. It is also an advantage to construct key-walls at right angles to the drain at intervals, especially where there is a curve in its course, to prevent water from outside from tearing away the earth supporting the side walls (Figs. 59, 60).

In the case of earth drains, if the flow of water is very swift, undermining of the banks may occur, or if there is some temporary obstruction excessive local scouring may ensue, removing soil from below the grade line of the bottom of the drain and causing a pot-hole. Subsequently, if the rest of the drain becomes dry, as in stormwater drains, pools will remain in such situations, which may become Anopheles breeding places. A small temporary channel should then be made to connect these pools and drain off the water.

The necessity for repeated regrading, cleaning and oiling of open earth drains makes their upkeep expensive. Lined drains last longer and are more easily cleaned; but these too require frequent inspection.

Subsoil drains. There are many varieties of underground drains. A primitive type of such drain may be made by half filling a deep trench with stones. A more useful method is to place a series of flat stones horizontally over smaller stones so arranged as to form a passageway for water. The best way is to place at the bottom of a deep trench three or four flat stones to form a triangle or a square; this construction, when continued, will result in a stone-lined underground channel. A method of drainage by stone packing of deep ravines has given good results in Malaysia, but this technique is applicable only where stones are abundant. A variant of primitive subsoil drains is that in which wooden poles, bamboo or faggots are used; the latter type refers to large twigs or tree-branches being laid at the bottom of a trench, the water draining through the interstices when the ditch is filled in with layers of coarse grass.

However, the very successful type of subsoil drainage evolved in Malaysia consists of using 'tile pipes'. The drain in this case is formed by a series of earthenware pipes laid end to end in trenches beneath the ground, the water entering from below at the joints between the pipes. If soft spots are found in the bottom of the trench (which must be properly graded), stones are rammed into place until a solid foundation is obtained. The laying of the pipes should commence at the outlet of the drain and continue upwards as the trench is made. Greasy water and house waste must not be allowed to discharge into any part of the system. Where pipes come near the surface, proper bridge crossings are necessary, to protect them from being crushed by wheeled vehicles. The pipes should be laid in an absolutely straight line, with as few changes in gradient as possible. Periodic inspections should be made to see that the outlets do not become clogged with silt or other deposit.

The space between lateral and central drains is levelled-up and turfed with growing grass. No cultivation is allowed on the cleared and grassed ravine space. The grass must be constantly kept short, or the roots will block the pipes and a careful lookout must be kept for washouts and seepages.

It has been claimed for subsoil drainage that it is self-cleaning, permits of rapid inspection, needs little attention, and requires no oiling. But the experience gained during the past thirty years has shown that it has many drawbacks; its main disadvantage is its high initial cost, added to the upkeep.

Vertical drainage. This method is sometimes used to drain swamps or marshes. The bed of the marsh is probably of silt or clay, which retain the water, but beneath this there may be permeable or fissured rock which will afford drainage. A shaft is sunk down to the permeable rock, the exposed surface of which is blasted. A vertical pipe surrounded with stone or gravel is carried up to the level of the marsh bottom. A strainer is placed at the mouth of each sink-hole and a certain amount of grading is required in the marsh leading up to the holes.

Tidal swamp drainage requires the construction of dikes (bunds) with sluices (tide gates) manually or mechanically operated in addition to the system of drains to remove the water collected within the bunded area (Fig. 62).

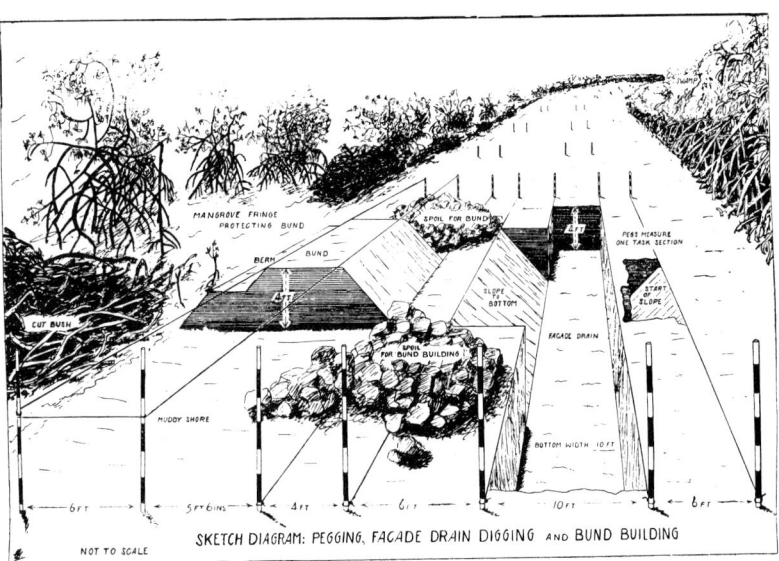

Fig 62 Diagram of the method of coastal swamp drainage as carried out in Nigeria. (Gilroy, 1948)

Construction of 'Lidos'. It often happens that for financial or other reasons it is impossible to drain off water from a particular area. Under these circumstances a useful method is to exclude extraneous water by embankments and dress the area within the embankment in such a way that all rain-water falling on it is directed into a single depression or 'lido', which is deepened and widened for the purpose to the required dimensions. In this way large numbers of pits are done away with, and the single potential breeding place remaining can easily be kept clean-weeded and treated with larvicides or stocked with larvivorous fish. This method is effective in areas where the annual rainfall is moderate in amount, and it can be carried out at a fraction of the cost required for filling operations in the same area.

Water management has been carried out to perfection by the Tennessee Valley Authority on the main reservoirs of this large engineering project. First of all a clean shore line was provided by cutting down the trees and bushes. Secondly, after the diking and de-watering of shallow areas, the water level of the main reservoirs was subjected to periodical combinations of cyclical fluctuations and surcharges to strand the larvae and pupae on the shore.

Sluicing and flushing methods are similar in principle and depend on a periodical discharge into the stream of a volume of water behind the dam to flush out the larvae and pupae from the edges and strand them on the banks as the wave passes downstream. This measure has been used extensively in tea-gardens and rubber estates in south-east Asia. The sluice gates may be operated by hand, or may be automatic.

Intermittent drying of irrigated rice-fields or fish-ponds consists of arranging that the surface water is removed from the field or pond for a few hours once a week or once every 10 days. During the dry period larvae or pupae of mosquitos will be destroyed in large numbers. The enforcement of a weekly 'dry day', on which all water containers, fountains, basins, etc., must be emptied and allowed to dry out, has a similar purpose.

Explosives have been successfully used in drainage and ditching operations with great saving of time and cost. Ditches varying from 1 to 10 metres wide and from 0.75 to 3.5 metres deep can be blasted using an appropriate amount of explosive and a precise method of placing the dynamite sticks.

Clearing of jungle or scrub. This may be of value because it removes sheltering places of adult mosquitos, promotes evaporation, and therefore speeds the drying up of water collections, and discloses breeding places which otherwise may be overlooked. Indiscriminate clearing of jungle may, however, favour the breeding of certain vector species of mosquito which lay their eggs in water exposed to bright sunlight.

Biological methods

These methods of control comprise so-called naturalistic measures. The meaning of this term covers all the ways in which natural limiting factors are deliberately intensified without any reliance on chemical or mechanical devices. This can be done by various means only a few of which can be indicated here.

In deltaic regions such as Lower Bengal, the annual flooding of the land by the rise of water-level in the great rivers provides a striking example of the natural control of malaria. The silty flood waters are inimical to the breeding of the local vectors, the extent of breeding edge is reduced, and the raising of the water-level above that of the aquatic vegetation exposes the larvae to the attacks of fish and other predators. Some of the dangerous Anopheles breed exclusively in brackish water. A method of dealing with such mosquitos, which include some of the most dangerous malaria vectors, is to *increase or diminish the degree of salinity* of their breeding places by the admission or complete exclusion of sea-water. The straightening and deepening of the central channels of streams and drains, and the maintenance of margins of breeding places free from pockets and bare of vegetation, allow the current to exert its greatest effect and to provide for larvivorous fish and other natural enemies. This measure of edging is a necessary complement to oiling, but even without the use of larvicide it has a marked effect in reducing the breeding of mosquitos.

The *growing of shade-giving plants* and trees over drains and small streams has been extensively practised in the tea-gardens of Assam and southern India. It is important that the plants used should give dense and complete shade, and that they shall be evergreen and if possible thorn-bearing. Under dense shade no vegetation can grow along the margins of a stream, so that the influence of the current extends right up to the bank and there are no longer any pockets of still water where mosquitos can deposit their eggs.

Other methods of biological control are based on the introduction into the environment of various pathogens and predators of insect vectors of disease. Such agents range from viruses, bacteria (*Bacillus thuringiensis*), protozoa (*Nosema*), fungi (*Coelomomyces*), and nematodes to natural predators such as larvivorous fish. Of all biological control methods the use of larvivorous fish has been the most successful in some parts of the world.

Larvivorous fish are natural enemies of mosquito larvae and have been utilised with advantage for malaria control in Spain, Italy, Greece and other countries in southern Europe and northern Africa, and also in Transcaucasia, India, New Guinea, Malaysia, Madagascar and many other countries. Naturally, the use of larvivorous fish is limited to some special situations where the water and other conditions are suitable. Cisterns, shallow ponds, small streams, ornamental pools etc. are ideal places for mosquito control by fish.

There are a number of species of fish that are particularly valuable in this respect. The most important and the best known is the top feeding minnow, *Gambusia affinis*, the guppy (*Lebistes reticulatus*), the goldfish (*Carassius auratus*) and several others of the families Poecilidae, Cyprinidae and Cyprinodontidae. Of the latter several species of 'annual fish' (e.g. *Nothobranchius* or *Cynolebias*) have been described and seem to hold considerable promise for control of mosquito larvae. The special merit of these small fishes lies in their capacity to survive and multiply in non-permanent waters, where other species would perish. 'Annual fishes' occupy tropical habitats with a wide range of temperature, where surface water disappears during the dry season (Fig. 63). They survive until the next rainy season in the form of eggs

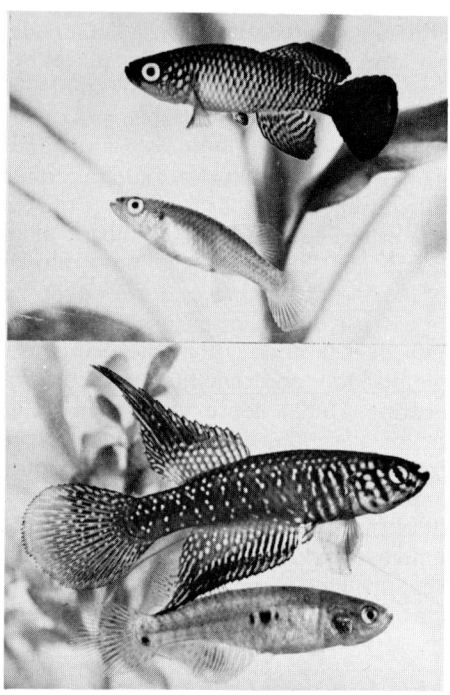

Fig 63 Larvivorous fish used in some malaria control programmes. These are two species of 'annual fish' of the family Cyprinodontidae: *Nothobranchius guentheri* (above), male and female (magnification × ca ⅓) and *Cynolebias whitei*, male and female (magnification × ca ½). (Hildemann & Walford, 1963)

buried in the soil. These eggs may be collected and transported in damp peat. Ripe eggs hatch within a few hours after being introduced into the water. The voracious young are hardy, mature rapidly and show high fertility. However, the most popular among larvivorous fish is still the *Gambusia affinis*, since it is small (30–65 mm), breeds rapidly and its rearing and transport are easy. It adapts itself to a wide range of waters, warm and cold, fresh and brackish. Such adaptation is slow and it is advisable to transport the fish in water taken from an original source and gradually adjust it to the type of water in which the fish are expected to thrive for a considerable time. There is now a considerable amount of technical literature on the breeding and introduction of larvivorous fish.

Disadvantages in the use of fish as a mosquito control measure are that they are only effective if present in very large numbers; they are less effective for control of Anopheles, especially in the presence of weed and floating debris; constant inspection is necessary to see that the fish are flourishing and are in sufficient numbers and that the water is free from horizontal vegetation.

Some species of fish have been found to have secondary uses for reducing the rooted aquatic vegetation and floating algae. These are the carp (*Cyprinus carpio*) and a species of *Tilapia*. Both species benefit larvicidal operations by ensuring a greater open water area in ponds and streams. However, both are very vulnerable to larvicidal compounds whenever the dosage of these substances exceeds the toxic threshold.

Genetic control is a special type of biological control; it has been defined as the use of any method that can reduce the reproductive potential of insects by altering the hereditary material of the vector species. Various methods of genetic control have been used, but the release of males sterilised by ionising irradiation or chemical compounds has received most attention. The principle of this method is that the sterilised males seek out and mate with the wild females in the natural population, thus preventing the hatching of their eggs and lowering their reproductive potential.

Chemosterilant compounds fall into two main categories; the alkylating agents (e.g. apholate) and the antimetabolites (e.g. methotrexate), used for treatment of tumours in man. A large number of the two groups were tested during the past ten years by the WHO in order to find the lowest concentration which produces complete sterility in male mosquitos without causing excessive mortality, so that they should be able to compete with normal males. About 40 of various compounds have given promising results but the toxicological and mutagenic implications for mammalian species including man prevented the setting up of any field trials.

Another method of genetic control is based on crossing two sibling species of an insect. This leads to hybrid male sterility and when very large numbers of sterile males are released, their competition with fertile males is so great that eventually the size of the succeeding generation decreases below the threshold when transmission of malaria is possible. The third method is that of incompatibility, in which the release of one sex of certain species, infertile with the opposite sex of another population of the same species, achieves the same effect.

These methods of genetic control based on cytoplasmic incompatibilities of two populations of the same species or on chromosome translocations are now the subject of much research. The main and difficult requirement for success of all genetic methods of mosquito control is the production of very large numbers of healthy, competitive though genetically different mosquitos and their release in the right place and at the right time to mate successfully with wild insects.

Although some of these methods have shown promise in field trials they have not come into practical use.

Chemical methods

The efficacy of chemical control measures depends on a number of factors: The species of vector involved; Efficacy of the pesticide; Type of its formulation; Thoroughness of its application; Nature of the surface treated and climatic conditions; Management of the control programme.

A detailed description of various chemical insecticides must be preceded by some knowledge of their classification.

Classification of insecticides

Insecticides can be classified: 1. According to their chemical composition, 2. By the way of their entry into the body of the insect, 3. By the method of their application, and 4. By the stage of the life cycle of the insect against which they are used.

1. *Classified by their chemical characters the most common insecticides applied in public health practice are:*
   1.1 Petroleum oils and their derivatives.
   1.2 Active constituents of flowers of Pyrethrum (pyrethrins) or some newer synthetic compounds of this group.
   1.3 Chlorinated hydrocarbons (DDT, HCH, dieldrin etc.).
   1.4 Organophosphorus insecticides (malathion, temephos, etc.).
   1.5 Carbamates (propoxur, carbaryl, etc.).
2. *Insecticides may be absorbed by the insect as follows:*
   2.1 By introduction into the plant or animal which is to be protected. These systemic insecticides are used mainly in agriculture and to some extent in veterinary medicine.
   2.2 By ingestion through the mouth (e.g. Paris green) of anopheline larvae. This is also the mode of action of various pesticides employed in agriculture (stomach poisons).

Rationale and Technique of Malaria Control

2.3 By inhalation through the tracheae. All highly volatile insecticides (e.g. methyl bromide, dichlorvos) act in this way. Some contact insecticides (HCH) also have this type of 'fumigant' action.

2.4 By contact with the cuticle and penetration into the body of the insect. Such contact insecticides are DDT, HCH, dieldrin; some of them may exert 'particulate' action through minute airborne particles without direct contact with the insect.

3. *According to the method of application insecticides may be:*
   3.1 Released into the surrounding air space *(space spraying)* in the form of vapour or aerosol such as fog, smoke etc., so that they are absorbed by inhalation or contact.
   3.2 Deposited on a surface, such as indoor walls and ceilings, for eventual contact with the insect. These long acting or *residual insecticides* are generally used for control of malaria and other mosquito-borne infections and include a wide range of compounds from DDT to the newer organophosphates.

4. *Insecticides may also be classified according to the action on the life cycle of mosquitos into:* larvicides and imagicides. (The use of the term adulticides for the latter is not recommended.)

In selecting a suitable insecticide the following factors should be taken into consideration:

1. Its effective toxicity towards the target insect. (The problem of specific resistance to one or another compound must be considered.)
2. Duration of action on a surface to which it will be applied.
3. Ease of application in existing conditions.
4. Toxicity towards man and domestic or wild animals.
5. Cost of insecticide and of transport and labour involved.

In the following section a simple classification by chemical composition will be used for convenience, though reference to the methods of application of these compounds is unavoidable.

Petroleum oils

Petroleum oil fractions have played an important part in mosquito control by larvicides since the beginning of this century. These oils are applied on the water in such a way as to produce a continuous thin film on the surface. When larvae come up to the water surface to breathe, the oil penetrates into their tracheae and kills them either by suffocation or by poisoning. For larvicidal work the mineral oil selected should have high toxicity to larvae and pupae, should spread easily and evenly over the water surface to form a stable film, penetrate quickly into the tracheal system of larvae, have no offensive odour, and be harmless to fish, waterfowl and livestock.

There are many grades of oils on the market which may be used for mosquito destruction, ranging from the very light oils such as kerosene to the heavier forms known as crude or fuel oils. The choice of oil is largely determined by local conditions. Thus, with high temperature a thicker oil is required, while in the presence of vegetation a lighter oil with great spreading power is necessary. Again, in still water a heavy non-toxic oil applied in sufficient quantity to form a complete film, will after some hours kill all the larvae; while in moving water a thin layer of rapidly spreading oil with a high toxicity is indicated.[1]

Larvicidal properties of mineral oils vary considerably in different consignments, according to the methods of refining. The addition of 1 to 2.5% of vegetable oil, such as castor or coconut oil, may increase the spreading power considerably. It is usually more satisfactory to use one of the proprietary oils (such as *Malariol*) which are specially designed for larvicidal work.

Good mineral oils must be homogeneous, fairly stable, free-flowing and easily spreading over the water surface. The approximate amount of oils used in practice is between 200 and 600 ml for each 100 square metres of water surface (20–60 l per hectare). Addition of 1% of synthetic insecticides such as DDT greatly increases the toxicity of ordinary oils.

Application of liquid larvicides can be carried out by simple oil-cans, by hand-operated continuous sprayers, by compression sprayers or by aerial spraying. However, oils are usually applied from a knapsack-sprayer, which must not be too heavy for its used in hot climate. The sprayer, fitted with a pump which has to be worked by hand, is preferable and less wasteful than a compression sprayer. All spraying requires supervision and regular, usually once a week, application.

Oil may also be applied from a garden watering-can or garden syringe, by used cotton waste soaked in oil and pegged into the ground for seepages and small pools, by means of a long stick with a bundle of old sacking attached, by balls of sacking tethered to the banks of streams or pools, by brushing over the surface with a sweeper's broom, by drip-cans placed over streams and drains, by oil-booms fixed across streams or irrigation channels, or it may be mixed with sawdust and thrown over breeding places after the manner of sowing grain.

---

[1] Full specifications for larvicidal oils are complex but the main points indicated in the WHO Manual on Larval Control Operations (1973) are: Specific gravity at 15.6°C 0.82–0.85; Viscosity at 37.8° C 33–45 cs; Spreading pressure not less than 23 dynes/cm.

The disadvantages of oiling are that it will not easily penetrate a barrier of grass, and to make it thoroughly effective all vegetation and floating debris must be removed; wind will break up an oil film and carry it to one side of a sheet of water; it is cumbersome and costly for transportation; it may kill fish and render them unfit for human consumption; and it renders water unfit for drinking purposes. On the other hand it kills the eggs and pupae of mosquitos as well as the larvae; it destroys culicine as well as anopheline mosquitos; it is easy to see whether it has been properly applied.

Mineral oils are not the cheapest materials that could be applied, especially at the present time when the cost of all petroleum products has sharply increased. However, the cost of oil is only a part of the total cost of operation and good results can be obtained with oils used in moderate amounts by experienced teams.

Paris Green. Paris green (copper aceto-arsenite) was first applied as a mosquito larvicide in 1921. Since then it has been extensively employed. It is a microcrystalline green powder, practically insoluble in water. It is so applied that small particles will float on water and be ingested by surface-feeding mosquitos, which subsequently die of poisoning. It should contain 50–55% of arsenious oxide and be fine enough to pass through a 200–300 mesh sieve. It is dispersed in the field in the form of dust mixed with a cheap diluent such as powdered soap-stone, talc, slaked lime, road dust, powdered charcoal or some other locally available material. The dilution varies between 1% and 30% and depends on the equipment used. For hand-operated dusters or blowers the dilution of 10 to 20% is adequate. Various liquid suspensions of Paris green with water have been used in compression sprayers with satisfactory results; other formulations of Paris green have been developed including granules and emulsion concentrates.

The application dosage of Paris green formulations ranges from 6 g to 15 g of the active chemical per 100 m^2 of water surface. Larger doses are needed where the vegetation is dense.

Advantages of Paris green are its comparatively low cost, its high toxicity for Anopheles larvae, its portability and ease of distribution by wind. There is no need to remove vegetation and no evidence of ill effects to domestic animals, fish or other natural enemies of larvae, or to crops. The water treated is not rendered unfit for domestic purposes and it is equally effective in fresh or brackish waters. On the other hand it has no effect on the eggs or pupae of mosquitos nor on any of the aquatic stages of culicines. It requires special apparatus for distribution for screening the diluent and for mixing; and its use requires constant supervision. It is difficult to see whether it has been applied properly or not except by dipping for larvae.

Pyrethrum is the oldest effective insecticide known and its main advantage is high immediate toxicity to insects while it is harmless to man. It is obtained from the flowers of the plant *Chrysanthemum cinerariaefolium* grown commercially in many parts of the world, and cultivated on a large scale in Kenya, Zaïre, Japan, India and South America.

Pyrethrum is used mainly in the form of a 10–25% extract of crushed dry flowers in kerosene or other organic solvents. This extract can be used when further diluted to 0.1%–0.5% with kerosene. If a suitable emulsifier is added this extract can be diluted with water. Pyrethrum contains from 0.7 to 3.0% of active principles. These are mainly esters of pyrethrins I and II which are rapidly oxidised and inactivated in sunlight with a loss of insecticidal activity.

Pyrethrins are nerve poisons, acting through the insect cuticle which is permeable to them. When sprayed, the droplets come into contact with the insect and their toxic action is fast. The addition of certain synergists increases the toxicity of pyrethrins to insects. Among these synergists piperonyl butoxide is most commonly used.

Pyrethrins in crude form have been used for control of various insects for many years. Their rapid 'knock-down' effect is of particular importance, though this action is relatively short lived and frequent applications are necessary. There is no evidence of mosquito resistance. Their use has greatly increased recently, because of the popularity of aerosol dispensers for rapid insect control at home and for disinfestation of aircraft. Pyrethrum was also the first insecticide used for large scale malaria control by attacking the adult Anopheles.

In malaria control programmes most common formulations of pyrethrum are: 0.2–0.4% dusts; 0.1–0.4% solutions in kerosene or petroleum distillate; as aerosol insect sprays (synergists are included in the formulations). The pattern of use of pyrethrum is very wide. It is applied as thermal fogs, mists for non-residual control by repetitive application in kitchens, food stores, factories, etc., where toxic residual insecticides cannot be used. Thermal fogs of 0.05% pyrethrins with 0.4% piperonyl butoxide are used for fly control. Ultra-low volume (ULV) sprays are used against mosquitos, houseflies, and tsetse flies. Pyrethrum is repellent to mosquitos; thus it is used in insect repellent creams and mosquito coils. Pyrethrins have a very low toxicity for warm blooded animals, but are toxic to fish. However, their persistence in water is brief.

Recently a number of synthetic compounds have been developed. They are as potent as pyrethrins and some of them present definite advantages over the natural products.

The first useful synthetic pyrethroid came from the USA in 1969; it was given the generic name of *allethrin*. Allethrin has 8 possible isomers depending on the position of the hydrogen atoms on the one (cis) or other (trans) side of the cyclopropane ring.

The chemical names of the new compounds now available commercially are: allethrin, dimethrin, resmethrin, tetramethrin, decamethrin, permethrin and others. The synthetic pyrethroids share with the natural product great safety in use. Acute toxicity to mammals of the various compounds is very low. The insecticidal activity (knockdown and kill) of synthetic pyrethroids is high, but each compound has a specific range of action, which is influenced by the formulation and the degree of synergism with other compounds. Synthetic pyrethroids are used as coarse space sprays, aerosols, and smokes in mosquito coils. The exceptional activity of synthetic pyrethroids against mosquitos and other insects is important because they are difficult to manufacture and must be used at dosage rates much lower than other insecticides. The new compounds are now available as usual formulations of solutions, emulsion concentrates and even as water dispersible powders. Some recent field tests in Africa showed that decamethrin at a dosage of 0.1 g/m^2 was effective as a residual spray for 2 months.

Chlorinated hydrocarbons. The three insecticides of this group most commonly employed in public health practice are DDT, HCH and dieldrin.

DDT. Dichloro-diphenyl-trichloroethane or DDT (known also under the name of dicophane or chlorophenothane) was originally synthesised in 1854, but its insecticidal properties were discovered in 1939 by Paul Muller of Switzerland. The first field trials of DDT took place during the Second World War. The abbreviated name DDT was given to this compound by the British Ministry of Supply.

DDT is still the most widely used insecticide in public health practice. The chemical structure of DDT is:

The two chlorine atoms attached to the benzene rings may be linked with other carbon molecules giving different isomers of the compound, but the most effective of these is the para-para isomer of DDT shown above.

Technical DDT is a mixture of isomers, but it must contain at least

70% of para-para isomer to be acceptable. The content of the para-para isomer is usually stated on the container.

DDT is a white, amorphous, waxy powder with an aromatic smell. It is soluble in oils and organic solvents, but not in water. It is very stable and on suitable impervious surfaces it may remain active for as long as a year, but normally, if the DDT deposit is not rubbed off or covered up, it is applied twice a year. On sorptive surfaces like mud (adobe) DDT loses its insecticidal effect somewhat faster. It has a certain irritant effect on insects, but its toxicity to most species of insects is high. Its toxicity to man is very low and there is no evidence that the millions of people whose houses were treated with DDT are at any risk from exposure to it. On the other hand it is true that DDT may adversely affect some animals (cats, chickens), predatory birds and fish. For this reason the use of DDT outdoors, when gross environmental contamination is likely, should be avoided. The amount of DDT for residual spraying of indoor surface is usually given in terms of technical DDT and the standard dosage is 2 g/m^2 of the treated surface every 6 months. DDT has also been used for its larvicidal properties mainly as an additional compound to fortify the toxic action of oils. The required dosage is very small. Two methods were used: a 2–5% solution of DDT in 'high speed' oil employed at 0.3 to 0.6 l to 1000 m^2 of water surface and an emulsion concentrate, to be diluted with water so that the final concentration of DDT is 0.1–0.15%, to be sprayed at a rate of 10–20 l per 1000 m^2 (about 10–20 gallons per hectare) of water surface.

Like all chlorinated hydrocarbons, DDT has a short effect when used as a larvicide: the insecticide is diluted or washed away or adsorbed by mud and vegetation. Thus for larvicidal control it must be applied relatively frequently. The use of all chlorinated hydrocarbons out of doors is today frowned upon because their adverse action on the environment: nevertheless in conditions where there is no danger to wild life DDT may still be used with caution.

The water dispersible powder of DDT for residual spraying of houses contains 50–75% of active substance; the higher content of the insecticide is preferable for a number of reasons, mainly economic.

Hexachlorocyclohexane (HCH). This compound, formerly called benzene hexachloride or BHC, was synthesised in 1825, apparently by Faraday. Its insecticidal action was discovered in the UK in 1942, when it was first known under the code name 666; it became widely used during the 1950s in agriculture, veterinary medicine and public health.

Its chemical constitution is remarkably simple ($C_6H_6Cl_6$) since it consists of a benzene ring with a chlorine atom attached to each carbon.

[Structure diagram: Hexachlorocyclohexane — cyclohexane ring with six Cl substituents]

The arrangement of the H and C atoms in space may vary, so that a number of optical isomers exist, the most active of which is the gamma isomer. This isomer when pure or at least 99% pure is called lindane. Technical HCH must contain at least 12% of gamma isomer. It is soluble in organic solvents. Technical HCH is a whitish or light-brown, granular or flaky substance with a characteric musty smell. It is relatively volatile and may kill insects fairly rapidly by fumigant action. However, because of this volatility, its residual action is generally half as long as that of DDT, though its toxic action is faster. HCH may be used in the form of water dispersible powder, containing 6.5% of gamma isomer, as a residual insecticide for indoor spraying of walls; other formulations (solutions, emulsions) exist for use as larvicides or as insecticidal smoke. The usual dosage of HCH for residual spraying is $0.3 g/m^2$ every three months or $0.5 g/m^2$ every 4–6 months.

Dieldrin. This insecticide, together with aldrin, belongs to a small group of compounds obtained by the cyclodiene synthesis discovered by Diels and Alder, whose names were given to the first two products.

The chemical structure of dieldrin is:

[Structure diagram: Dieldrin]

The active principle is hexachloro-octahydro-epoxy-dimethano-naphthalene or HEOD which comprises some 80% of technical product soluble in organic solvents but not in water. Formulations of dieldrin may comprise powders, emulsions, granules or briquettes. Dieldrin is more toxic than DDT and HCH both to insects, to animals and to man. Its residual activity at the dosage of $0.5 g/m^2$ was expected to be of six months' duration, but it was found that it is shorter, being not more than four to five months. Dieldrin is less excito-repelling to mosquitos than DDT and its action is faster. However, it has two main disadvantages: fairly high toxicity to man or animals and proneness rapidly to produce resistance to cyclodiene compounds and to HCH. Dieldrin has been responsible for poisoning spray operators, domestic animals and poultry. Because of this and other factors, its use in public health practice has now greatly decreased. Wherever its use is justified the field operations should be well supervised.

Other chlorinated hydrocarbon insecticides comprise such compounds as chlordane, methoxychlor, heptachlor and many more. The increased trend of resistance to this group of chemicals has now led to a progressive search for and use of alternative compounds.

Organophosphorus compounds. This group of insecticides, widely used in agriculture (e.g. parathion) is now commonly employed in public health practice, mainly because several insect vectors of disease have become resistant to chlorinated hydrocarbons. Most of the organophosphorus insecticides are esters or amides of organically bound phosphoric or pyro-phosphoric acid. Their general mode of action is due to the inhibition of the enzyme cholinesterase in arthropods as well as in mammals. The normal mechanism of transmission of nerve impulses is through the liberation of acetylcholine, which acts on the effector cells of a muscle or a gland. Cholinesterase present in the nerves stops the effect of acetylcholine by hydrolising it; organophosphorus compounds neutralise the enzyme and cause an accumulation of acetylcholine. This results in a blockage of the nervous system with consequent muscle paralysis, excessive gland secretion and finally death. Atropine is a specific antidote which counteracts these effects of organophosphorus poisoning. The suitability of organophosphorus compounds for use in public health programmes depends on their toxicity to the target insects and their danger to man, but also on their properties of persistence, tendency to produce resistance in mosquitos, ease of formulation and cost. Generally speaking organophosphorus insecticides are more volatile than chlorinated hydrocarbons and their activity is shorter. This also increases the cost of application of these compounds. The following organophosphorus compounds are in use for malaria control as imagicides or larvicides.

Malathion is now much favoured. It is an ester of dimethyl phosphorodithioate; the technical product is a brownish liquid with an unpleasant garlicky smell that can be masked by various additives. Its chemical structure is:

$$(CH_3O)_2 \overset{\overset{S}{\|}}{P}-S-\underset{\underset{\overset{\|}{O}}{CH_2-C-OC_2H_5}}{CH}-\overset{\overset{O}{\|}}{C}-OC_2H_5$$

Malathion

Its formulation consist of emulsifiable 60–90% concentrates or of water dispersible powders containing 50% of the active compound. Thus malathion can be used either for outdoor space spraying or for indoor residual applications. The duration of residual action of malathion depends on the substrate on which it is used but averages about 3–4 months when the dosage of the active substance is at the standard 2 g/m² of sprayable surface.

While most of the organophosphates are very toxic to man the toxicity of malathion is relatively low and this compound has been widely used for indoor spraying of human dwellings and animal shelters. However, some formulations undergo rapid chemical degradation on storage in tropical conditions and their toxicity can be much higher than expected. Thus even with malathion very strict safety precautions should be observed.

Fenthion (Baytex) another derivative of phosphorothioate has a higher toxicity to insects and to mammals than malathion but it was used with some success in Africa and Iran as water-dispersible powder at a target dosage of 1.5 g/m². However, because of its toxic hazards to spraymen fenthion is not suitable for routine indoor spraying though its value as a larvicide is being assessed in field trials.

Fenitrothion is an ortho-dimethyl-nitro-tolyl-phosphorothioate known under proprietary names of Sumithion or Folithion. It has been widely used in agriculture, but recent trials showed that it can be of value for residual control of malaria vectors when used as a water-dispersible powder for house spraying. At a dosage of 2 g/m² this insecticide gave good results for about 4 months. The conclusions of the WHO expert committee were that this insecticide can be used for spraying of houses providing that various precautionary measures are observed for protection of spraymen and domestic animals.

Dichlorvos (DDVP) a dichlorovinyl dimethyl phosphate is a liquid product with a high volatility; the vapours thus produced are highly toxic to flying insect pests and of low toxicity to man. The compound is now widely used when incorporated into various plastic resins (e.g. Vapona) for control of domestic flies. Despite many field trials carried out in Africa and elsewhere dichlorvos has not found its utility for control of malaria vectors.

Temephos (Abate) is a tetramethyl-thio-diphenylene phosphorothioate, highly active against aquatic larvae of mosquitos and other insects. It has been formulated into fine granules impregnated with 1% of the compound. The granules are applied on water surfaces at monthly intervals, in doses aiming at 1 part per million of the active product. This compound is highly effective against various species of mosquito larvae including those resistant to other insecticides. Its toxicity to fish, birds, and mammals is very low and it is also used in liquid form as an emulsion at a rate of 37 to 100 ml per hectare and in granular form of 2% concentration at between 5 and 20 kg per hectare, depending on the type of water and the amount of aquatic vegetation. This treatment can be repeated at 2–3 months' intervals, viz. much less frequently than any other larvicide.

Various other organophosphorus compounds (phenthoate, chlorphoxim etc.) have been developed and tested in field trials but showed no or only relative improvement in comparison to existing insecticides or were less acceptable for other reasons.

Carbamates. This fairly recent class of carbamic acid esters resembles in some ways the organophosphorus insecticides since they also affect the enzyme cholinesterase.

Carbaryl (Sevin) – an alpha naphthyl methylcarbamate is in use as an agricultural pesticide. Field trials carried out in Haiti showed some promise at the dosage of 1–2 g/m^2 but the persistence of the compound was not as long as had been expected. Further trials may be needed.

Propoxur (Arprocarb) – an isopropoxy-phenyl methylcarbamate underwent a number of field tests in various parts of the world. The results showed that at the dosage of 2 g/m^2 in the form of a water-dispersible powder propoxur remains highly active against Anopheles mosquitos for up to 3 months. It is generally agreed that this compound, of low toxicity to man, is an acceptable alternative to DDT and other insecticides to which malaria vectors have become resistant. However, the high cost of propoxur greatly limits its wider use in tropical developing countries.

Landrin – a trimethyl phenyl methyl carbamate is a new compound of this group with high effectiveness against malaria vectors. Further evaluations of it are planned when this insecticide becomes commercially available at a competitive price.

For a number of years the WHO conducted an intensive research programme to develop new insecticides for mosquito control. This research work has grown in complexity because of the problem of safety of new compounds and their effects on the environment. Increasing costs of such research have led to a gradual fall in the number of new insecticides available for field evaluation. Only a few compounds (bromophos, iodfenphos, chlorphoxim and pirimiphos-methyl) out of some 1500 possibles have been selected for future field testing.

Formulations of insecticides

Formulations of chemical compounds for mosquito control are numerous, ranging from fogs to fluid oils to solid briquettes. *Solutions* are either in oil or kerosene, solvent naphtha or white spirit with concentrations of 10–15%; aromatic hydrocarbons such as benzene and cyclohexane permit higher concentrations up to 25–40% which can be diluted to the required spray concentration.

Insecticide solutions can be used either for larviciding or as imagicides for control of adult mosquiotos by space- or residual spraying. The latter method has been used when spraying some types of houses in which the staining of walls by unsightly deposits of water-dispersible powder had to be avoided. However, this method has been replaced by the introduction of water-emulsion concentrates.

Emulsions are made up from two immiscible liquids, one of which is broken up into globules and scattered in the other liquid. To prevent the separation of the two, various emulsifying agents are added. Emulsions are prepared from emulsifiable concentrates containing 10–35% of a chemical compound by dilution with water. Pastes are special types of emulsion concentrates.

Water-dispersible (or wettable) *powders* are composed of an active insecticide diluted with an inert carrier, to which various wetting, suspending and anti-caking agents are added. Commercially available water-dispersible powders contain between 50% and 75% of the technical product. When mixed with water and stirred these powders form a suspension i.e. a mixture of the liquid and of the insoluble small particles, which tend to settle more or less rapidly. This depends on various physical factors related to the composition of the water-dispersible powder, its amount, the type of water used and, naturally, the agitation of the suspended powder. Particle size and suspensibility are important factors in residual insecticide spraying. In standard formulations of water-dispersible powders the WHO specifications require that at least 50–70% of the insecticide content should have a particle size of less than 10–20 microns.

Other *solid formulations* of insecticides are powders, granules, pellets or briquettes. All of these preparations used as larvicides are designed to disintegrate slowly in the water while releasing the toxic agent.

A new type of formulation is that of *granules*. These are produced from inorganic materials such as clays or organic polymers. The choice of carrier, solvent and binder provides some control over wetting and breakdown with subsequent release of the active ingredient. They are safe to handle, convenient and with little hazard of drifting away from the target. Another new procedure is that of microcapsulation. The tiny capsules containing the insecticide can be stored as suspensions in water and diluted for spraying. Like the granules microcapsules are designed to provide controlled release of the insecticide.

Space spraying formulations range from fumigants, through fogs, mists, and other aerosols, to fine droplets.

Some insecticides (such as dichlorvos) have a low vapour pressure and volatilise spontaneously. This fumigant action has been proposed for aircraft disinsectisation.

Coarse sprays which consist of droplets over 400 microns in volume median diameter (VMD) have a space spraying effect if the relevant liquid evaporates. *Fine sprays* in which the droplets are between 100 and 400 microns VMD have also this effect in addition to direct impact on flying mosquitos. When the droplets are between 50 and 100 microns VMD they are classified as *mists*. Finally true aerosols or fogs have their particles less than 50 microns in volume median diameter; the latter type of aerosol remains suspended in the still air for about one hour.

Aerosols are produced from containers, through the action of a compressed liquefied inert gas; for large scale use various thermal or rotary generators are available.[1]

EQUIPMENT FOR VECTOR CONTROL OPERATIONS

Equipment for application of methods of chemical control of mosquitos can be classified in many different ways. The following arbitrary classification is convenient and widely used.

1. *Equipment for application of liquids*
    1.1 Hydraulic energy propulsion
    1.2 Gaseous energy propulsion
    1.3 Centrifugal energy propulsion

    Hydraulic- or gaseous energy propulsion equipment may be either manually or power operated; centrifugal energy propulsion is always power-operated

2. *Equipment for application of solids*
    2.1 Dusting equipment

    Manual or power-operated

    2.2 Granules or pellets dispersing equipment

---

[1] For WHO specifications of insecticide formulations see section G of the list of references.

3. *Aerosol dispersing equipment*
   3.1 Mechanical aerosol generators
   3.2 Thermal aerosol generators
   3.3 Gaseous energy aerosol generators

The type of application of liquids depends in the first instance on the design and construction of the nozzle. There are many different types of nozzles (e.g. impact, cone, fan etc.) for different purposes. The equipment may range from hand-carried, through knapsack type, shoulder-carried, barrow wheeled, vehicle mounted, to aircraft or helicopter fitted types.[1]

The choice of equipment depends on the knowledge of the habits of the vector involved and must be consistent with the recommended method of control. It will also depend on the physical nature of the formulation of the pesticide. Moreover one has to bear in mind: (1) the frequency and duration of control measures, (2) the extent and accessibility of the target area, (3) the ease of use of the equipment by the operator, (4) the amounbt of maintenance and (5) initial and recurring cost. Only the briefest description of conventional equipment can be given here.

EQUIPMENT AND ITS USE FOR MALARIA CONTROL BY LARVICIDAL METHODS

The technique of application of larvicides to water surfaces depends on both the type of compound used and on the type of mosquito-breeding place (Table 17). *Liquid larvicidal* compounds such as oils may be applied from simple garden watering-pot or a hand sprayer on small pools or drains. Alternative simple methods such as using an ordinary sweeper's broom dipped into oil, drip-cans improvised from tins with a hole in the bottom, sawdust mixed with oil and broadcast by hand etc. have been employed with reasonably good results providing that the water surfaces are still and not too extensive. However, more commonly knapsack sprayers are used, as by this means the oil can be distributed 5–10 metres from the operator. Various designs of knapsack- or shoulder-slung larvicide sprayers exist but their general design is the same. It consists of a container with a 7–9 litres capacity, with a lever operated plunger- or diaphragm-pump, connected by a rubber or plastic hose to a cut-off valve, lance and nozzle. The pressure developed by the hand operated lever is low and the semi-continuous pumping can be maintained without much effort while the operator points the lance towards the target of the spray.

Various hand operated or motor driven modifications of these

---

[1] See WHO (1974) Equipment for Vector Control, 2nd edition.

Table 17

Selected insecticides suitable for larvicidal application in mosquito control

Insecticide	Dosage per hectare	Remarks
Diesel oil (fuel oil) and other petroleum oils	140–190 l in open ponds to cover water surface	With an addition of a spreading agent the amount can be decreased 5 times or more
Larvicidal oil	19–47 l (with special spreading agents)	Various proprietary formulations
Paris green	ca 800–1000 g of pure toxicant diluted at 1–5% in dust	Pellets containing 5% of Paris green may be applied at about 17 kg per hectare using ground based machines or aircraft
DDT	ca 200 g	Outdoor application of chlorinated hydrocarbons is not advised. In some conditions a limited use may be permissible as oil or water emulsion formulations on waters with little vegetation. Granular formulations are available
HCH (Lindane)	ca 110 g	
Dieldrin	ca 110 g	
Malathion	200–700 g	Usually as emulsion concentrate. Avoid overdoing which may injure fish
Temephos (Abate)	50–200 g of pure compound. 2 kg–20 kg of granular formulation	As emulsion concentrate or granular formulation. The latter are available in 1%, 2% and 5% concentration and higher dosages are used for polluted waters
Fenitrothion	200–300 g	Not to be applied to waters containing fish
Fenthion	20–100 g	

sprayers, mounted on wheels, on boats, or now on small hovercraft, are available but their description exceeds the bounds of this book.

Larvicidal dusts such as Paris green may be broadcast by hand, by small bellows-operated blowers, by pump-type hand dusters, by knapsack- or front-carried rotary blowers and by power operated, wheel mounted dusting machines.

For application of granulated compounds several modifications of standard equipment have now been developed and are increasingly used.

For large-scale application of larvicidal measures either in the form of large-droplet sprays or as granulated insecticide formulations, fixed wing aircraft and helicopters are the best solution. In general aerial spraying produces a broad spectrum of droplets so that the resulting effect is due to direct action on larvae and adults of mosquitos as well as to some residual action on the vegetation.

Applications of larvicides must be repeated at intervals corresponding to the development cycle of Anopheles species. Generally the relevant period is between 7 and 14 days; longer periods are possible with some newer compounds.

IMAGICIDAL MEASURES AIMED AT CONTROL OF ADULT MOSQUITOS

Although individual protection from bites of adult mosquitos by smoke or various fumigant devices ('joss-sticks') was well known in the past, large scale malaria control projects by indoor spraying with pyrethrum solutions proved to be unexpectedly successful some 40 years ago in southern Africa and India.

However, the introduction of DDT and other synthetic insecticides resulted in the revolutionary concept of malaria control by residual action of the new compounds. In contrast to the immediate knockdown effect of pyrethrum, which lasts only for a short time, the new synthetic insecticides retain their toxic action for a considerable period, when applied to a surface with which adult Anopheles (and other mosquitos) may come into contact.

Residual insecticides are almost invariably applied in some liquid form which, on drying, leaves a crystalline deposit on the wall. Some wall surfaces absorb the original fluid which is put on, and if this is a solution or an emulsion, much of the active insecticide is drawn into the inner part of the wall where the insect cannot come into contact with it. This causes some loss of insecticidal power on mud and porous plaster walls. Surfaces such as wood may not absorb much of the insecticide which remains on the surface in an active form for many months.

These insecticides act slowly, and some of them irritate the mosquitos, leading to their flight towards the light and usually out of the house. Their fate after that depends on whether or not they take away a small quantity of insecticide on their feet. Crystals formed after the evaporation of the solvents used in solutions and emulsions vary in size but the range of insecticide particles in a wettable powder formulation is determined in the course of manufacture and is standardised to a specification that can be checked by suitable suspensibility tests to ensure optimum size for biological effectiveness. Volatility is important since a volatile product disappears in time whatever the quality of the wall, but exerts some fumigant effect which will kill insects not in actual contact.

The irritant effect, which occurs with DDT, nullifies the value of counts of mosquitos in treated houses as an index of efficacy since it always leads to the mosquito avoiding the house as a shelter, though it may still use it as a feeding place. The only reliable checking mechanism consists in trapping mosquitos leaving the house and noting the proportion of them dying in the next 12 or 24 hours. This demands the use of special traps and a rather elaborate technique which cannot be universally applied.

Obviously large scale application of residual insecticides will have a particularly marked effect on those species of mosquitos which feed preferentially on man inside his dwelling or which shelter in human houses or sheds for domestic animals.

When it comes to the choice of residual insecticide the factors to be considered are: the susceptibility of the relevant Anopheles species to the compound, the type of its formulation in relation to the surface to be applied, the feasibility of its correct application and, last but not least, the cost involved.

The duration of residual activity of insecticidal compounds and their formulations depends not only on the intrinsic persistency of the chemical but also on its effectiveness viz. the biological action on the target insect. The latter varies considerably in relation to the type and composition of the sprayed surface. Thus on porous walls made of unbaked clay or mud (adobe) the phenomenon of sorption interferes with the effectiveness of some insecticides incorporated into water-dispersible powders. This is the case of DDT which lasts much longer on non-porous surfaces (e.g. wood) than on mud; on the other hand HCH may be effective even after sorption through its fumigant action. Organophosphorus insectides formulated as water-dispersible powders may be less effective on sorptive walls after a few weeks.

All houses within the area to be protected should receive the appropriate dose of the insecticide before the start of the transmission season and at agreed intervals. The usual doses of insecticides (e.g DDT at 2 g/m^2 every 6 months) though widely applicable, may vary somewhat depending on local conditions. The insecticide must be applied to the indoor walls and ceilings surfaces of all inhabited rooms and also animal shelters. Heavy furniture in the rooms must also be sprayed, particularly the back of it, close to the walls. Where wall surfaces and furniture are of good quality, emulsions or solutions of insecticides should be used rather than suspensions of water-dispersible powders, which leave a whitish deposit (Tables 18 and 19).

Space spraying

In spite of the tremendous success of the technique of residual insecticide spraying the method of space dispersion of fast acting compounds is still of value. A degree of local control of mosquitos (and other flying insects) may be achieved by 'space-spraying', viz. by releasing the insecticides into the air as smoke, fumigants or as fine droplets. Naturally such measures of protection must be frequently repeated to result in any significant effect. However, in epidemics of insect-borne diseases the 'space spraying' technique can rapidly reduce the numbers of mosquitos not only in dwellings but also in outside breeding grounds.

Table 18

Insecticides suitable as residual spray applications for control of Anopheles vectors of malaria

Insecticide	Dosage in grams per m^2	Average duration of effectiveness in months	Remarks
DDT	2.0	6–12	In some conditions 1.0g/m^2 may be used
HCH (Lindane)	0.5	3	In special conditions
Dieldrin	0.5	6–12	Now rarely used
Malathion	2.0	3	Widely used
Propoxur	2.0	3	More expensive than other compounds
Fenitrothion	2.0	3	Reasonably safe when usual precautions are observed. Expensive.

EQUIPMENT FOR MALARIA CONTROL BY IMAGICIDAL METHODS

Space-spraying equipment

The simplest hand operated atomisers (e.g. Flit-guns), used for space spraying of pyrethrum solutions of bedrooms in the evening, need no elaborate description. They are composed of a pump, container and nozzle; they are often crudely made and easily damaged. The spray they produce is usually coarse and much of the insecticidal solution is wasted. Some better sprayers have, instead of an intermittent, a continuous action which produces finer droplets, and are more effective. In using the simple sprayers it is important to keep the nozzle upward during the operation and to start with the corners of the room, finishing in the centre. If there is a mosquito net over the bed of the treated room, the net should be fitted over the bed before spraying; a few strokes should also be directed over the sides of the bed-net. Moreover one should be certain that the solution of insecticide (usually about 0.05–0.1% of pyrethrum extract in kerosene with various synergists) is of good quality. The number of strokes required depends on the size of the room and the type of insecticide solution but on the average about 10 ml per 30 m^3 (about 1000 cubic feet) of space are generally adequate. To obtain the best effect of space-spraying the room should be closed during application and for 10–15 minutes after.

Pressurized aerosol dispensers and smokes

At the present time the hand operated pumps have been largely replaced by aerosol dispensers, which contain liquid insecticides under pressure of a liquefied gas. The amount of pressure and the size of the orifice of the container determine the rate of discharge of the liquid and its droplet size. The time required to produce an effective dosage of the insecticidal solution for a given volume of space is indicated by the manufacturers, though it averages 3–5 seconds per 30 m^3. The aerosol dispensers must be always operated in an upright position and kept away from excessive heat.

Smokes are special types of aerosols produced by a chemical mixed with an insecticide compound. Mosquito coils containing pyrethrum are produced in large numbers in eastern Asia. Each coil consists of a flat spiral of material which will smoulder slowly when lit; it releases smoke which deters mosquitos from entering the room and prevents them from biting. These coils are made of a vegetable filler, a starch binding agent and contain 0.1–0.4% of natural or synthetic pyrethrins.

Other smoke generators such as 'HCH bombs' for outdoor use are of limited value since a proportion of the insecticide is decomposed by the heat.

Aerosol generators and mist-blowers

There are several types of machines for production of insecticidal aerosols. In some of them the atomised insecticide solution is introduced into a hot stream of air and further dispersed to produce thermal aerosols. One of these machines (Swingfog) is portable and operates on a pulse jet system (Fig. 64). Other types use the principle of dispersion of liquid by discs rotating at a very high speed. The centrifugal force thus created breaks up the solution of the insecticide into very fine droplets about 10–20 microns of volume median diameter (VMD). Vehicle mounted aerosol generators are particularly useful in reducing the numbers of adult mosquitos in urban and suburban areas with adequate access roads. Where roads are inadequate hand-carried or knapsack type aerosol generators are available. For adequate

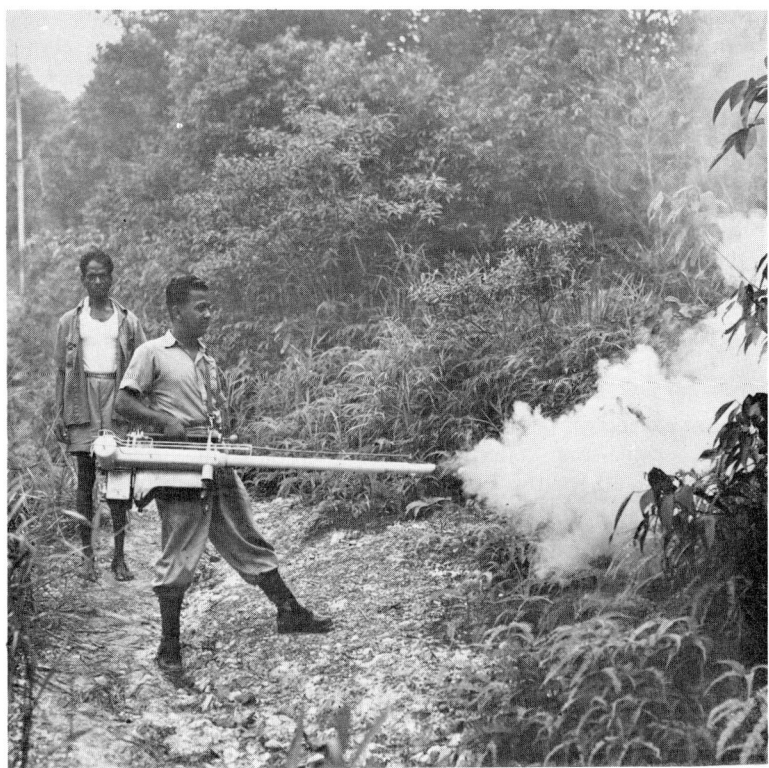

Fig 64 Outdoor control of mosquitos by space spraying in a rural area of Singapore, using dieldrin and a portable 'Swingfog' fogging machine. (Shell Co. photograph)

coverage inside open houses and other buildings the vehicle mounted equipment should be capable of discharging an aerosol cloud on either side of the vehicle; this discharge should extend more than 8 metres from the vehicle. For outdoor space treatment a swath at 100 metres interval should be achieved by wind dispersal of the cloud. Great strides have now been made in the design of motorised knapsack mist-blowers, in which a 2-stroke engine drives a blower to produce a high velocity airstream into which the insecticide is introduced. The spray operator walks along the street directing the lance of the mist-blower through the doors or windows.

Recently the ultra low volume (ULV) technique of applying insecticides proved to be a useful and economical method of temporary control of adult mosquitos. This method is based on the production by special machines of insecticide droplets of 5–10 microns diameter for ground aerosols and 10–25 microns diameter for aerial sprays.

The great advantage of the ULV technique is that the total amount of insecticide distributed per unit area is the same as or slightly less than used in thermal fogging, while the total volume of the carrier is very much less. Thus about 0.5–1.0 litres of the liquid carrier per hectare are sufficient and this results in great savings in materials and labour involved.

Both thermal fogging and ULV spraying should be undertaken preferably at dawn or in the late evening because of thermal currents that build up during the day. The area to be treated should be divided into sections related to the desired frequency of spraying. ULV methods can cover a much greater area in a given time than a thermal fogging unit.

Aircraft

Aerial space sprays are commonly used in agricultural practice and also occasionally in malaria control. There are a number of aircraft specially suited for this purpose. Two different principles are employed. The solution of insecticide may be pumped or gravity-fed into a boom with nozzles along it. The spray so produced is further broken up by the slipstream of the aircraft or by a rotary atomiser. An alternative system, in which the insecticide is introduced into the exhaust of the aircraft's engine to produce a thermal aerosol, is less favoured because of some decomposition of the active compound. At the present time the use of ULV atomisers has been generally adopted. Helicopters are increasingly used because of the downdraught of this aircraft and better distribution of the spray. As mentioned before aerosol generating machines and aircraft are of particular value when rapid elimination of mosquitos from a relatively small area is needed, as in the case of epidemic outbreaks of a vector borne disease.

Several types of atomisers are used for ULV spraying. The most widely employed consist of a metal gauze cylinder rotating around a fixed spindle, which is attached to a bracket on the aircraft wing or to a boom designed for helicopter operation. The rotating power comes from the slipstream through a fan clamped in a hub that carries the bearing assembly. The pitch of the fan blades is adjustable and this controls the particle size of the insecticide solution, introduced through the hollow spindle under pressure and dispersed by a diffuser tube over the rotating gauze of the cylinder. Normally 4–6 of such units are mounted on the aircraft. Another type of ULV atomiser uses an electrically driven rotating multi-disc. In this type the particle size is independent of the speed of the aircraft; such atomisers are particularly suited for low speed helicopter operations.

Aircraft have been used for aerial application of pesticides for the past 50 years but only recently on a larger scale. The early aircraft used principally for agricultural spraying were standard military or commercial planes fitted with a tank and a boom. In the USA the Stearman (PT-17), in the UK and Canada the DHC-2 (Beaver) and in the USSR the Antonov (An-2M) were commonly employed. Except in an absolutely flat country four-engined piston-driven aircraft have to fly much higher than twin-engined planes. Spraying at high levels produces a wide but uneven dispersion of insecticide and a relatively small aircraft designed specifically for pesticide spraying is greatly superior. The Piper Pawnee (PA-25) is now the most popular but further developments in this field are in progress. The present technique of aerial spraying tends to decrease the size of the spray drops while maintaining the concentration in order to get the spray to drift across wide swaths (ULV drift-spraying). For large size spraying programmes such as the tsetse and locust control the Avro Anson was widely used, but now Piper Aztec, Beechcraft Baron, Cessna 310 and Britten-Norman Islander are increasingly popular. For vector control aircraft need higher operating speeds (80–120 m.p.h. = 130–190 km.p.h.) than for agricultural work and thus must have special navigational instruments, flow meters and a 'black box' to record all the information on airspeeds and height. The spraying equipment should be an integral part of the aircraft. Trials of small size hovercraft are in progress.

Residual spraying equipment

Most of the residual insecticidal spraying for control of Anopheles is carried out now by means of compression sprayers. However, in some parts of the world the much simpler and cheaper *stirrup-pumps* or bucket-sprayers have been extensively used in the past and may still be of value. These pumps consist of a bucket containing the liquid to be sprayed and a pump with a double-acting piston operated manually. A hose attached to the pump leads to the spraying lance ending with a nozzle (Fig. 65). Obviously this equipment must be operated by two persons: one working the pump and the other directing the spray lance. Moreover the pressures are highly erratic and do not make for even application. Nevertheless stirrup-pumps are adequate for use in malaria control if no other sprayers are available.

The *compression sprayer* is universally regarded as standard equipment for residual insecticide spraying (Fig. 66). This type of sprayer consists of a cylindrical tank about 9–13 litres (2–3 gallons) capacity in which the liquid insecticide formulation (usually a suspension of water-dispersible powder) is contained. The internal pressure in the tank is raised by a hand-operated pump incorporated in the sprayer. It is fitted with a hose, a cut-off valve, a lance and a nozzle. Some types of sprayers have also a constant pressure valve and a pressure gauge. One or more straps are attached for carrying the sprayer. This equipment is designed to produce a uniform insecticide dosage on sprayed surfaces and to be simple, robust and durable so that it can be used by spraymen

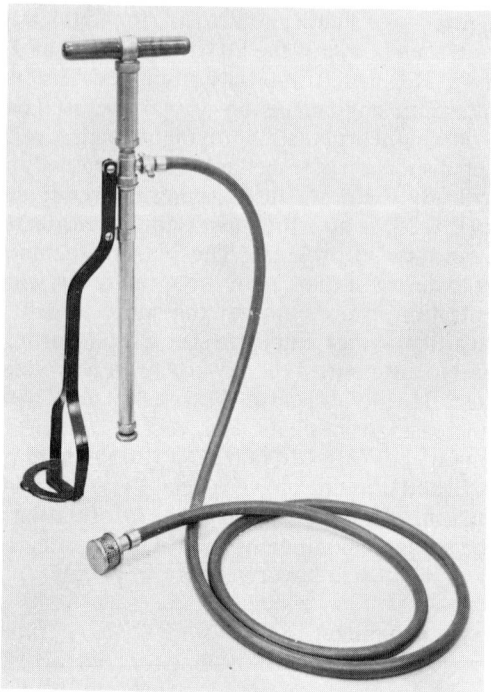

Fig 65 Stirrup pump, a simple and robust type of sprayer used for residual indoor spraying of insecticides. (Wellcome Museum of Medical Science)

with elementary technical knowledge. The important requirement is a controllable and uniform nozzle discharge rate. Nozzle spray patterns of different forms have been tried, the flat-fan shape being favoured because it facilitates the application of parallel, vertical spraying swaths on interior surfaces.

In practice the rate of application of an insecticide is regulated by three controlling factors: its concentration in the liquid carrier, the nozzle discharge rate and the speed of spraying.

The generally recommended operating pressure in the delivery lance and nozzle to give the most efficient application is 2.8 kg/cm^2 (40 lb per in^2). To maintain this pressure until the sprayer is empty, after a single filling and pumping, involves a higher pressure in the tank and a pressure control valve in the lance. The required cylinder pressure may be achieved by a given number of strokes of the pump or more accurately-read from a pressure gauge (Fig. 67).

The ideal nozzle to ensure uniformity of application is one delivering a fan-type spray, with a spray angle of 80° and an output of 0.76 litres

Rationale and Technique of Malaria Control

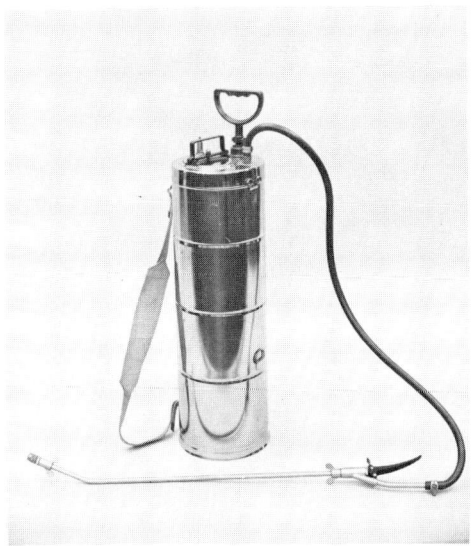

Fig 66 Compression sprayer, a standard type of equipment for residual insecticide spraying in malaria control and eradication programmes. (Wellcome Museum of Medical Science)

(0.18 gallons) per minute at the standard pressure. Held at a distance of 45 cm (18 inches) from the surface to be sprayed, such a nozzle will deposit a swath of spray 75 cm (30 inches) wide, of which the middle half is effective. In practice, therefore, the marginal 18–20 cm of one swath should be overlapped by the margin of the next swath to produce a uniform deposit.

Important from the standpoint of spraying efficiency is frequent and regular maintenance of sprayers, in particular the replacement of worn washers, pressure hose, nozzles and hose clips.

Irregularities in spraying and uneven dosage are due in part to faults of the operator, and in part to faults of apparatus. The first can be overcome by thorough training in which the operator is taught how to apply a standard dose, usually 4.5 litres to 100 m^2 (1 gallon to 1000 ft^2) of surface, with complete regularity. The training having been given, supervision must continue to ensure its maintenance. The principal faults in maintenance are wear in the nozzle, and fall of pressure as the quantity of fluid in the tank decreases. The ordinary brass nozzle may wear very quickly, particularly when wettable powders are used because their composition may be abrasive. The nozzle should be made of very hard material, for which various metal alloys and ceramic materials are used.

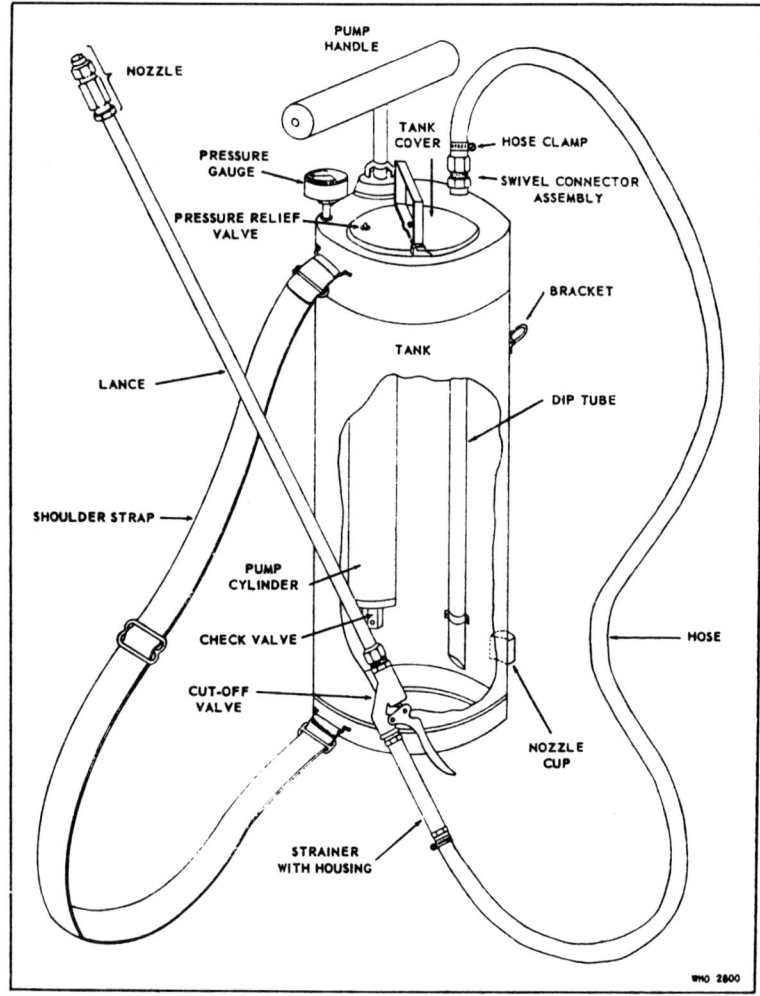

Fig 67 Standard type of compression sprayer and its component parts. (WHO, 1963)

An essential requirement of spraying equipment is that it should be of a standard type, constructed of durable materials, with a standard lance and a cut-off valve which does not leak, thus ensuring uniform application of insecticide with minimal risks of toxicity to spraymen. It is also important to make provision ahead for sufficient supplies of equipment and for ample spare parts and replacements to be available at all field depots. At least one man in each spraying team should be trained in the maintenance of equipment.

Rationale and Technique of Malaria Control

TECHNIQUE OF RESIDUAL SPRAYING

In view of the importance of correct technique for the successful application of residual insecticides some details of the relevant practice may be of value.

The basic field unit for carrying out a spraying operation is a *spraying squad* which consists of two to six spraymen and a squad leader. The pre-determined area of work and itinerary must be established in advance. The task of the spraymen consists of proper application of the insecticide formulation to all sprayable surfaces of all the dwelling units and other premises in the locality. This must often include animal sheds and temporary field shelters, away from the centre of the village. Knowledge of the number, location and accessibility of the houses and field shelters is of great importance and this is the real aim of *geographical reconnaissance*, which should be carried out during the preparatory phase of the programme and kept up to date as much as possible. This activity should also take care of the numbering of houses and of measuring their average sprayable surface, to estimate the requirement of insecticide and manpower (Fig. 68).

In applying residual spraying the indoor surface must be covered

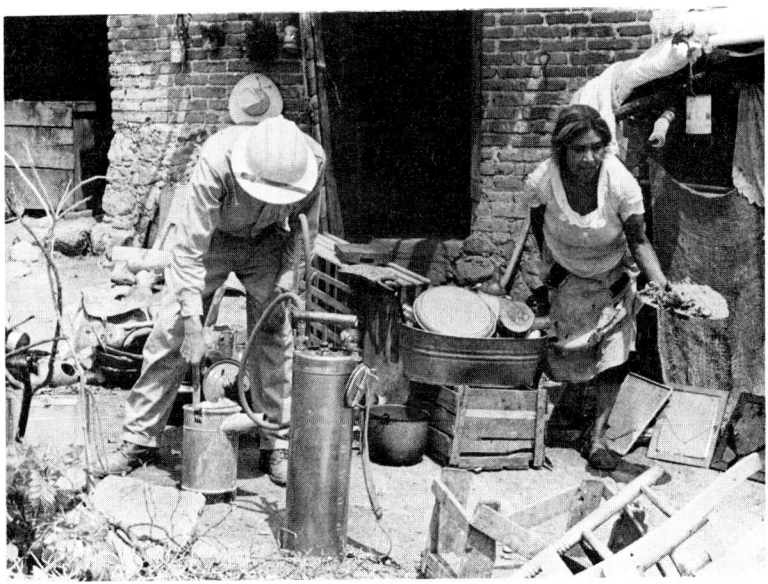

Fig 68 Temporary removal of part of the furniture and food supplies from dwellings before residual spraying begins. The assistance of local inhabitants in this procedure is an important factor of co-operation with the spraying squad. (WHO photograph by E. Schwab)

Table 19

Quantities of formulations for standard residual spraying[1]

Insecticide	Formulation	Active insecticide content	Dilution required for field use[2]	Remarks
DDT	Water-dispersible powder	50%	90 g per litre (14 oz per gallon)	Imperial gallons (4.5 litres) throughout
DDT	Water-dispersible powder	75%	60 g per litre (9.5 oz per gallon)	
DDT	Liquid concentrate	20%	1 part to 3½ parts of kerosene or water	Kerosene for solutions, water for emulsion concentrates
Hexachloro-cyclohexane (HCH)	Water-dispersible powder	25%	40 g per litre (6 oz per gallon)	
Hexachloro-cyclohexane (HCH)	Water-dispersible powder	50%	20 g per litre (3 oz per gallon)	
Hexachloro-cyclohexane (HCH)	Liquid concentrate	20%	1 part to 22 parts of kerosene or water	Kerosene for solutions, water for emulsion concentrates
Dieldrin	Water-dispersible powder	50%	26 g per litre (4.2 oz per gallon)	Now rarely used
Malathion	Water-dispersible powder	50§	90 g per litre (14 oz per gallon of water)	
Malathion	Water-dispersible powder	25%	180 g per litre (28 oz per gallon)	For dosage of 1 g per m² add twice the amount of water
Malathion	Emulsion concentrate	20%	1 part to 4 parts of water	

[1] This table indicates the quantity of different formulations required to prepare one gallon (4.5 litres) of spray dilution applied using a sprayer with the average application rate of one gallon per 1000 square feet of surface (4.5–5.0 litres per 100m²) to obtain the usual application rates of DDT 2 g per m², HCH 0.5 g per m², Dieldrin 0.5 g per m² and Malathion 2 g per m².

[2] The generally used standard type of sprayer operating at the recommended pressure and with the usual nozzle aperture allows the sprayman to cover 1000 square

evenly at the required dosage. The spray should be applied so that there are no gaps in the treated surface. The walls and the ceiling should be thoroughly wetted but not so much as to cause the suspension to run down.

The spraying is done at stated intervals. The operation of spraying in one locality is known as the *spraying round*, while the spraying of all houses in a given area, repeated at regular intervals, is known as the *spraying cycle*. Focal spraying is limited to a group of houses forming a distinct focus of transmission. The progress of spraying operations is measured by comparing the number of houses sprayed and localities with the totals included in the programme. Special measures are put into action to ensure the complete spraying of all houses, localities and the area involved. This objective of '*total coverage*' is of particular importance in malaria eradication campaigns.

Proper spraying depends on good training and is best carried out by men continuously employed at it; men working in a squad produce the best results. Much of the successful work is done by squads carried by a truck together with their supplies. The extent of the population which

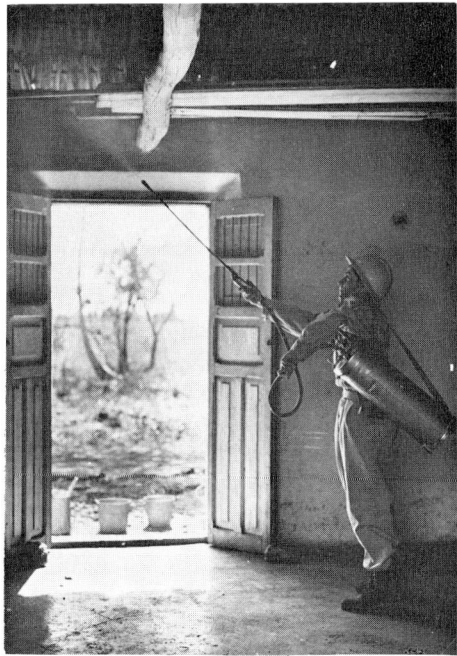

Fig 69 Residual house spraying as carried out in the state of Yucatán in Mexico. (WHO photograph by P. Almasy).

can be protected by a squad varies with local conditions, such as distance and nature of housing, but is commonly of the order of 20 000 to 30 000 people. After preliminary planning and trial each successive day's work is followed precisely. The average area which can be sprayed comfortably in one day by one sprayman appears to be of the order of 2500 square metres, or 10 sprayer charges of 10 litres each. However, this limit may extend to near 4000 square metres per day in areas with favourable field conditions (with high population concentration, good roads and communications) or to around 1000 square metres in areas with adverse field conditions. The support of local population is essential; the people in an area to be treated are usually given adequate warning of the day and time of spraying, being asked to arrange that houses are open, foodstuffs removed or covered, and furniture pulled out into the middle of the rooms. Spraymen must be accompanied by a responsible local resident whose main function is to secure co-operation and vouch for the safety of persons and property in the houses treated as without their support future work may be hampered by misunderstandings. After spraying, a printed form should be left on the indoor wall of the house, with the date of spraying and the date of next visit, which gives needed information to inspectors checking the work and to the householder about provision for the next spraying (Fig. 69).

The public response may be that of suspicion in the early stages, but this soon gives way to active co-operation when the benefits of treatment become apparent, and for the most part such schemes run smoothly.

RESISTANCE OF MOSQUITOS TO INSECTICIDES

General considerations

Resistance to insecticides has been defined as the 'ability of a population of insects to tolerate doses of an insecticide which would prove lethal to the majority of individuals in a normal population of the same species'. It is understood that this biological phenomenon develops as a result of selection pressure by the relevant insecticidal compound or its analogue.

The above definition refers to what is known as *physiological resistance* affecting the direct mortality of a proportion of a population of insects exposed to the toxic compound. Another, different, aspect of this phenomenon is the change of behaviour pattern of a population of insects, so that they acquire the ability to avoid contact with the insecticide. This phenomenon is known under the term '*behaviouristic resistance*' or '*insecticide avoidance*'.

Both types of resistance may interfere with the results of malaria control measures, especially when the main method comprises residual insecticide spraying. However, the 'physiological resistance' is by far the most important of the two and more easily measurable.

Although the resistance of Anopheles to DDT was recognised as a potentially serious problem already 25 years ago, the impact of this phenomenon on malaria control and eradication has become fully obvious only during the past decade. It is now fully acknowledged that insecticide resistance is one of the major obstacles in the struggle against vector borne diseases. The extension of resistance from DDT to other chlorinated hydrocarbons (HCH and dieldrin) led to giving up these efficient and cheap compounds in many parts of the world. The alternative use of organophosphorus and carbamate insecticides proved to be expensive and few developing tropical countries are able to afford it without external help. Moreover, in some countries mosquito vectors have developed a degree of resistance to several newer insecticides, and particularly those widely used in agriculture. Research on and development of new insecticidal compounds is expensive and increasingly difficult so that the possibility of having in the immediate future a vast array of valuable compounds is not very likely. Nevertheless even in the present, less than satisfactory, situation the available insecticides, if properly used, can still play a major role in the decrease of malaria transmission.

Nature and cause of resistance

Much research in the laboratory and in the field has been devoted to our understanding of the nature and mechanism of the development of resistance. Only the briefest review of this complex problem can be given here.

The multiple factors that influence the development of resistance to insecticides in a population of mosquitos can be classified into genetic (e.g. presence of a specific genes and their frequency), operational (e.g. type of insecticide and its method of application) and biological (e.g. size and characteristics of the insect population).

Resistance to insecticides arises not through a process of gradual adaptation of mosquitos to a toxic compound. It is a speeded up process of selection, which can occur only when in the original population of mosquitos there was a small proportion of individuals genetically endowed with the capacity to withstand, at least partly, the toxic action of the insecticidal compound. Individuals within the relevant mosquito population which are susceptible to the insecticidal action are gradually killed off and thus the proportion of resistant mosquitos is able to increase, often very rapidly. At one stage there are only two groups within the mosquito population under insecticidal pressure: pure resistant individuals and hybrids between the resistant and susceptible strains. Finally almost all individuals within the given population are resistant.

Some types of resistance are due to one single gene while other types are related to several genes. Studies which revealed that certain types of resistance can be assigned to specific loci on chromosomes of relevant mosquitos, allowed to distinguish between different biochemical mechanisms of resistance. While some such mechanisms involve detoxification by enzymatic processes of the chemical compound, other mechanisms are due to the change of the site of the toxic action or reduced penetration.

A distinction between monogenic resistance and the more complex polygenic type is important as the former type is more amenable to countermeasures such as the addition of synergists or change to a different insecticide.

There appear to be two main forms of the capacity of resistance mosquitos to break down or otherwise to neutralise certain groups of chemical insecticides. DDT and some closely allied compounds is in one group, while HCH and dieldrin are in the other. The selection of a strain of mosquito species which is resistant to dieldrin results in that strain being resistant to HCH and vice versa. Conversely a strain resistant to DDT is initially susceptible to HCH and dieldrin. However, some strains of mosquito have appeared which are resistant to both groups of insecticides and even to the newer organophosphorus compounds.

When resistance due to the selection of one or more genes by a certain insecticide extends to other chemical compounds we are dealing with the phenomenon of *cross resistance*. The spectrum of cross-resistance may be narrow as in the case of the cyclodiene group (HCH – dieldrin) or it may be wide, covering also other groups (e.g. organophosphorus compounds).

Resistance to dieldrin (and HCH) is more common and develops more rapidly than does DDT resistance, because the former is of a higher degree and since the gene for dieldrin resistance is fully or partially dominant. On the other hand the DDT resistance is of a lower degree and recessive in its genetic expression. If the type of resistance in the anopheline population to be controlled is unknown it is preferable to use DDT rather than dieldrin or HCH. Even if DDT resistance in Anopheles is confirmed, its development may be slow and the continued use of DDT may still have a sufficient impact on the mosquito population to achieve a fair degree of control. In any case of suspected resistance a definite proof of it by competent specialists should be sought.

When resistance to both groups of chlorinated hydrocarbons occurs it may be necessary to change either to one of the organophosphorus compounds or to a carbamate. Although there are some cases of cross-resistance between these two groups this is uncommon and usually one may employ one or the other of these compounds as an

Table 20

Insecticide resistance in some important species of Anopheles vectors of malaria as reported by the WHO in 1977

Species	DDT	Dieldrin-HCH	Organophosphorus compounds	Carbamates
A. aconitus	+	+	−	−
A. albimanus	+	+	+	+
A. albitarsis	+	+	−	−
A. annularis	+	+	−	−
A. aquasalis	−	+	−	−
A. atroparvus	−	+	−	−
A. culicifacies	+	+	+	−
A. farauti	−	+	−	−
A. flavirostris	−	+	−	−
A. fluviatilis	+	+	−	−
A. funestus	−	+	−	−
A. gambiae	+	+	−	−
A. hyrcanus	+	+	+	−
A. labranchiae	+	+	−	−
A. messeae	+	+	+	−
A. minimus	−	+	−	−
A. multicolor	+	+	−	−
A. pharoensis	+	+	−	−
A. philippinensis	+	+	−	−
A. pseudopunctipennis	+	+	−	−
A. pulcherrimus	+	+	−	−
A. quadrimaculatus	+	+	−	−
A. sacharovi	+	+	+	+
A. sergenti	−	+	−	−
A. sinensis	+	+	+	−
A. stephensi	+	+	+	−
A. subpictus	+	+	−	−
A. sundaicus	+	+	−	−
A. vagus	+	+	−	−

Note: This list based on the data provided in the WHO Technical Report Series No 585 (1976) refers only to the most important Anopheles species, vectors of malaria. It should be remembered that in each of species quoted the phenomenon of resistance and its degree do not cover the whole geographical area of distribution of the species concerned.

alternative insecticide, although its effectiveness may be time-limited.

In spite of our fair knowledge of the problem, the nature of the possible extension of resistance to various insecticides cannot be predicted.

Determination of resistance

The standardised WHO method entails a comparison of mortality of a number of female Anopheles of a known species exposed in special tubes to filter papers impregnated with various concentrations of a given insecticide dissolved in mineral oil (Fig. 70). After a determined time of exposure the mosquitos are transferred to a clean tube. Their mortality is checked after 24 hours and the results are plotted on a graph. A simplified method of monitoring for early detection of resistance uses a pre-determined diagnostic concentration of a given insecticide which has the high probability of killing all susceptible mosquitos. On this basis the proportion of survivors indicates the degree of resistance.

Appropriate test kits for determination of susceptibility or resistance are issued by the World Health Organization, which also circulates periodically the latest reports on findings in the field.

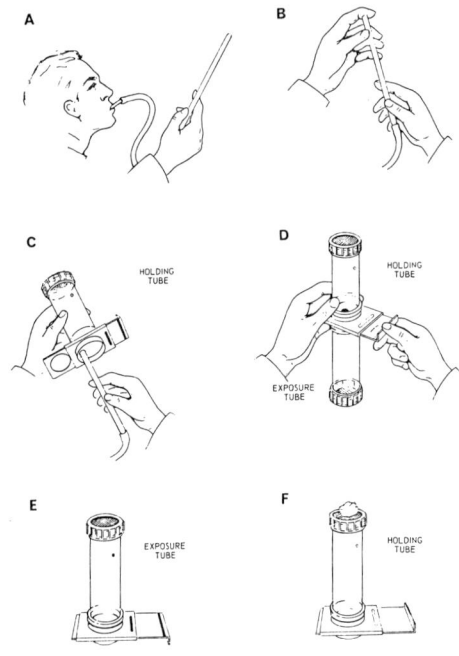

Fig 70 Method for determining the susceptibility or resistance of adult mosquitos.
Note: Mosquitos are collected by means of an aspirator (A) and (B); they are then transferred to a special plastic holding tube (C); a plastic exposure tube lined with insecticide-impregnated paper is then connected with the holding tube and the mosquitos are transferred to the exposure tube through a hole in the slide between the two tubes (D). The slide is closed and the exposure tube is allowed to stand upright for the determined period (E); after the exposure period the mosquitos are transferred back to the holding tube, which should stand upright for 24 hours, with a piece of moist cotton wool on the gauze end (F). Counts of dead mosquitos killed by the contact with the insecticide are made at the end of this recovery period. (WHO 1970 Technical Report Series, No. 443)

PRESENT STATE OF RESISTANCE TO INSECTICIDES IN MALARIA VECTORS

In 1946 only two species of Anopheles were resistant to DDT, but by 1976 a total of 43 anopheline species showed a degree of resistance to one or more insecticides. Forty-two were resistant to dieldrin and 24 to DDT, 21 of the latter having developed double resistance. A disquieting development is the appearance in six species of some resistance to one or more organophosphorus compounds. Table 20 indicates the present pattern of resistance in some of the most important vectors of malaria. However, it should be emphasised that usually the resistance does not extend over the whole geographical area of natural distribution of the Anopheles vector and in many cases the available insecticides are still of value in many parts of the world. None the less the status of resistance is changing faster in some countries, slower in others (Fig. 71).

The most important areas of insecticide resistance are at present in West Africa and the Sudan where *A. gambiae* is resistant to DDT and dieldrin, in Central America where *A. albimanus* is resistant to chlorinated hydrocarbons and to malathion, in several countries of western and south-eastern Asia where *A. culicifacies* and *A. stephensi* are resistant to chlorinated hydrocarbons and in Asian Turkey where *A. sacharovi* developed resistance to most of the commonly used compounds (Table 20).

Tactics of malaria control to counteract insecticide resistance

As mentioned previously the development of resistance to insecticides was related to two causal factors: 1. The biological characteristics of the species and population of Anopheles and 2. The type and degree of selection pressure of the insecticide. Our knowledge of all aspects of the first factor is inadequate to have much effect on alternative methods of control. On the other hand there are a number of ways in which operational measure may be of considerable usefulness.

In view of the fact that contamination of mosquito breeding sites by extensive use of agricultural pesticides often leads to marked resistance of Anopheles vectors, the co-ordination of antimalaria activities with other schemes, based on the outdoor use of pesticides, is desirable.

The next objective is the judicious use of alternative methods of vector control such as source reduction, environmental or biological means, in preference to relying on the use of synthetic insecticides. Such selection and alternation of various types of mosquito control is often defined as *integrated control*: this approach is most likely to succeed over long periods. In several countries, and particularly in Japan, Hawaii and in Italy larvicidal treatment of ponds with an

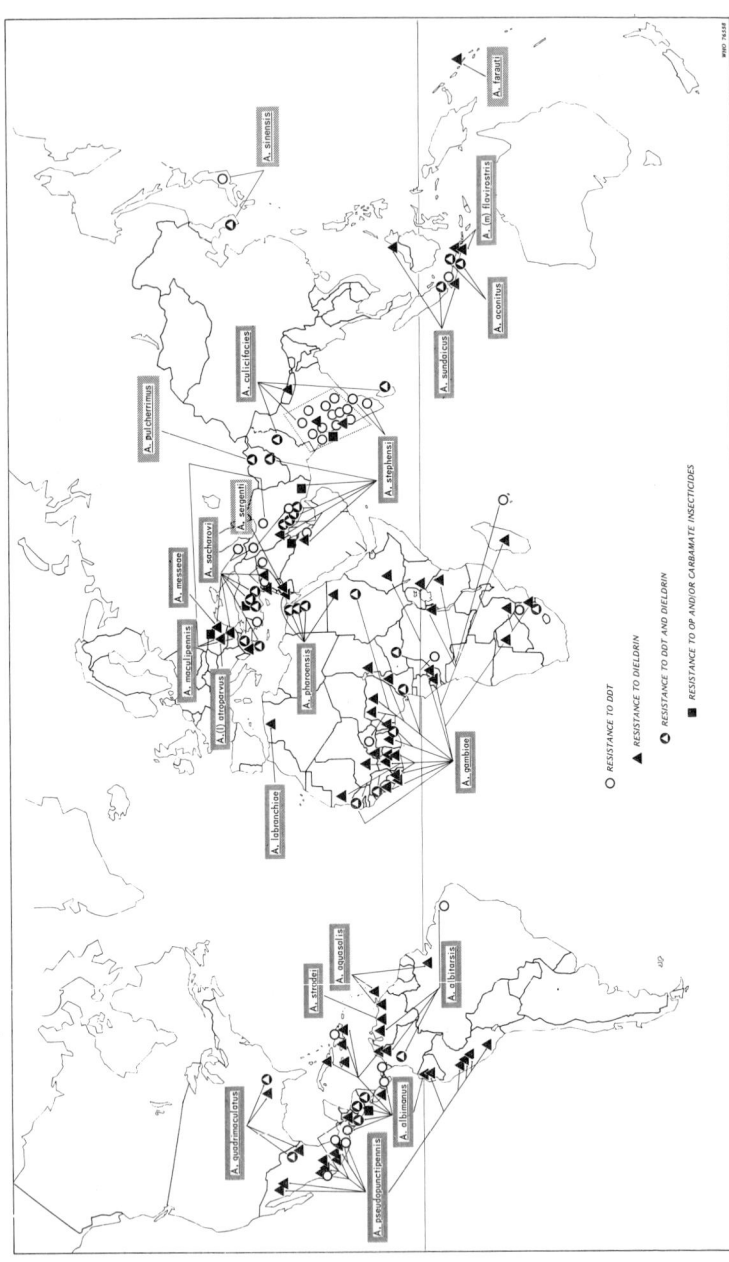

Fig 71 Geographical distribution of resistance of main vectors of malaria to four groups of insecticides, according to WHO data

appropriate insecticide is sequentially combined with naturalistic control methods including the use of larvivorous fish.

Thirdly, whenever the use of insecticides is unavoidable, the type, dosage and cycle of their application should be such that only the vector population involved in the transmission of malaria is affected.

When the presence and degree of resistance of malaria vectors in the area have been confirmed, the only solution is to change to a different insecticide, taking into account the operational and financial consequences of this decision. These could be considerable since in some cases the substitution of malathion for DDT may increase the cost of the spraying campaign about 4 times.

The importance of consequent monitoring the progress of malaria control by entomological methods (including testing for resistance by the standardised WHO tests) is obvious. But not less important is the epidemiological evaluation of the impact of the new insecticide on the transmission of malaria and the application of chemotherapeutic measures whenever necessary and feasible.

Alternative insecticides

The great increase of resistance of mosquitos and other disease vectors to chlorinated hydrocarbons and lately also to organophosphates and carbamates has stimulated some attempts to produce compounds of different chemical structure or a new mode of action. However, the rising costs of research and development as also the possibility of resistance against these new insecticides have undermined the confidence of the chemical industry and limited the scientific and industrial effort in this field.

Until now the alternative method of control of anopheline vectors resistant to chlorinated hydrocarbons was to change to malathion or propoxur as imagicides and to use fenthion or temephos as larvicides. However, the substitute compound may not remain useful for very long especially in areas where various insecticides are widely applied in agriculture. This has happened already in cotton growing areas of Central America and in other parts of the world.

Much progress has been achieved in the development of synthetic pyrethroids (e.g. allethrin, resmethrin, tetramethrin etc.) with high toxicity to insect vectors of disease and low toxicity to man. The stability of these compounds has greatly improved and they may soon match the 6-months duration of residual activity of chlorinated hydrocarbons. In some insects such as houseflies resistance to these new compounds has already been observed. Among the new group of chemicals that underwent a series of laboratory trials one should mention the insect development inhibitors. These compounds seem to mimic the action of juvenile hormones of insects and cause death by preventing the metamorphosis of larvae into pupae; other compounds interfere with chitinisation of insects at any instar. Two groups of such chemicals (Dimilin and methoprene) have undergone various tests and are of some promise but their practical value is still uncertain.

SAFE USE OF INSECTICIDES

General principles

All pesticides are in some degree toxic to man and animals. Care in handling them should form an integral part of all public health programmes involving the application of insecticides. Proper precautions must also be observed by anyone handling insecticidal compounds for protection of their houses and immediate environment from mosquitos.

It should be emphasised that there is a difference between the *toxicity* of a given insecticide and the *hazard* that it presents. A measure of potential toxicity of a compound to man and other mammals is the oral or dermal LD_{50} value, viz. the estimate of the amount of the toxicant per kg of body weight required to kill 50% of experimental animals (usually rats) used for testing (Table 21).

The degree of hazard is estimated by the dangers involved when the insecticide is used under the particular conditions of employment.

Thus the factors relevant to hazard depend not only on the intrinsic toxicity of the compound but also on the type of formulation used, concentration of the pesticide in the formulation, method of use,

Table 21

Acute oral and dermal LD_{50} values for female white rats of most common pesticides used in agriculture and public health practice

Compound	Type	Oral LD_{50} in mg/kg	Dermal LD_{50} in mg/kg
DDT	CH	118	2510
Dichlorvos	OP	56	75
Dieldrin	CH	46	60
Fenitrothion	OP	570	350
Fenthion	OP	245	330
HCH (lindane)	CH	91	900
Malathion	OP	1000	>4000
Parathion	OP	3	6.8
Propoxur	C	86	>2400
Pyrethrum	B	200	—
Temephos (Abate)	OP	13 000	>4000

Note: The type of insecticide is indicated by abbreviations: B – botanical, C – carbamate, CH – chlorinated hydrocarbon, OP – organophosphorus compound.

possible contact of pesticide with man or animals, and other practical aspects.

According to Table 21 parathion (an agricultural pesticide) is the most toxic and temephos the least toxic compound when taken by mouth. The apparently low toxicity of malathion may be misleading since some formulations may become toxic in tropical conditions.[1]

Precautions to be observed

In the first instance any vector control campaign must include provision for the safe transport and secure storage of pesticide concentrates. These should not be stored in rooms in which people live or in which food is kept. Protection against theft, misuse, and accessibility to children must be provided. Safe disposal of empty insecticide containers must be taken care of. All pesticide containers should be adequately labelled in a form or language understood by the local operators. All equipment used for distribution of pesticides should conform to the WHO recommendations with regard to design and manufacture. There should be regular systematic inspection of all equipment to ensure that it is adequate.

Training in the safe use of pesticides should be provided for the supervisory medical and other personnel so that they should recognise the signs and symptoms of accidental poisoning and be able to give immediate treatment in an emergency. Equally important is the training of the foreman and other responsible field operators in the technique of proper spraying, safety precautions and maintenance of protective equipment.

Any extensive spraying should be carried out under adequate supervision. Spraymen should wash, using soap or detergent, at the end of each working day and whenever the insecticide is spilled in quantity on the skin or clothes. Spraymen should not smoke or eat while on duty, or after duty unless they first wash their hands. Insecticide should be scooped out with proper implements and not by hand.

Protective equipment

There are various items of protective equipment that should be used

---

[1] The increased use of malathion coincided with the increase of the number of manufacturers of this insecticide and as a result of this certain formulations of malathion underwent some changes, which gave rise to the presence of iso-malathion, a modified component with high toxicity to man. This led to serious toxic effects on the personnel handling the product, and underlined the fact that certain compounds can potentiate the toxicity of malathion in mammals by inhibiting the normal detoxification mechanism. The incident was caused by prolonged storage of some malathion formulations in tropical conditions and stressed the need to observe all the usual precautionary measures, even with insecticides of relatively low toxicity.

by field staff directly involved in insecticide spraying. The most important of these are the following:

Hats – these should be of impervious material with a broad brim to protect face and neck.

Veils – a plastic mesh net loosely attached to the hat will give protection from large drops of spray and permit sufficient visibility.

Overalls – should be of light, durable cotton fabric; they should be washed regularly with soap or detergent.

Aprons – of rubber or plastic will protect from liquid concentrates.

Impervious gloves, capes, respirators and rubber boots are often advised but they are seldom acceptable in tropical countries (Fig. 72).

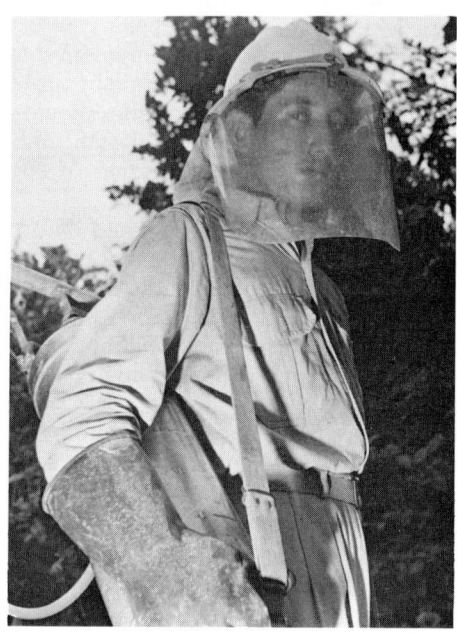

Fig 72 Sprayman employed by the Malaria Eradication Programme in Mexico wearing full protective clothing. (WHO photograph by E. Schwab)

Greater risk occurs when handling oil solutions, such as concentrates or emulsions, which should be poured through threaded taps, or by pumps arranged to prevent contact of the solution with the skin.

Emergency treatment of poisoning by insecticides

With careful handling there is little real risk to the occupants of treated houses, but as a safety measure all foodstuffs should be removed or carefully covered before a house is sprayed. There is some risk to domestic animals, especially with dieldrin, and casualties have occurred amongst cats, which lick their contaminated fur, and chickens which have pecked along the floor near the sprayed walls.

As with all other types of poisoning the emergency treatment of accidental poisoning of human subjects comprises: (a) removal of the toxicant and (b) administration of specific antidotes and maintenance of vital functions such as artificial respiration.

In poisoning by ingestion rapid gastric lavage is needed. Clear the mouth and pharynx of vomit and maintain a patent airway. Place the patient flat on his stomach with his head down and to one side, the tongue pulled forward. Use endotracheal intubation if airway obstruction persists.

If the body is soiled with the insecticide, clothes must be removed and skin cleaned with soap and water. Contamination of eyes must be dealt with by washing with water.

The symptoms of acute poisoning by *chlorinated hydrocarbons* such as DDT, HCH, dieldrin include convulsions followed by an adverse effect on the liver tissue. Acute poisoning due to ingestion should be met by emetics, e.g. a tablespoon of salt in a glass of warm water. Chronic poisoning due to the continued intake of smaller quantities is heralded by nervous symptoms which include hyperexcitability, anxiety and tremors. In addition, there is a very marked loss of appetite which quickly leads to loss of weight. Convulsions should be controlled by high doses of injectable barbiturates, diazepam or paraldehyde. Blood samples for organochlorine levels may be necessary for confirmation of the cause of poisoning but this is a complex analytical procedure. Treatment must not be delayed pending the results of laboratory tests.

Any person who is thought to have suffered toxic effects due to handling chlorinated hydrocarbon insecticides should be removed from risk of contact with the insecticide for a long period – dieldrin is known to persist in the body in toxic amounts for many months, and six months' freedom from further risk should be ensured.

Symptoms of poisoning by *organophosphorus insecticides* are similar in many respects to those of chlorinated hydrocarbon poisoning, but include also giddiness, nausea, vomiting and diarrhoea; excessive sweating and salivation may be present. In severe cases respiratory difficulties, convulsions and loss of consciousness may follow. In such cases artificial respiration by mechanical means may be necessary before the administration of atropine sulphate (2–4 mg) and 1–2 g of a soluble salt of pralidoxime by slow intravenous injection. More atropine (up to 20–50 mg) may be given depending on the severity of symptoms and the response to the first dose. If the patient is cyanotic because of respiratory difficulty, this must be dealt with before further atropine injections are given. Morphine and tranquillizers *must not* be given to persons poisoned by anti-cholinesterase compounds. Organophosphorus insecticides inhibit cholinesterase, one of the vital body enzymes, and blood samples should be taken for cholinesterase determinations before and after the treatment of a case of poisoning. Supplies of atropine should be available in first-aid kits when organophosphorus or carbamate insecticides are being applied and the spraying supervisor should be trained to administer atropine in emergencies. Medical help should be sought immediately if poisoning is suspected. It is advised that people habitually handling these insecticides should have their blood cholinesterase activity checked periodically. Operators should be withdrawn from exposure if this activity decreases by 25% or more from a well-established pre-exposure value.

The insecticidal carbamates give rise to a more rapidly reversible cholinesterase-inhibition complex. This makes it impossible to use estimates of cholinesterase activity as an accurate index of the levels of this enzyme in the tissues. In cases of poisoning by carbamates all the methosed used for treating poisoning by organic phosphorus compounds are useful with one exception: pralidoxime and other oximes are not recommended for routine use. Recovery from carbamate poisoning is usually quite rapid.

Pesticides and the environment

The application of residual insecticides and especially of DDT has been the main factor responsible for eradication of malaria from large parts of the world and the most important method for control of this disease in the tropics. However, anxiety about the pollution of the environment by pesticides increased during the past few years to such an extent that all the virtues of these compounds tend to be forgotten, while their disadvantages receive much sensational publicity.

While it may be true that indiscriminate use of DDT in some parts of the world has had an adverse effect on certain species of wild fauna, several exaggerated restrictions on the use of this and other insecticides have been followed by resurgence of malaria and have jeopardised the search for new compounds.

Naturally, one should reduce as much as possible the contamination of the environment by long lasting insecticides but control of malaria and other insect-borne diseases must be carried out by technical means that are both reliable and economical.

The predominant use of DDT in public health programmes is for control and eradication of malaria. Although over 1500 million people live now in areas where endemic malaria has disappeared not less than 500 million are still exposed to this disease. The continued availability of DDT for malaria control is imperative. Studies carried out under the auspices of the WHO have shown that even high degrees of continuous exposure of DDT in factory workers have not led to any obvious adverse effects.

In human populations where extensive malaria control has been carried out for several years there was an increased amount of DDT storage in fat but no evidence of any deleterious influence on health.

Thus in the final account, in spite of the difficulty of long term studies, there is no indication that the use of DDT should be banned, providing that for malaria control it is limited, as much as possible, to indoor residual spraying which avoids the contamination of the environment.

Other insecticides which are more toxic than DDT undergo much faster degradation and are more acceptable to the ecologist. Their immediate toxicity to man is often very much higher and great attention should be given to the prevention and treatment of accidental poisoning by pesticides.

SELECTION OF METHODS OF MALARIA CONTROL

Malaria control methods vary from the simplest to the most elaborate but the success of the former and the failure of the latter are equally likely if they are applied with what Paul Russell, the great American malariologist, called 'prejudice of experience' due to the blind belief in cherished fetishes.

Sound practice involves consideration of each local problem to determine the logical solution in the light of available knowledge.

This view expressed nearly 30 years ago are of even greater significance today, when as a result of disappointments with some over-ambitious goals of malaria eradication the need for a more flexible though not less important approach to malaria control has become increasingly urgent.

The classification of control measures in relation to the chain of infection includes those that aim at the prevention of the contact of man with the Anopheles vector or at the reduction of the vector population in its larval or adult form. Finally chemotherapeutic means are designed to eliminate malaria parasites in the human host.

Most of these measures can be also considered from both the individual and collective angles (Table 22).

In planning malaria control measures one must not be bound by any standardised methodology but adopt a flexible approach related to local conditions and circumstances. In general we should be guided by the following objectives:

1. Reduction of sickness and mortality to a defined threshold.
2. Organisation of anti-malarial activity according to well defined tasks and management procedures.

3. Maintenance of manpower resources and their training.
4. Provision of financial resources for the setting up and continuation of efficient malaria control.
5. Involvement of the population in anti-malaria activities and assurance of their active co-operation.

A point made in Table 22 and concerning 'man-made malaria' deserves some amplification. It refers to the creation of breeding places of malaria vectors and other mosquitos as a result of human activities. The list of such potential breeding places, which are usually close to human habitations, is very long. It comprises barrels, badly designed or blocked soakaway pits, garden pools, cisterns, disused wells, borrow-pits left by building projects, obstructed drains etc. Much malaria has been due to bad handling of water in irrigation

Table 22

Classification of malaria control measures

Type of measures	Individual protection	Community protection
Prevention of man/vector contact	Repellents, protective clothing, bednets, screening of houses	Site selection, screening of houses
Destruction of adult Anopheles vectors	Use of domestic space sprays including aerosols	Space spraying, ultra low volume sprays, residual insecticide spraying
Destruction of mosquito larvae	Peri-domestic sanitation, intermittent drying of water containers	Larviciding of water surfaces, intermittent drying, sluicing, biological methods
Source reduction of mosquitos	Filling, small scale drainage and other forms of water management	Prevention of man-made malaria, environmental sanitation, water management, drainage schemes, naturalistic methods of control
Measures against the malaria parasites	Diagnosis and early treatment, chemoprophylaxis	Diagnosis and early treatment, mass drug administration
Social participation	Motivation for personal and family protection	Community involvement, health education, expansion of rural health services. Training of staff.

channels, poorly sited ditches, culverts, leaking sluice gates, seepages and fallow rice-fields. No major operations involving water supply should be undertaken without considering their possible impact on malaria and other water-related diseases and requesting appropriate advice on the malaria situation of the area involved and on methods of prevention and control of the disease.

Three principles should be adhered to in all engineering projects in the tropics: the *first* is not to make additional breeding places of mosquitos, the *second* is to know how to correct the errors once made and the *third* is to involve the health authorities from the very beginning of the project.

Malaria control in development projects

Development projects and industrial undertakings in the tropics are often a rife ground for outbreaks of malaria due to the fact that many among a large labour force, comprising newcomers to the area, are either non-immune to the local strains of plasmodia or introduce strains to which local population is particularly susceptible. Moreover, since the living conditions of the labour force may be often less than adequate and the construction activity contributes to the creation of breeding places of mosquitos, conditions for serious epidemics readily exist.

The duty of the resident medical adviser is to foresee the potential dangers, to protect the health of the working force as well as their families and to be ready to act in an emergency.

Selection of a suitable site for new housing, temporary or permanent, may avoid much subsequent difficulty. The principles of this have been described in the earlier section. Such site selection may be vital to the success of many projects, though better methods of control, if available, should be fully used.

Existing breeding places may be dealt with by the use of larvicides, by drainage, or by biological modification of the water to make it unsuitable as a breeding place. It must be carried out within the radius of flight of the local vector, commonly a mile (1.6 km) but more in some places, and throughout the entire transmission season. It must be based on a knowledge of the local vector and particularly of its breeding habits, and on a detailed survey of the area showing all water of the potentially dangerous type within the radius prescribed.

If malaria is prevalent on any scale among the labour force the right policy is to reduce its transmission as soon as possible and at the same eliminate the source of the infection. The best way of doing this is by large scale distribution of appropriate drugs such as proguanil, pyrimethamine, chloroquine or amodiaquine. In parts of the world where resistance of plasmodia to 4-aminoquinolines exists sulphones or sulphonamides with pyrimethamine may be used.

For distribution of chloroquine the work force will have to be mustered and each adult should receive and swallow 2 tablets representing 300 mg base of drug on each of two days during the first week and 300 mg base once a week thereafter. In areas of pronounced seasonal transmission it may be prudent to institute twice weekly administration of the drug during the relevant weeks or months.

An alternative to this regimen is the daily taking of 100 mg of proguanil, but this can be advised mainly for employees who can be trusted to take the drug regularly without supervision. An addition to the standard daily proguanil, a regimen of daily dose of 25 mg of dapsone during the peak transmission period has been successful in south-east Asia. As an alternative pyrimethamine, at the usual single dose of 25 mg, or a combination of pyrimethamine with dapsone may be given once a week in areas where resistance to this compound is absent.

The use of space-spraying of pyrethrum or its synthetic analogues is of limited practical value and the expense of this method is considerable. However, at times noisy and clearly visible applications of thermal or other aerosols has some value, in addition to having a psychological effect which may inspire confidence in the health authorities and increase the co-operation of the population and of administrative echelons.

The regular use of commercial low pressure aerosol containers for disinsectisation of premises of the technical and managerial staff (usually at their own expense) should be encouraged.

For more permanent malaria control residual insecticides should be used. This does not make great demands on manpower; several small schemes could be amalgamated into one. The most economical working unit is a population of between 20 000 and 30 000 people. When amalgamation into units of such size is possible, one skilled assistant can be employed full time on organisation and management. In smaller schemes supervision must be part time, but should not be, for that reason, of minor importance. For the initial rounds of spraying the choice will in most cases be DDT at a dose of 2 g/m^2. This application should be repeated every six months or more often in case of interference with the insecticide deposit on the walls.

Workers should be carefully trained in their use of sprayers and should be practised in the regular and even application of given quantities of fluid, using water only for this training. Even dosage of the spray can be attained by practice, provided that the supervisor himself has taken the trouble to become competent at it. All houses and all animal sheds in the area should be treated, and the whole of the interior surfaces of each should be sprayed unless reliable local experience shows that discrimination between different dwellings is possible

After establishing full control by such means, a revision of pro gramme can be considered. The chief intention will be to prolong the interval between insecticide applications, but before this is contemplated the frequency with which walls are replastered should be carefully examined. If they are often whitewashed or replastered, frequent re-sprayings are essential. In this case the insecticide of choice is DDT at a standard dose or half of it, according to local conditions, to be applied at intervals never exceeding 3–4 months during the malaria transmission season.

After the initial treatment has been operative for one year, transmission of malaria within the treated area should greatly decrease. The size of the treated area and the extent to which people move out of it at nights will clearly affect the resulting incidence of malaria, but in a labour group of 10 000 or more people, the amount of malaria should be reduced to negligible proportions. Prophylactic drugs should be continued until the end of the malaria season. Unless the residual insecticides are properly applied, drugs should be used again during the following season.

Managerial and senior staff should be also protected by residual insecticide spraying. As they normally occupy houses in which the discoloration caused by wettable powders would be objectionable, solutions or emulsions of insecticides should be used. Such houses may well be screened or provided with some screened rooms, and for this purpose it is best to use plastic screen cloth. The use of bed-nets even in screened houses should be encouraged and the importance of regular drug prophylaxis emphasised.

COST OF MALARIA CONTROL IN DEVELOPMENT PROJECTS

The cost of eradication programmes varies considerably in relation to a number of factors such as the type of insecticide, the method involved in its use, the degree of surveillance, the cost of labour, transport, administration etc. Thus it is difficult if not impossible to give any idea of an average cost of a time-limited programme. Nevertheless the cost of activities, which by definition aim at a substantial reduction of the amount of malaria, is more predictable. Thus it should be possible to plan malaria control measures which are within the economic possibilities of the project and could be expanded as economic development proceeds. Malaria control depends for its effectiveness on the regular carrying out of appropriate procedures. This can be assured only if a regular budget is provided and maintained over the whole duration of the project, which should also be so planned that its eventual extension may be beneficial for the future development of the country concerned.

On the basis of available data for a number of countries of Africa and Asia it appeared in the early 1970s that the cost of malaria control was between US $0.30 and US $1.50 per head per year depending on the measures employed and on the degree of supervision required. At the time of this estimate the proportional distribution of costs of the main items of expenditure was as follows: wages and salaries 50%, insecticide (DDT 75% wdp) 33%, transport, fuel, repairs and depreciation 10%, spraying equipment, laboratory and contingencies 7%. The WHO experts who presented this estimate pointed out that unforeseen changes in the cost of materials and labour may alter these proportions considerably. They also indicated that the annual cost of minimal adequate antimalaria measures in tropical Africa calculated for a population of 1 million persons of whom three quarters live in rural areas would come (in 1973) to approximately US $345 000 or US $0.34 per person per year. Of this sum about 60% would have to be spent on rural areas. This calculation comprises vector control measures and distribution of antimalarial drugs.

However, antimalaria activities aiming at interruption of transmission of malaria would be more expensive. Sustained vector control alone in urban areas would cost at least US $0.54 per person per annum while in rural areas the cost would be nearly three times higher.

Generally speaking the average expenditure in extensive programmes involving the protection of a million people is not comparable with the estimation of costs of antimalaria activities aimed at protection of a few thousand people over a limited period, depending on the construction phase of a development project. In the latter case the cost per head per annum would be higher, because of the need for a high degree of performance over a relatively short time. Estimates for such an expenditure depend on the constantly rising cost of imported materials and on local wages and salaries which constitute not less than 50% (and may reach 80%) of total expenditure. Obviously the cost will also depend on the insecticide employed and in areas of DDT resistance the substitution of malathion would double the cost. The method of application is not less important in this respect, ground based simple equipment being much less expensive than aerial spraying. However, where local salaries are high, technically more advanced methods may compare favourably with other ways.

Larviciding operations are uneconomical in areas where the Anopheles breeding is extensive. In these conditions mass drug administration supplemented by residual spraying of houses is the method of choice in development projects or in localities with a sudden influx of settlers. It should be remembered that drug administration to a large population is not the cheapest method. The cost of antimalaria drugs (e.g. 300 mg of chloroquine per adult per week) over a 6 month transmission period would amount to not less than US $0.30 pe person; operational costs may increase this sum by a factor of 2 or 3 per year.

In estimating overall expenditure on malaria control in developing projects the cost of drainage, filling, water management and other semi-permanent measures should not be included in the calculation of the per capita expenses on repetitive measures such as drug distribution or spraying. It goes without saying that the proper organisation of antimalaria activities for a development project demands the availability of competent technical supervisory and executive personnel. Unreasonable budgetary restrictions on trained and experienced staff are a false economy as they jeopardise the very aim of some development projects.

Chapter 10

Malaria Eradication

Soon after the Second World War the World Health Organization recognised that malaria not only killed more people than any other disease but also interfered with the development of agriculture and industry, especially in the new independent countries. The intensive control methods carried out in some western countries and in certain colonial territories gave satisfactory results but could not be applied in many rural tropical areas. The advent of DDT presented the world with a new method of interrupting the transmission of malaria infection by attacking the adult Anopheles vector during its epidemiologically most important stage, when it feeds on man in his dwelling or when it shelters indoors in the nearest house or animal shelter.

The epidemiological concept of the interruption of malaria transmission by residual insecticide spraying is simple. After taking her blood-meal the female Anopheles usually rests on a nearby indoor surface such as a wall, ceiling, etc. for several hours while the blood meal is digested and the batch of eggs matures. Spraying of all inside surfaces of dwellings with a long-lasting insecticide creates conditions in which a substantial proportion of Anopheles would be killed before they could transmit the disease.

This concept proved to be correct as shown on several examples of early campaigns in Italy, Cyprus, Greece, Guyana and Venezuela. It appeared that the widespread use of DDT and other residual insecticides was the most reliable, feasible and economical method for the interruption of transmission. Any remaining foci of malaria could be detected by proper surveillance and eliminated by distribution of antimalarial drugs and local application of insecticides.

This simplified description of the principle of malaria eradication gives only a perfunctory idea of the operational complexity of a large scale programme (Pampana, 1969).

The malaria eradication programme has been defined as an operation aimed at cessation of transmission of malaria and elimination of the reservoir of infected cases in a campaign limited in time and carried to such a degree of perfection that, when it comes to an end, there is no resumption of transmission.

Three main epidemiological principles of malaria eradication can be tersely summarised as follows:
1. Female Anopheles of vector species feed preferably on man, who is the only host of human malaria parasites. Frequency of feeding is

related to the gonotrophic cycle of mosquito (usually every 2–3 days). After feeding the female mosquito rests on surface inside the house to digest the blood.
2. Duration of cycle of development of malaria parasites in the mosquito depends on the temperature. For *P. falciparum* at 26°C about 12 days. During that period there are 4–6 mosquito feeds on man and this increases the chance of mortality of female mosquitos alighting on indoor surfaces with an insecticide deposit.
3. Residual insecticides maintain their toxicity for several months and, as a result of this, the local population of Anopheles decreases its mean longevity to a point when maintenance of transmission becomes impossible and the malaria infection of the community is gradually eliminated. Any remaining foci of infection are dealt with by case detection and treatment.

The substantial differences between malaria control and malaria eradication are given succinctly in Table 23.

Table 23

Differences between malaria control and eradication

	Control	Eradication
Objective	Reduction of incidence until no longer a major public health problem	Cessation of transmission and elimination of the human reservoir of infection
Duration	Indefinite	Limited in time
Area of operation	Only where transmission is intense	All areas where transmission occurs
Total coverage (by spraying and surveillance)	Not necessary	Indispensable
Operational standards	Good	Perfect
Cost	Recurring	Capital investment; after completion no recurring annual cost except for surveillance
Assessment of results	Sampling of population for parasite rates and spleen rates (malariometric surveys)	Case detection (active and passive) in advanced stages. Surveillance procedure
Imported cases	Not relevant	Of concern in advanced stages of the programme

Because of the size and cost of the undertaking a malaria eradication programme is usually organised on a national scale. The planning of a full scale programme presupposes that its practical feasibility has been assured. If there is doubt that the proposed attack measures will stop transmission it must be first tested in a pilot project on a limited scale

The programme is usually carried out over 8 or more years, in four phases (Fig. 73). The phases of the programme are: 1. *Preparatory phase* of one to two years' duration is devoted to geographical reconnaissance of the area, training of field staff, identification and numbering of sprayable houses, collection of equipment and vehicles etc. 2. *The attack phase* during which residual house spraying and other measures aimed at the vector population are instituted so that the principle of 'total coverage' of all premises and areas is observed. The dosage and frequency of spraying depend on local epidemiological conditions. This may be supplemented by chemotherapy. The duration of the attack phase is 4 years or longer.

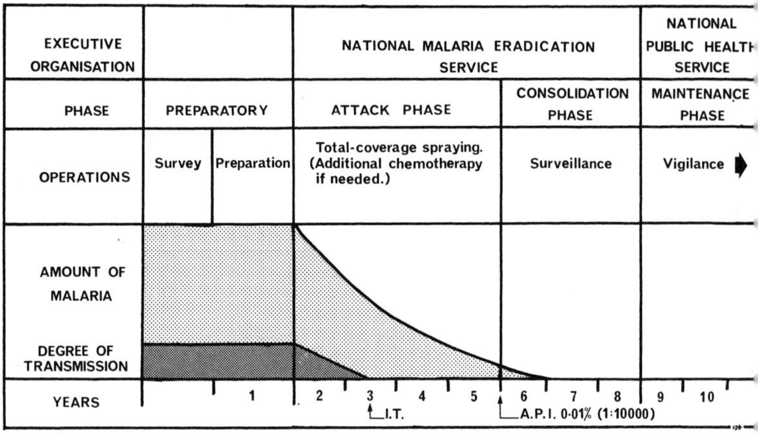

EXECUTIVE ORGANISATION			NATIONAL MALARIA ERADICATION SERVICE		NATIONAL PUBLIC HEALTH SERVICE
PHASE	PREPARATORY		ATTACK PHASE	CONSOLIDATION PHASE	MAINTENANCE PHASE
OPERATIONS	Survey	Preparation	Total-coverage spraying. (Additional chemotherapy if needed.)	Surveillance	Vigilance ▶
AMOUNT OF MALARIA DEGREE OF TRANSMISSION					
YEARS	1	2	3 4 5 ⌊_I.T.	6 7 8 ⌊_A.P.I. 0·01% (1:10000)	9 10

Fig 73 Diagram of theoretical sequence of phases in malaria eradication programmes

The progress of the decrease of transmission is followed by taking blood slides from samples of population to determine the parasite rate according to age-groups. When the parasite rate is below 5% case finding and treatment are instituted. Active case detection is carried out by house-to-house visits at fortnightly intervals; passive case detection is based on reporting from static medical units such as dispensaries and hospitals. For every fever case, a blood slide is taken and presumptive (single dose) treatment is given.

The number of blood slides examined from fever cases in any given area should be not less than 1% of the population for each month of transmission. As the parasite reservoir falls full surveillance is instituted; this comprises, besides case-finding, epidemiological investigation and remedial measures such as radical treatment, focal spraying and mass drug administration.

3. *The consolidation phase* of malaria eradication may begin when the surveillance activity shows that the annual parasite incidence (AIP), which is the proportion of positive slides per 1000 population, is below 0.1 per 1000. However, the receptivity and vulnerability[1] of the area to introduced infections must be considered.

The main activity during this phase is the continuation of surveillance and remedial action to eliminate any foci of transmission. When the results of this activity show that there has been no indigenous case of malaria for three consecutive years the area is ready for entry into the 4. *Maintenance phase* of malaria eradication, providing that there is an adequate organisation capable of undertaking the vigilance activity to prevent the resurgence of endemic malaria. Thus, normally the maintenance of malaria eradication is the responsibility of general health services.

Certification of malaria eradication by the WHO can be and has been requested by several countries. The inspection and review of the accomplishments of the programme are vested in a special certification team acting on behalf of the World Health Organization and subject to its confirmation.

THE PROGRESS OF GLOBAL MALARIA ERADICATION

The worldwide programme of malaria eradication was formally endorsed by the Eighth World Health Assembly in 1955 and in 1957 the WHO took over the coordinating activities and the provision of technical assistance.

The concept of malaria eradication was accepted by all the member governments of the WHO. Previous control programmes were converted to eradication programmes and these were initiated in all malarious countries in the Americas and Europe, and in the majority of countries in Asia and Oceania. But only pilot projects were attempted in Africa.

Today, after two decades of this unique international endeavour in the field of public health, the overall results are of great interest; they justify the original concept and yet show that under some conditions it cannot be put into practice.

---

[1] The WHO definitions of these two terms are as follows: *Receptivity* – abundant presence of vector Anopheles in the area and the existence of ecological and climatic factors favouring the transmission of malaria; *Vulnerability* – proximity to malarious areas or liability to frequent influx of infected individuals or groups and/or of infective Anopheles vectors.

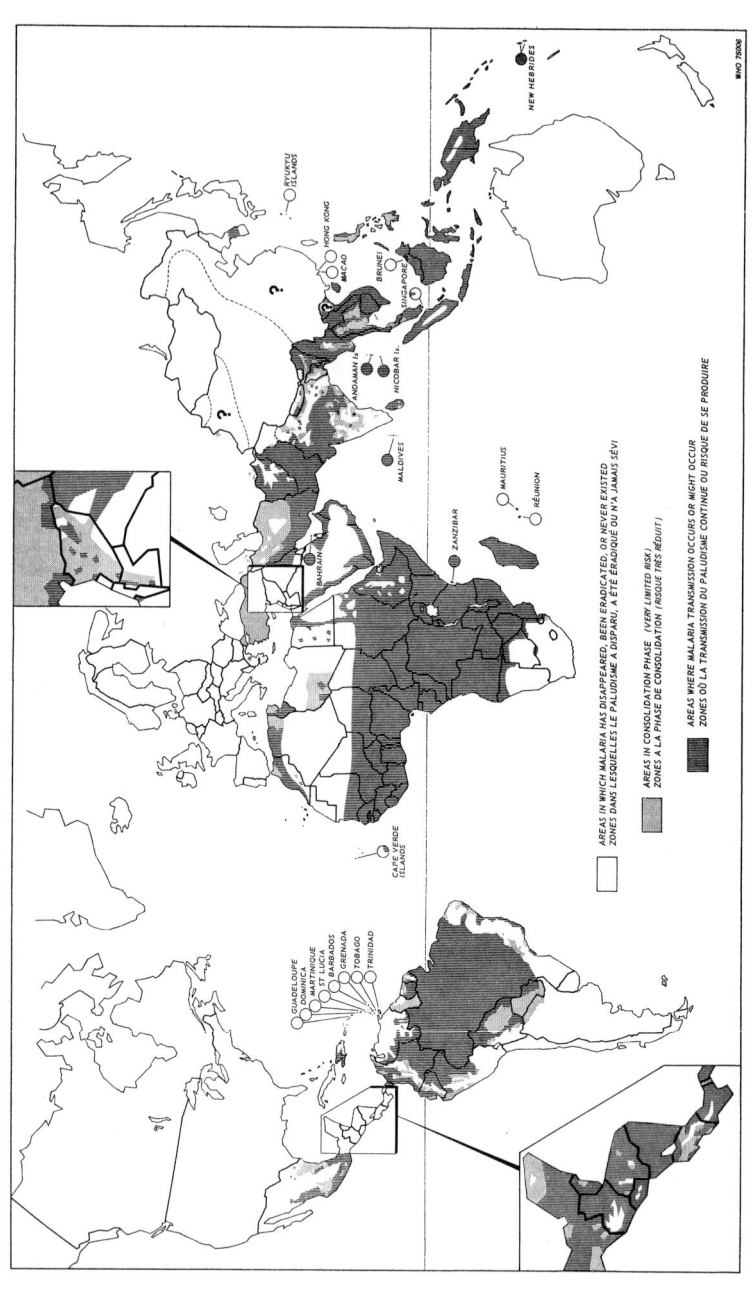

Fig 74 State of malaria eradication in 1976 according to data available to the World Health Organization. (From WHO 1976 Weekly

By the early 1970s malaria had been eliminated from the whole of Europe, the Asian part of the USSR, several countries of the Near East, most of North America including the whole of the USA, most of the Caribbean, large areas of the northern and southern portions of South America, Australia, Japan, Singapore, Korea, and Taiwan. There is little official information about China, but it seems that malaria has been greatly reduced in most of that country.

In African countries south of the Sahara various malaria-control activities, especially the distribution of drugs for prevention and treatment of the infection, are being carried out in urban and some rural areas but the overall situation has not greatly improved. On the other hand, in northern and southern Africa malaria is definitely on the retreat, while its eradication has been accomplished on the islands of Mauritius and Réunion.

The progress of antimalaria activities during the period 1961–76 is shown in Table 24 and Fig. 74.

Table 24

Progress of malaria eradication and control in 1961 and 1976, in terms of millions of population according to WHO

Description of area	Population in millions (approx.) 1961	1976
Areas freed from endemic malaria (under vigilance)	317	436
Areas under surveillance	75	809
Areas under mosquito control or protection by drugs	576	451
Areas without specific antimalaria measures	452	352
Grand total of the population in originally malarious areas	1420	2048

The global malaria eradication campaign had succeeded within the first 15 years in increasing the population freed from malaria transmission from 400 million to over 1200 million. The proportion of the world population previously at risk and subsequently freed from it rose from 40% to 73%. The effect of this campaign on the incidence of malaria and on the mortality from it has been much greater, though the exact figures for morbidity are difficult to obtain.

However, the world malaria situation in 1976–79 gives cause for anxiety for a number of reasons. While the endemic conditions in Africa south of the Sahara remained unchanged, the number of reported malaria cases in some areas of southern Asia and Middle America continues to increase. The situation either remained the same or showed some improvements in several parts of South America, south-east Asia, the Western Pacific, and the Mediterranean area, but there was an epidemic outbreak in the southern plains of Asian Turkey. The deteriorating situation since 1976 led a number of countries to intensify their efforts to curb the advance of malaria by trying to adapt their stategies to the epidemiological situation and to the available resources.

Because of serious technical problems (multiple resistance of vectors to insecticides, exophilic behaviour of vectors, or population migration), administrative limitations (in financial resources or organisational structure), or the consequences of natural disasters (earthquakes, cyclones, or floods), several Middle American malaria eradication programmes have been converted into long-term malaria control programmes. In southern and south-eastern Asia the deterioration in the epidemiological situation and the scarcity of resources have led some countries to adapt the antimalaria programme objectives to the existing means. Programme revisions have also been made by several countries in the eastern Mediterranean and South America regions.

The tropical African countries are experiencing enormous difficulties in implementing the simplified antimalaria strategy, i.e. protection of the most vulnerable groups and those of socio-economic importance. However, the decision by Nigeria to launch a countrywide malaria control programme may stimulate other African governments to develop antimalaria activities in their countries.

Many developing countries are determined to embark on major antimalaria efforts despite the consequences of the current economic crisis and worldwide inflation; this reflects the growing concern of governments about the serious deterioration in the malaria situation.

A more detailed review of the present situation is presented here in relation to regional surveys of the World Health Organization at the end of 1978. It should be remembered that the administrative regions of WHO do not necessarily correspond with the geographical location of several countries.

African Region

Although malaria had been eradicated from Mauritius and Réunion, a few indigenous malaria cases continued to be reported from Mauritius following a small outbreak in 1975.

The Chagos archipelago, Lesotho, the Seychelles, St Helena and the western Sahara are naturally malaria free. Malaria risk is minimal in Cape Verde, South Africa and Swaziland while the risks of malaria are high in remaining countries, with the exception of mountainous areas above 2000 m.

In the mainland areas south of Sahara, mosquito control measures continued to be limited to the large towns and to the southern fringe areas of malaria distribution. These measures were intensified in the areas around international ports and airports. Mass drug administration was carried out in several countries (Cameroon, Congo, Malagasy Republic, Senegal, Sierra Leone, United Republic of Tanzania, and Upper Volta) for the protection of particularly vulnerable population groups. Efforts are being made in these and some other countries to make antimalaria drugs available to the population through an expanding network of self-help projects. No important changes in the susceptibility of vectors to insecticides were reported from the countries of the region. Investigation of alleged foci of drug resistance has so far failed to substantiate reports by clinicians suggesting the presence of chloroquine-resistant falciparum malaria, though a few recent observations from the field are less optimistic in this respect.

Region of the Americas

Twelve countries and areas from where malaria was eradicated have maintained a malaria-free status (Chile, Cuba, Dominica, Grenada and Carriacou, Guadeloupe, Jamaica, Martinique, Puerto Rico, St Lucia, Trinidad and Tobago, USA, Virgin Islands). The malaria risk is minimal in Argentina, Panama Canal Zone, Dominican Republic, Paraguay and Venezuela. In the other 17 countries or areas of this region the malaria risk is considered to be between moderate and high. Further progress was reported from Argentina, Panama, and Paraguay. Belize, Costa Rica, the Dominican Republic, and French Guiana have reported limited outbreaks of malaria after massive influxes of imported malaria cases and a lesser efficacy of the surveillance mechanism. In a third group, comprising 15 countries and areas, the objectives of the programme are a) the preservation of gains achieved in areas where malaria transmission was previously interrupted, and b) the development of an effective system of malaria control in areas where extensive control measures have produced limited results. In this group, the general epidemiological situation has improved in Brazil, Haiti, Mexico, and Venezuela. In other countries, the malaria situation has deteriorated at various levels, especially in the areas where previous control measures were not sufficiently effective.

Although lack of progress in most instances is mainly due to administrative and operational problems, technical problems (e.g. resistance of vectors to insecticides, *P. falciparum* resistance to chloroquine, and social factors related to human behaviour and activities) have been found to play an increasingly important and adverse role.

At present, approximately 20% of the population of malarious areas are living in zones where the vectors are resistant to current insecticides. The situation has become serious in four countries of Central America where resistance to alternative insecticides, especially malathion and propoxur, continues to increase in intensity and extent. This is due to the use of the same type of insecticides for both health and agriculture. In addition to Brazil, Colombia, Guyana, Panama, Surinam, and Venezuela, French Guiana and Ecuador also reported the presence of chloroquine-resistant strains of *P. falciparum* in limited areas.

South-East Asia Region

The malaria situation deteriorated in 5 out of 8 countries: Bangladesh, Burma, India, Indonesia, and Thailand. From the other 3 countries – Maldives, Nepal, and Sri Lanka – limited progress was reported compared with 1976. The population of the originally malarious areas in all countries of the region, except for a very few areas, should again be considered under malaria risk. Although the coverage of case detection activities has decreased in most programmes, the number of detected and confirmed malaria cases continued to increase and exceeded 7 million by the end of 1976.

Realising the seriousness of the present situation, the Government of India has decided to double the funds allotted to the programme and has begun to revise and reorientate programme activities. The new plan aims at preventing malaria mortality by supplying antimalaria drugs free to all persons with fever, by intensifying antimalaria measures in areas of great economic importance, and by maintaining the gains achieved through extending insecticide spraying operations to all areas with an annual parasite incidence exceeding 2 per 1000. In order to ensure the active participation of the general health services in the antimalaria activities, the government is planning a partial integration of malaria and health services at peripheral and intermediate levels. At the same time, the government is encouraging the active involvement of the population and of panchayats (village councils), village leaders, and notables in antimalaria activities.

Resistance of malaria vectors to DDT and of *P. falciparum* to chloroquine is a serious problem in some countries of the region (including Burma and parts of Indonesia).

European Region

The 14 countries of continental Europe continued to be malaria-free with the exception of a few minor foci of introduced malaria transmission in Greece and areas in the USSR bordering on malarious countries. During the last five years there has been a steady increase in the number of malaria cases imported into malaria-free or malaria-freed areas of the continent. As before, many of the imported cases originated in Africa. However, as a result of the progressive deterioration in the malaria situation in Asia, the number and the proportion of malaria cases imported from Asia show a marked upward trend. The annual fatality rate of imported cases of falciparum malaria ranged between 2 and 5%. This underlines the risk of the re-establishment of malaria endemicity should there be a relaxation of the surveillance system.

Outside the continent of Europe progress in malaria control was reported by Algeria and Morocco. However, in the south-eastern part of Turkey, which is battling with serious technical and operational problems, the number of malaria cases has greatly increased. The considerable population movements in Asian Turkey make emergency measures imperative to limit the extension of the epidemic outbreak and to stop the spread of infection inside and outside this country, especially to Greece.

Eastern Mediterranean Region

No indigenous malaria cases were reported from Cyprus, Israel, and Lebanon, the countries in which malaria had been eradicated, although the unsettled conditions in the Lebanon have increased the potential risk and reduced the vigilance activities. The malaria risk is minimal in Egypt. Three out of six countries with malaria eradication programmes (Jordan, Libya, and Tunisia) have continued to make satisfactory progress. In the other three (Iran, Iraq, and Syria), some limited malaria foci were detected in areas previously freed from malaria.

The malaria risk is moderate to high in the remaining 15 countries of this region (Afghanistan, Bahrain, Yemen, Djibouti, Ethiopia, Iran, Iraq, Oman, Pakistan, Qatar, Saudi Arabia, Somalia, Sudan, United Arab Emirates).

Population movements between malarious and malaria-free areas, relaxation of surveillance operations, and mounting technical and administrative problems are responsible for the deterioration of the situation particularly in Ethiopia and Pakistan. However, an improvement was observed in some areas of Sudan and Pakistan where spraying operations with malathion were carried out. The integration of malaria activities within the general health services continued to be pursued in all countries. In Pakistan and Ethiopia it was a short-term objective, in Sudan and Afghanistan a medium-term objective, and in other countries (e.g., Saudi Arabia) a long-term objective. A coordinated malaria control programme in the Arabian peninsula is at present in the planning stage.

The status of vector resistance to chlorinated hydrocarbon insecticides remained unchanged and no resistance of *P. falciparum* to 4-aminoquinolines has been reported so far from countries in this region.

Western Pacific Region

Six countries or areas have been freed of malaria: these are Australia, Brunei, Hong Kong, Japan, Macao and Taiwan. The risk is minimal in the Republic of Korea, and in Singapore. There is no full information from mainland China but it seems that the malaria eradication programme in that huge country has been largely successful. The risk is considered high in Cambodia, East Timor, Laos, Malaysia, New Hebrides, Papua New Guinea, Philippines, Solomon Islands and Viet-Nam.

Further progress was reported from Peninsular Malaysia where malaria eradication activities were extended to the entire population. Extensive antimalaria measures have brought about a further amelioration in the malaria situation in Sabah and Sarawak (Malaysia), the Philippines, and the Solomon Islands. Some improvement in the organisation of antimalaria measures was reported from Papua New Guinea.

More information on the distribution of *P. falciparum* strains resistant to 4-aminoquinolines was collected from the Philippines and the Lao People's Democratic Republic. The presence of chloroquine-resistant strains of *P. falciparum* extends to the Indo-Chinese peninsula, the Philippines, and was reported for the first time from Papua New Guinea.

Thus, on a world scale the health gains of malaria eradication are immense; this can be judged from the fact that the previous annual malaria morbidity rate of about 250 million has now declined to about 100 million. The corresponding mortality rate has decreased from 2.5 million to less than one million per annum. However, there is no denying that in spite of the great achievements of the global programme, in large areas of the world, particularly in the tropical countries, malaria remains one of the most prevalent diseases. The present resurgence of malaria indicates how far we are from the conquest of this disease. It also emphasises the role of malaria as one of the many factors at the core of the great issue of socioeconomic development of the Third World.

THE FUTURE OF MALARIA ERADICATION

The reasons for the present lack of progress and possible further reverses of the global malaria eradication programme are complex. Technical obstacles such as the exophilic habits of some anopheline species, resistance of malaria vectors to insecticides, resistance of plasmodia to antimalarial drugs, inaccessibility of outlying groups of houses, the primitive structure of dwellings, and other factors are of undoubted importance.

Serious difficulties that have stopped the striking advance of global malaria eradication refer to administrative, socioeconomic, financial, and political problems which affect the improvement of health conditions in countries with inadequate basic health services and short of trained manpower.

The importance of the latter point will be fully understood when we remember that in the attack phase, but especially in the consolidation phase, there is great need for a reliable and complete surveillance, with the object of monitoring the interruption of transmission. In this phase adequately developed public health services should carry out much of their task of case detection of malaria. This also explains why the proper organisation and country-wide coverage of public health services are necessary for the transition from the consolidation phase to the maintenance phase of malaria eradication.

The conditions seen in tropical Africa explain why the eradication of malaria from the whole of that continent is now considered unlikely as long as basic health services are qualitatively and quantitatively inadequate.

A re-examination of the global strategy of malaria eradication was carried out during the 1960s and the results were presented at the 22nd World Health Assembly in 1969.

The main conclusions of this report stressed that malaria eradication should remain the final aim: a long-term investment because of its overall impact on health and its socioeconomic benefits. Wherever malaria eradication programmes have good prospects they should be pursued with vigour towards their defined goal. In countries where eradication does not appear to be feasible because of the inadequacy of financial resources, manpower requirements, or shortcomings of basic health services, malaria control operations may form a transitional stage toward the future launching of an eradication programme. The 31st World Health Assembly, meeting in 1978, approved a revised strategy of malaria control and recommended four tactical variants of it, ranging from reduction of malaria mortality to a comprehensive country-wide antimalaria programme.

Within the general agreement on the urgency of malaria control as a prerequisite for eventual eradication two needs emerge: the improvement of basic health services in developing countries and better technical means of controlling the transmission of the infection.

Our technical means of controlling, let alone eradicating, malaria from any endemic areas of the world are still inadequate. A concentrated research effort may find new ways to attack the malaria parasite and its vector. Fields in which research is felt to be particularly important include the improvement of immunological surveillance techniques, study of the behaviour of mosquito vectors and their resistance to insecticides, better and more acceptable insecticides, and the development of new antimalarial drugs.

The place of chemotherapy in malaria eradication depends on both the local epidemiology of the disease and operational facilities. The use of drugs for large-scale treatment is difficult since all those in use at present are rapidly excreted and have to be administered very frequently to be effective. Another handicap is the appearance of drug resistance due to the modified response of the parasite to the chemical compound. Such instances of resistance have been reported in various parts of the world and the spread of this phenomenon causes much concern.

There is also the possibility of a prospective malaria vaccine, but the present experimental results, however encouraging, show the practical difficulties of this method. It seems that synthetic antimalarial drugs will be our most reliable weapon for many years.

The need for an increased research effort for more effective fight against malaria is now reflected in the activity of the Special Programme for Research and Training in Tropical Diseases recently set up by the World Health Organization and supported generously by the United Nations Development Programme and the World Bank. The bilateral assistance of the USA Agency for International Development deserves special mention.

As the resurgence of malaria in many parts of the world gives cause for anxiety, a number of countries intensify their efforts by adapting their health policies to the epidemiological situation and mustering their resources. The World Health Organization aims at merging the antimalaria activities at the peripheral level with the work of expanding health services. Promotion of international and bilateral assistance for application of environmental methods of malaria control and stimulation of training courses for all cadres of medical and health personnel are long term programmes which are closely related to the pace of socio-economic advance of developing tropical countries where malaria will remain a serious health problem for many years.

In several resolutions passed at recent World Health Assemblies the member states of the World Health Organization have stressed the need to improve the number and qualifications of antimalaria personnel at all levels. In the past various excellent centres for such training were available. However, many of these centres have closed down and the staff already trained went to other fields of activity. There is now the opportunity of reviving or extending training activities specifically orientated towards malaria control.

According to expert opinion the various aspects of malariology should not be taught in isolation but in the context of varying priorities of national public health programmes and in relation to the needs of the community. Modern teaching methods should be introduced and the participants must be directly involved in the training process. Learning by doing and practical field work must be emphasised.

The subject of malaria in its epidemiological, parasitological, clinical and public health aspects should be reflected in the undergraduate and postgraduate curricula of medical schools in developing countries. The concept of the community orientated health team should be in the centre of training activities. Ways and means must be found to train a large number of primary health workers and medical auxiliaries having sufficient knowledge and skills with regard to treatment of malaria and its prevention.

Every health project in a developing country, which is supported by an advanced country or by an international agency, should contain a training component. Moreover every one of such projects should be co-ordinated with the relevant country's overall health programme.

The general consensus is that training facilities for the diagnosis of malaria, its treatment and its control should be provided for medical professional and auxiliary personnel involved in clinical and public health aspects of communicable disease in developing and developed countries. The old generation of 'blood, mud and sweat' malariologists has nearly disappeared and much of their experience has been largely forgotten. The author of the present book hopes that he has contributed to forging a link between the not so distant past and the new generation of specialists in tropical community health.

Selected References

The bibliography on malaria is immense and the following list of selected references concentrates on publications of the past 10 years although it comprises some important books of the previous period. The most extensive list of references up to about 1946 will be found in Boyd M.F. (1949), *Malariology*, 2 volumes, W. B. Saunders, Philadelphia. For those interested in parasitology of malaria, P. C. C. Garnham's *Malaria Parasites and other Haemosporidia* (1966), published by Blackwell, Oxford, provides a rich source of references. Many basic references on various aspects of malaria up to 1962 are quoted at the end of each chapter of the fundamental (and still valuable) *Practical Malariology* by Russell P. F., West L. S., Manwell R. D. and Macdonald G. (1963), Oxford University Press, London.

For chemotherapy of malaria the following four books are a mine of bibliographical data: Findlay G. M. (1951), *Recent Advances in Chemotherapy* Vol. II (Third edition) J. A. Churchill, London; Peters W. (1970) *Chemotherapy and Drug Resistance in Malaria*, Academic Press, London and New York; Thompson P. E. and Werbel L. M. (1972), *Antimalarial Agents*, Academic Press, New York and London; Pinder R. M. (1973), *Malaria*, Scientechnica, Bristol. Finally a comprehensive list of references on most aspects of malaria eradication is available in *A Textbook of Malaria Eradication*, by E. J. Pampana (1969), Oxford University Press, London, 2nd edition.

For keeping abreast of the large volume of publications on all subjects directly or indirectly related to research on and control of malaria the *Tropical Diseases Bulletin*, issued monthly by the Bureau of Tropical Diseases in London, is invaluable.

In the present book particular attention has been given to the sources of authoritative and abundant information on all problems of malaria and its control, provided over the past two decades by the World Health Organization. Two series of cyclostyled documents dealing with various aspects of research on and control of malaria are distributed by the World Health Organization to institutes and individual scientists or public health workers. Current issues of these series known as WHO/Mal and WHO/VBC reports can be forwarded on request to interested professional persons by writing to the World Health Organization, Documents Distribution Section, 1211, Geneva, Switzerland. Catalogues of WHO publications are produced periodically by the Organization's Headquarters in Geneva and by the Regional Offices.

Furthermore, the complete 'Bibliography of World Health Organization's Publications, 1973–1977' has become available in 1979.

A. GENERAL AND HISTORICAL

Andrews J. M. and Langmuir, A. D. (1963), The philosophy of disease eradication. *American Journal of Public Health,* **53,** 1–6.

Barlow R. (1968), *The Economic Effects of Malaria Eradication.* School of Public Health, University of Michigan, Ann Arbor, Michigan.

Benenson A. S., Ed. (1970), *Control of Communicable Diseases in Man*, 11th edition. American Public Health Association, New York.

Black R. H. (1972), *Malaria in Australia*. Service Publication No. 9, School of Public Health and Tropical Medicine, University of Sydney.

Boyd M. F., Ed. (1949), *Malariology*, Vols. I and II. W. B. Saunders Co., Philadelphia.

Boyd M. F. (1930), *An Introduction to Malariology*. Harvard University Press, Cambridge, Mass.

Bradley D. J. (1978) New epidemiological and environmental approaches to tropical infections. In Wood C. Ed. *Tropical Medicine – From Romance to Reality*. Academic Press London; Grune & Stratton, New York.

Bradley D. J. (1979) Prevention of disease in the tropics: questions in health economics. *Epidemiology and Community Health*. **33**, 66–73.

Bruce-Chwatt L. J. (1959), Malaria research and eradication in the USSR. *Bulletin of the World Health Organization*, **21**, 737–72.

Bruce-Chwatt L. J. (1971), Malaria, in *Textbook of Medicine* (Beeson P. and McDermott W., Eds.), 13th edition. Saunders, Philadelphia and London.

Bruce-Chwatt L. J., Southgate B. A. and Draper C. C. (1974), Malaria in the United Kingdom. *British Medical Journal*, **2**, 707–11.

Cahill K. M., Ed. (1969), *Symposium on Malaria. Bulletin of the New York Academy of Medicine*, **45**, No. 10, 997–1086.

Christophers S. R., Sinton A. J. and Covell G. (1941), *How to do a Malaria Survey*. Government of India Press, Delhi.

Clyde D. F. (1967), *Malaria in Tanzania*. Oxford University Press, London, New York, Toronto.

Cockburn A., Ed. (1967), *Infectious Diseases: Their Evolution and Eradication*. Charles Thomas, Springfield, Illinois.

Cohn G. J. (1973), Assessing the costs and benefits of anti-malaria programs: the Indian experience. *American Journal of Public Health*, **63**, 1086–96.

Conly G. N. (1975), *The Impact of Malaria on Economic Development: A Case Study*. Pan-American Health Organization Publication No. 297, Washington DC.

Field J. W., Ed. (1951), *Fifty Years of Medical Research in Malaya*. Government Press, Kuala Lumpur.

Gonzalez C. L. (1965), *Mass Campaigns and General Health Services*. Public Health Papers No. 29, World Health Organization, Geneva.

Hackett L. W. (1937), *Malaria in Europe*. Oxford University Press, London.

Harrison G. (1978), *Mosquitoes, Malaria and Man*. John Murray, London.

International Cooperation Administration (1961), Report and recommendations on malaria: A summary. *American Journal of Tropical Medicine and Hygiene*, **10**, 451–502.

Janssens P. G. (1974), Le procés du paludisme. *Journal of Tropical Medicine and Hygiene*, **77** (Suppl.), 47–53.

Jeffery G. M. (1975), Malaria control in the twentieth century. *American Journal of Tropical Medicine and Hygiene*, **25**, 361–70.

Jones W. H. S. (1909), *Malaria and Greek History*. Manchester University Press, Manchester.

Knowles R. and Senior-White R. (1927), *Malaria, Its Investigation and Control with Special Reference to Indian Conditions*. Thacker, Spink and Co., Calcutta.

Lepeš T. (1972), Research related to malaria: A review of achievements and further needs. *American Journal of Tropical Medicine and Hygiene*, **21**, 640–47.

Lepeš T. (1974), Review of research on malaria. *Bulletin of the World Health Organization*, **50**, 151–57.

Logan J. A. (1953), *The Sardinian Project*. Johns Hopkins Press, Baltimore.

Maegraith B. G. (1973), *One World*. Athlone Press, London.

Manson-Bahr R. (1963), The story of malaria: The drama and actors. In *International Review of Tropical Medicine* (Lincicome R. D. Ed.) Academic Press, London and New York.

National Academy of Sciences – National Research Council (1962), *Tropical Health: A Report on a Study of Needs and Resources*. Publication No. 996, Washington DC.

New York Academy of Medicine (1969), Symposium on malaria. *Bulletin of the New York Academy of Medicine*, **45**, 997–1101.

Noguer A., Wernsdorfer W., Kouznetsov R. and Hempel J. (1978), The malaria situation in 1976. *WHO Chronicle* **32**, 9–17.

Ross Institute of Tropical Hygiene (1974), *Preservation of Personal Health in Warm Climates*, 7th edition. Ross Institute, London.

Russell P. F. (1943), Malaria and its influence on world health. *Bulletin of the New York Academy of Medicine*, **19**, 599–630.

Russell P. F. (1952), *Malaria: Basic Principles Briefly Stated*. Blackwell Scientific Publications, Oxford.

Russell P. F. (1955), *Man's Mastery of Malaria*. Oxford University Press, London, New York, Toronto.

Russell P. F., West L. S., Manwell R. D. and Macdonald G. (1963), *Practical Malariology* (2nd edition). Oxford University Press, London, New York, Toronto.

Sadun E. H., Ed. (1966), *Research in Malaria* (An International Panel Workshop). *Military Medicine*, **131** (Suppl.), 847–1272.

Sadun E. H., Ed. (1969), *Experimental Malaria* (A Panel Workshop). *Military Medicine* (Special issue) No. 10, **134**, 729–1306.

Sadun E. H. Ed. (1972), *Basic Research in Malaria. Proceedings of Helminthological Society of Washington* (Special issue), **39**, 3–583.

Sandosham A. A. (1965) *Malariology, with Special Reference to Malaya.* University of Malaya Press, Singapore.

Scholtens R. G. and Najera J. A., Eds. Proceedings of the Inter-American Malaria Research Symposium, San Salvador. *American Journal of Tropical Medicine and Hygiene*, **21**, 607–850.

Scott H. H. (1939), *A History of Tropical Medicine*, Vols I and II. Edward Arnold, London.

Sergiev P. G., Ed. (1968), *Multivolume Manual on the Microbiology, Clinical Aspects and Epidemiology of Infectious Diseases*, Volume 9 'Malaria' (in Russian). Medicina, Moscow.

Sergiev P. G. and Yakusheva A. I. (1956), *Malaria and the Fight Against it in the USSR* (in Russian). Medgiz, Moscow.

Société de Pathologie Exotique (1966), Réunion d'information sur le paludisme. *Bulletin de la Société de Pathologie Exotique*, **59**, 459–685.

Soper F. G. (1970), *Building the Health Bridge.* Indiana University Press, Bloomington and London.

Sotiroff-Junker J. (1978), *A Bibliography on the behavioural, social and economic aspects of malaria and its control.* WHO Offset Publications No. 42, Geneva.

Swellengrebel N. H. and de Buck A. (1938), *Malaria in the Netherlands.* Scheltema and Holkema Ltd., Amsterdam.

Weller T. H. (1974), World Health in a Changing World. *Journal of Tropical Medicine and Hygiene*, **77** (Suppl.), 54–61.

Wood C. Edit. (1978), *Tropical Medicine: From romance to reality.* Academic Press, London; Grune and Stratton, New York.

WHO (1951), *Report on Malaria Conference in Equatorial Africa.* Technical Report Series No. 38, Geneva.

Selected References

World Health Organization (1954–72), Reports on the World Health Situation: First Report (1954–56), No. 94; Second Report (1957–60), No. 122; Third Report (1961–64), No. 155; Fourth Report (1965–68), No. 192; Fifth Report (1969–72), No. 225, Geneva.

World Health Organization (1957), *Malaria. Sixth Report of the Expert Committee*. Technical Reports Series No. 123, Geneva.

World Health Organization (1958), *The First Ten Years 1948–57*. WHO, Geneva.

World Health Organization (1959), *Malaria: Seventh Report of the Expert Committee on Malaria*. Technical Reports Series No. 162, Geneva.

World Health Organization (1961), *Malaria: Eighth Report of the Expert Committee*. Technical Reports Series No. 205, Geneva.

World Health Organization (1962), *Malaria: Ninth Report of the Expert Committee*. Technical Reports Series No. 243, Geneva.

World Health Organization (1963), *Terminology of Malaria and of Malaria Eradication*. Monograph Series No. 13, Geneva.

World Health Organization (1964), *Malaria: Tenth Report of the Expert Committee*. Technical Reports Series No. 272, Geneva.

World Health Organization (1964), *Malaria: Eleventh Report of the Expert Committee*. Technical Reports Series No. 291, Geneva.

World Health Organization (1965), *Integration of Mass Campaigns against Specific Diseases into General Health Services*. Technical Reports Series No. 294, Geneva.

World Health Organization (1966), *Malaria: Twelfth Report of the Expert Committee on Malaria*. Technical Reports Series No. 324, Geneva.

World Health Organization (1967), *Malaria: Thirteenth Report of the Expert Committee on Malaria*. Technical Reports Series No. 357, Geneva.

World Health Organization (1968), *Malaria: Fourteenth Report of the Expert Committee*. Technical Reports Series No. 382, Geneva.

World Health Organization (1968), *The Second Ten Years 1958–67*. Geneva.

World Health Organization (1969), *Re-examination of the Global Strategy of Malaria Eradication*. Official Records of the WHO No. 176, Annex 13, Geneva.

World Health Organization (1971), *Malaria: Fifteenth Report of the Expert Committee*. Technical Reports Series No. 467, Geneva.

World Health Organization (1972), *Human Development and Public Health*. Technical Reports Series No. 485, Geneva.

World Health Organization (1973), *Interrelationship Between Health Programmes and Socioeconomic Development*. Public Health Papers No. 49, Geneva.

World Health Organization (1974), *Malaria: Sixteenth Report of the Expert Committee on Malaria*. Technical Reports Series No. 549, Geneva.

World Health Organization (1974), Proceedings of the symposium on malaria research (Rabat, Morocco, April 1974). *Bulletin of the World Health Organization*, **50**, 143–372.

World Health Organization (1975), *A Special Programme for Research and Training in Tropical Diseases: Strategy*. Cyclostyled document TDR/75.4, Geneva.

World Health Organization (1977), Synopsis of the world malaria situation in 1976. *WHO Weekly Epidemiological Record*, **52**, 41–46.

B. PARASITOLOGY

Aikawa M. (1971), Plasmodium: the fine structure of malarial parasites. *Experimental Parasitology*, **30**, 284–320.

Aikawa M. and Sterling C. R. (1974), *Intracellular Parasitic Protozoa*. Academic Press, New York.

Aikawa M. and Ward R. H. (1974), Intraspecific variation in *P. falciparum*. *American Journal of Tropical Medicine and Hygiene*, **23**, 570–73.

Bray R. H. (1957), *Studies on the Exo-erythrocytic Cycle of the Genus Plasmodium*. London School of Hygiene and Tropical Medicine, Memoir No. 12, H. K. Lewis, London.

Selected References

Bray, R. S. (1963), The exoerythrocytic phase of malaria parasites, in *International Review of Tropical Medicine* (Lincicome R. D., Ed.) Academic Press, London and New York.

Bruce-Chwatt L. J. (1961), *Manual for Processing and Examination of Blood-slides in Malaria Eradication Programmes* (2nd edition). WHO (Cyclostyled document MHO/PA/262.61), Geneva.

Coatney G. A., Collins W. E., Warren McW. and Contacos P. G. (1971), *The Primate Malarias*. US Department of Health, Education and Welfare, National Institute of Health, Bethesda, Maryland, USA.

Field J. W. (1948), *The Microscopic Diagnosis of Human Malaria*, Part I. A short descriptive atlas of thick-film diagnosis. Institute for Medical Research, Federation of Malaya, Kuala Lumpur.

Field J. W. and Shute P. G. (1956), *The Microscopic Diagnosis of Human Malaria*, II. A morphological study of the erythrocytic parasite. Government Printer, Kuala Lumpur.

Field J. W., Sandosham A. A. and Fong Y. L. (1963), *The Microscopical Diagnosis of Human Malaria*, Parts I and II. Institute for Medical Research, Federation of Malaya, Kuala Lumpur.

Garnham P. C. C. (1948), Exo-erythrocytic schizogony in malaria. *Tropical Diseases Bulletin*, **45**, 831–44.

Garnham P. C. C. (1966), *Malaria Parasites and Other Haemosporidia*. Blackwell Scientific Publications, Oxford.

Gutteridge W. W. and Coombs G. H. (1977), *Biochemistry of Parasitic Protozoa*. Macmillan Press, London.

Hoare C. A. (1949), *Handbook of Medical Protozoology*. Baillière, Tindall and Cox, London.

Killick-Kendrick R. and Peters W. (1978), *Rodent Malaria*. Academic Press, London and New York.

Mitchell G. H., Butcher G. A., Langhorne J. and Cohen S. (1977), A freeze dried merozoite vaccine effective against *P. knowlesi* malaria. *Clinical and Experimental Immunology*, **28**, 276–79.

Rieckmann K. H., Campbell G. H., Sax G. J. and Krema J. E. (1978), Drug sensitivity of *P. falciparum*. *Lancet*, **1**, 22–23.

Sinden R. E., Canning G. V., Bray R. S. and Smalley M. E. (1978), Gametocyte and gamete development in *P. falciparum*. *Proceedings of the Royal Society*, **B 201**, 375–99.

Shute P. G. and Maryon M. (1960), *Laboratory Technique for the Study of Malaria*. J. A. Churchill, London.

Trager W. and Jensen J. B. (1977), *In vitro* cultivation of malaria parasites. *Bulletin of the World Health Organization*, **55**, 363–64.

Trager W, and Jensen J. B. (1978), Cultivation of malarial parasites. *Nature*, **273** (Suppl.), 621–22.

Van den Bossche H., Ed. (1976), *Biochemistry of Parasites and Host-parasite Relationships*. North Holland, Amsterdam.

Walker A. J. (1960), *Manual of the Microscopic Diagnosis of Malaria*. Scientific Publications No. 46, Pan-American Health Organization, Washington DC.

Wilcox A. (1960), *Manual for the Microscopical Diagnosis of Malaria in Man* (2nd edition). US Department of Health, Education and Welfare, Public Health Service, Washington DC.

Wilcocks Ch. and Manson-Bahr P. E. C. (1972), *Manson's Tropical Diseases* (17th edition). Baillière, Tindall, London.

World Health Organization (1969), *Parasitology of Malaria*. Technical Reports Series No. 433, Geneva.

World Health Organization (1977), USAID/WHO Workshop on the biology and in vitro cultivation of malaria parasites. *Bulletin of the World Health Organization*, **55**, No. 2–3, 121–427.

C. CLINICAL ASPECTS AND PATHOLOGY AND IMMUNOLOGY

Adams R. A. D. and Maegraith B. G. (1958), *Clinical Tropical Diseases*. Blackwell, Oxford.

Bourdais A., Monnier A., Lartisien D., Derrien J.-P. and Thomas J. (1978) Insuffisance aigue rénale provoquée par le paludisme à P. falciparum en fin de grossesse. *Médecine Tropicale*, **38**, 35–42.

Bruce-Chwatt L. J. (1974), Transfusion malaria. *Bulletin of the World Health Organization*, **50**, 337–46.

Carter R. and Chen D. H. (1976). Malaria transmission blocked by immunisation with gametes of the malaria parasite. *Nature*, **263**, 57–60.

Christophers S. R. (1924), The mechanism of immunity against malaria in communities living under hyper-endemic conditions. *Indian Journal of Medical Research*, **12**, 273–94.

Covell G. (1950), Congenital malaria. *Tropical Diseases Bulletin*, **47**, 1147–67.

Cohen S. (1979) Immunity to malaria, *Proceedings of the Royal Society*, **203**, 323–45.

Cox F. E. G. (1978), Specific and nonspecific immunisation against parasite infections. *Nature*, **273** (Suppl.), 623–26.

Edington G. and Gilles H. M. (1976), *Pathology in the Tropics* (2nd edition). Edward Arnold, London.

Fairley N. H. (1947), Sidelights on malaria in man obtained by sub-inoculation experiments. *Transactions of the Royal Society of Tropical Medicine and Hygiene*, **40**, 621–76.

Garnham P. C. C. (1949), Malaria immunity in Africans; Effects in infancy and early childhood. *Annals of Tropical Medicine*, **43**, 47–61.

Garnham P. C. C., Pierce A. E. and Roitt I., Eds. (1963), *Immunity to Protozoa*. Blackwell, Oxford.

Garnham P. C. C. (1967), Relapses and latency in malaria. *Protozoology* **2**, 55–64.

Garnham P. C. C. (1977), The continuing mystery of relapses in malarias. *Protozoological Abstracts* **1**, 1–12.

Gentilini M., Duflo B., Lagardère B. and Davis M (1972), *Médecine Tropicale*. Flammarion, Paris.

Gilles H. M., Lawson J. B., Sibelas M., Voller A. and Allan N. (1969), Malaria, anaemia and pregnancy. *Annals of Tropical Medicine and Parasitology*, **62**, 245–63.

Hall A. P. (1977, The treatment of severe falciparum malaria. *Transactions of the Royal Society of Tropical Medicine and Hygiene*, **71**, 367–79.

Le Bras M., Gekra A., Beda B., Martine J. and Bertiand E. (1974), L'insuffisance rénale aigue du paludisme à *P. falciparum*. *Médecine d'Afrique Noire*, **21**, 491–98.

Lepeš T. (1973), Advances in malaria immunology. *Acta Parasitologica Yugoslavica*, **4**, 13–24.

Luzzato L. (1974), Genetic factors in malaria. *Bulletin of the World Health Organization* **50**, 195–202.

Lysenko A. Y., Belaev A. E. and Rybalka V. M. (1977). Population studies of P. vivax, Parts I and II. *Bulletin of the World Health Organization*, **55**, 541–49 and 551–56.

Kortmann H. F. (1972), *Malaria and Pregnancy*. Thesis, University of Utrecht, Elinkwijk, Utrecht.

Maegraith B. G. (1948), *Pathological Processes in Malaria and Blackwater Fever*. Blackwell, Oxford.

Maegraith B. G. (1965), *Exotic Diseases in Practice*. Wm Heinemann Medical Books, London.

Maegraith B. G. (1977), Interdependence: The pathology of malaria. *American Journal of Tropical Medicine and Hygiene*, **26**, 344–54.

Marsden P. D. and Bruce-Chwatt L. J. (1975), Cerebral malaria in *Topics on Tropical Neurology* (Hornabrook R. W. Ed.). Davis, Philadelphia.

Marsden P. D. and Crane G. G. (1976), The tropical splenomegaly syndrome: A current appraisal. *Revista de Instituto de Medicina Tropical de São Paulo*, São Paulo, **18**, 54–70.

McGregor I. A. (1964), Studies in the acquisition of immunity to P. falciparum infections in West Africa. *Transactions of the Royal Society of Tropical Medicine and Hygiene*, **58**, 80–92.

McGregor I. A. (1972), Immunology of malarial infection and its possible consequences. *British Medical Bulletin*, **28**, 12–17.

Meuwissen J. H. (1975) Serological diagnosis of malaria. *Annales Société Belge de Médecine Tropicale* **55**, 585–591.

Miller L. H. (1977), Current prospects and problems for a malaria vaccine. *Journal of Infectious Diseases*, **135**, 855–64.

Payet M. and Coulaud J. P. (1976), *Les Maladies d'Importation*. Masson, Paris.

Ranque J. (1976). Le paludisme post-transfusionnel en France. *Revue Française de Transfusion et Immunohematologie*, **19**, 315–24.

Reid A. M. Goldsmith H. J. and Wright F. K. (1967), Peritoneal dialysis in acute renal failure following malaria. *Lancet* **2**, 436–39.

Richards W. H. G. (1977), Vaccination against sporozoite challenge: A review. *Transactions of the Royal Society of Tropical Medicine and Hygiene*, **71**, 279–80.

Roitt I. (1971), *Essential Immunology*. Blackwell Scientific Publications, Oxford.

Royal Society of Tropical Medicine and Hygiene (1971), Symposium: The role of serum antibodies in malarial immunity. *Transactions of the Royal Society of Tropical Medicine and Hygiene*, **65**, No. 2.

Schneider J. J. (1962), *Les Maladies Tropicales dans la Pratique Médicale Courante*. Masson, Paris.

Sheehy. T. W. and Reba A. C. (1967), Complications of falciparum malaria and their treatment. *Annals of Internal Medicine.* **66**, 807–809.

Sulzer A. J. and Wilson M (1971) The fluorescent antibody test for malaria. *CRC Critical Reviews in Clinical Laboratory Sciences*, **9**, 601–619

Taliaferro W. H. and Mulligan H. W. (1937), *Histopathology of Malaria*. Indian Medical Research Memoirs No. 23, Delhi.

Trigg P. I. (1976), Parasite cultivation in relation to research on chemotherapy of malaria. *Bulletin of the World Health Organization*. **53**, 399–406.

Toro G. and Roman G. (1978), Cerebral malaria. *Journal of the American Medical Association*. **35**, 271–76.

Vachon F. *et al.* (1973), Insuffisance rénale aigue du paludisme pernicieux. *Presse Médicale* **2**, 1035–39.

Voller A. (1976), Applications of immunofluorescence to sero-epidemiology of malaria. *Annals of the New York Academy of Sciences* **254**, 326–30.

Voller A. (1976), Immunopathology of malaria. *Bulletin of the World Health Organisation*. **50**, 177–86.

Voller A., Bartlett A. and Bidwell S. E. (1976), Enzyme immunoassays for parasitic diseases. *Transactions of the Royal Society of Tropical Medicine and Hygiene*, **70**, 98–106.

Williamson W. R. and Greenwood B. M. (1978), Impairment of the immune response to vaccination after acute malaria. *Lancet* **1**, 1328–29.

Woodruff A. W., Ed. (1974), *Medicine in the Tropics*, Churchill Livingstone, Edinburgh and London.

World Health Organization (1965), *Immunology and Parasitic Diseases*. Technical Reports Series No. 315, Geneva.

World Health Organization (1966). *Haemoglobinopathies and Allied Disorders*. Technical Reports Series No. 338, Geneva.

World Health Organization (1967), *Standardization of Procedures for the Study of Glucose 6-phosphate dehydrogenase Deficiency*. Technical Reports Series No. 366, Geneva.

World Health Organization (1968), *Immunology of Malaria*. Technical Reports Series No. 396, Geneva.

World Health Organization (1968), *Genetics of the Immune Response*. Technical Reports Series No. 402, Geneva.

World Health Organization (1969), *Cell-mediated Immune Responses*. Technical Reports Series No. 423, Geneva.

World Health Organization (1970), *Factors Regulating the Immune Response*. Technical Reports Series No. 448, Geneva.

World Health Organization (1972), *Clinical Immunology*. Technical Reports Series No. 496, Geneva.

World Health Organization (1972), *Treatment of Haemoglobinopathies and Allied Disorders*. Technical Reports Series No. 509, Geneva.

World Health Organization (1973), *Cell-mediated Immunity and Resistance to Infection*. Technical Reports Series No. 519, Geneva.

World Health Organization (1974), Serological testing in malaria (Memorandum). *Bulletin of the World Health Organization*, **50**, 527–35.

World Health Organization (1975), *Developments in Malaria Immunology*. Technical Reports Series No. 579, Geneva.

World Health Organization (1976), *Immunological Adjuvants*. Technical Reports Series No. 595, Geneva.

World Health Organization (1977), *The role of Immune Complexes in Disease*. Technical Reports Series No. 606, Geneva.

D. CHEMOTHERAPY

Black R. H. (1977), The prevention and treatment of malaria. *Medical Journal of Australia* **1**, 929–33.

Bruce-Chwatt L. J. (1970), Resistance of P. falciparum to chloroquine in Africa: True or false? *Transactions of the Royal Society of Tropical Medicine and Hygiene*, **64**, 776–84.

Bruce-Chwatt L. J. (1974), *Antimalarial Drugs*. Ross Institute's Bulletin No. 2. Ross Institute, London.

Burger A., Ed. (1970), *Medicinal Chemistry*, 3rd edition. Wiley: Interscience, New York.

Canfield C. J. and Rozman. A. S. (1974), Clinical testing of new antimalarial compounds. *Bulletin World Health Organization* **50**, 203–12.

Center for Disease Control (1978), Chemoprophylaxis of malaria. *Morbidity and Mortality Weekly Report*, **27**, No. 10 (Suppl.), US Dept. of Health, Education and Welfare, Atlanta.

Clyde D. F., McCarthy V. C., Miller R. M., and Hornick R. B. (1976), Suppressive activity of mefloquine in sporozoite-induced human malaria. *Antimicrobial Agents and Chemotherapy* **9**, 384–86.

Contacos P. G. (1969), Treatment of malaria infection, *Bulletin of the New York Academy Medicine Public Health Reports*, **45**, 1077–1085.

Covell G., Coatney G. A., Field J. W. and Singh J. (1955), *Chemotherapy of Malaria*. Monograph Series No. 27, World Health Organization, Geneva.

Dunschede H. B. (1971), *Tropenmedizinische Forschung bei Bayer*. Michael Triltsch Verlag, Düsseldorf.

Findlay G. M. (1951), *Recent Advances in Chemotherapy*, 3rd edition, Vol. II. J. & A. Churchill Ltd., London.

Hall A. P. (1976), The treatment of malaria. *British Medical Journal*, **1**, 323–28.

Jaramillo-Arango J. (1950), *The Conquest of Malaria*. Wm. Heinemann Medical Books, London.

Peters W. (1970), *Chemotherapy and Drug Resistance in Malaria*. Academic Press, London and New York.

Peters W. (1974), Recent advances in antimalarial chemotherapy and drug resistance. *Advances in Parasitology* **12**, 69–114.

Peters W. (1977), Malaria. *New England Journal of Medicine*. **297**, 1261–64.

Pinder R. M. (1973), *Malaria: the Design, Use and Mode of Action of Chemotherapeutic Agents*. Scientechnica, Bristol.

Rollo I. M. (1964), Chemotherapy of malaria. In *Biochemistry and Physiology of Protozoa*, Vol. III (Hutner S. H., Ed.). Academic Press, New York.

Schmidt L. H. (1969), Chemotherapy of drug resistant malaria *Annual Reviews of Microbiology* **23**, 427–47.

Schmidt L. H. (1978), *Plasmodium falciparum* and *Plasmodium vivax* infections in the owl monkey (*Aotus trivirgatus*). I. The courses of untreated infections. *American Journal of Tropical Medicine and Hygiene* **27**, 671–702.

Schmidt L. H. (1978), *Plasmodium falciparum* and *Plasmodium vivax* infections in the owl monkey (*Aotus trivirgatus*). II. Responses to choroquine, quinine, and pyrimethamine. *American Journal of Tropical Medicine and Hygiene* **27**, 703–17.

Schmidt L. H. (1978), *Plasmodium falciparum* and *Plasmodium vivax* infections in the owl monkey (*Aotus trivirgatus*). III. Methods employed in the search for new blood schizonticidal drugs. *American Journal of Tropical Medicine and Hygiene* **27**, 718–37.

Selected References

Schmidt L. H., Crosby R., Rasco J., and Vaughan D., (1978), The antimalarial activities of various 4-quinolinemethanols with special attention to WR-142, 490 (mefloquine). *Antimicrobial Agents and Chemotherapy* **13**, 1011–30.

Schnitzer R. Y. (1963), Drug resistance of protozoa. In *International Review of Tropical Medicine* (Lincicome R. D., Ed.). Academic Press, London and New York.

Schnitzer R. Y. and Hawking F. (Eds.) (1963), *Experimental Chemotherapy*. Academic Press, New York.

Steck E. A. (1972), *The Chemotherapy of Protozoan Diseases*. US Govt. Printing Office, Washington DC.

Taylor N. (1945), *Cinchona in Java*. Greenberg Publications, New York.

Thompson P. E. and Werbel R. M. (1972), *Antimalarial Agents*. Academic Press, New York and London.

Trenholme G. M. *et al.* (1975), Mefloquine. *Science* **190**, 792–94.

Van den Bossche H. (1978), Chemotherapy of parasitic infections. *Nature* **273** (Suppl.), 626–29.

Von Brand T. (1966), *The biochemistry of parasites*. Academic Press, New York.

Wilson T. and Edeson J. F. B. (1957–58), Studies on the chemotherapy of malaria VI and VII. *The Medical Journal of Malaya*, **11**, 190–200, **12**, 472–99.

Wiselogle F. Y., Ed. (1946). *A Survey of Antimalarial Drugs*, 1941–45, Vols. I and II. Edwards, Ann Arbor, Michigan.

World Health Organization (1961), *Chemotherapy of Malaria*. Technical Reports Series No. 226, Geneva.

World Health Organization (1965), *Resistance of Malaria Parasites to Drugs*. Technical Reports Series No. 296, Geneva.

World Health Organization (1967), *Chemotherapy of Malaria*. Technical Reports Series No. 375, Geneva.

World Health Organization (1973), *Chemotherapy of Malaria and Resistance to Antimalarials*. Technical Reports Series No. 529, Geneva.

E. ENTOMOLOGY

American Geographical Society (1951), Distribution of malaria vectors. Atlas of distribution of diseases. *Geographical Revue* **41**, Plate 3.

Bates M. (1949), *The Natural History of Mosquitoes*. Macmillan Company, New York.

Belkin Y. N. (1962), *The Mosquitoes of the South Pacific* (Diptera, Culicidae), University of California Press, Berkeley.

Bonne-Webster J. and Swellengrebel, N. H. (1953), *The Anopheline Mosquitoes of the Indo-Australian Region*. Amsterdam.

Brown A. W. A. and Pal R. (1971), *Insecticide Resistance in Arthropods*, 2nd edition. Monograph Series No. 38, World Health Organization, Geneva.

Bruce-Chwatt L. J. and Goeckel C. W. (1960), A study of blood feeding patterns of Anopheles mosquitoes. *Bulletin of the World Health Organization* **22**, 685–730.

Bruce-Chwatt L. J. (1970), Global review of malaria control and eradication by attack on the vector. *Miscellaneous Publication of the Entomological Society of America*. **7**, 7–23.

Busvine Y. (1951), *Insects and Hygiene*. Methuen and Co., London.

Causey O. R., Deane L. M. and Deane M. P. (1946), *Studies on Brazilian Anopheles from the Northeast and Amazon Regions*. Johns Hopkins Press, Baltimore.

Clements A. N. (1963), *The Physiology of Mosquitoes*. Pergamon Oxford.

Cova-Garcia P. (1946), *Notas sobre los Anofelinos de Venezuela y su Identificacion*. Editorial Grafolit, Caracas, Venezuela.

Davidson G. (1964), Anopheles gambiae, a complex of species. *Bulletin of the World Health Organisation*. **31**, 625–34.

Davidson G. (1972), Alternative measures to insecticides for mosquito control. *Pesticide Science* **3**, 503–14.

Davidson G. (1974), *Genetic Control of Insect Pests*. Academic Press, London and New York.

Davidson G. and Zahar A. R. (1973), The practical implications of resistance of malaria vectors to insecticides. *Bulletin of the World Health Organization.* **49**, 475–83.

Davidson G. (1978), Prospects of genetic control for medically important insects. In *Medical Entomology Centenary Symposium.* Royal Society of Tropical Medicine and Hygiene, London.

De Meillon B. (1947), *The Anophelini of the Ethiopian Geographical Region*. South African Institute for Medical Research, Johannesburg.

Detinova T. S. (1961), *Age-grouping Methods in Diptera of Medical Importance: with Special Reference to some Vectors of Malaria*. Monograph Series No. 47, World Health Organization, Geneva.

Doucet J. (1951), *Les Anophélines de la Région Malgache*. Institut de Recherches Scientifiques, Tananarive, Madagascar.

Elliott R. (1970), The influence of vector behaviour on malaria transmission. *American Journal of Tropical Medicine and Hygiene.* **21**, 755–63.

Farmer D. S., Dicke, R. J., Sweet G. and others (1946). *The Distribution of Mosquitos of Medical Importance in the Pacific Area*. US Bureau of Medicine and Surgery, Washington DC.

Gad A. M. (1956), Mosquitos of the oases of the Libyan desert of Egypt. *Bulletin of the Society of Entomology of Egypt*, **40**, 131–36.

Gillies M. T. and De Meillon B. (1968), *The Anophelinae of Africa South of the Sahara*. South African Institute for Medical Research, Johannesburg.

Hamon J., Adam J. P. and Grzebine A. (1956). Distribution maps of anophelines of West Africa. *Bulletin of the World Health Organization*. **15**, 549–91.

Hamon J. and Garrett-Jones C. (1963), La résistance aux insecticides chez les vecteurs majeurs du paludisme. *Bulletin of the World Health Organization.* **28**, 1–24.

Hamon J., Mouchet J., Brengues Y. and Chauvet G. (1970), Vector ecology and behaviour before, during and after application of control measures. *Miscellaneous Publications of the Entomological Society of America*. **7**, 28–41.

Horsfall W. H. (1955), *Mosquitoes: Their Bionomics and Relation to Disease*. Ronald Press, New York.

Hoskins W. M. (1963), Resistance to insecticides. in *International Review of Tropical Medicine* (Lincicome R. D., Ed.). Academic Press, London and New York.

King W. V., Bradley G. H., and McNeel T. E. (1939), *A Handbook of the Mosquitoes of the South-eastern United States*. US Department of Agriculture. No. 336.

Laird M. (1977), Enemies and diseases of mosquitoes. *Mosquito News* **37**, 331–39.

Lee D. J. and Woodhill A. R. (1944), *The Anopheline Mosquitoes of the Australian Region*. Sydney University, Zoological Publication No. 2.

Leeson H. S., Lumsden W. H. R., Yofe J. and Macan T. T. (1950), *Anophelines and Malaria in the Near East*. London School of Hygiene and Tropical Medicine Memoir No. 7, H. K. Lewis & Co. London.

Lewis D. J. (1956), The anopheline mosquitoes of the Sudan. *Bulletin of Entomological Research* **47**, 475–94.

Mattingly P. F. and Knight K. G. (1956), The mosquitoes of Arabia. *Bulletin of the British Museum (Natural History) Entomology Series*. **4**, 91–141.

Mattingly P. F. (1969), *The Biology of Mosquito-borne Disease*. George Allen and Unwin, London.

Muirhead-Thomson R. C. (1951), *Mosquito Behaviour*. Edward Arnold, London.

Muirhead-Thomson R. C. (1968), *Ecology of Insect Vector Populations*. Academic Press, London and New York.

National Society of India for Malaria and other Mosquito-borne Diseases, (1957), *Vectors of Malaria in India*. Delhi.

Pal. A. and La Chance G. D. (1974), The operational feasibility of genetic methods for control of insects of medical and veterinary importance. *Annual Review of Entomology* **19**, 269–96.

Pinotti M. (1951), The biological basis for the campaign against vectors of Brazil. *Transactions of the Royal Society of Tropical Medicine and Hygiene*. **44**, 663–82.

Puri I. M. (1957), *A Practical Entomological Course for Students of Malariology*. Health Bulletin No. 18, Government of India Press, Delhi.

Raffaele G., Ed. (1964), Symposium on A. gambiae. *Rivista di Malariologia* **43**, 165–275.

Reid J. A. (1968), *Anopheline Mosquitoes of Malaya and Borneo*. Studies from the Institute for Medical Research, No. 21, Government of Malaysia, Kuala Lumpur.

Russell P. F., Rozeboom L. E. and Stone A. (1943), *Keys to the Anopheline Mosquitoes of the World*, American Entomological Society, Philadelphia.

Senevet G. and Andarelli G. (1955), *Les Anophèles de l'Afrique du Nord et du Bassin Méditerranéen*. Maloine, Paris.

Smith K. G. V. (1978), *Insects and Other Arthropods of Medical Importance*. J. Wiley and Sons, Chichester.

Stone A., Knight K. G. and Starcke H. (1959), *A Synoptic Catalogue of the Mosquitoes of the World*. Th. Say Foundation Vol. 6, Entomological Society of America, Washington DC.

Stone A. (1961, 1963, 1967, 1970), A Synoptic Catalogue of the Mosquitoes of the World, Supplements I–IV. *Proceedings of the Entomological Society of America*. Washington **63**, 29–52; **65**, 117–40; **69**, 197–224; **72**, 137–76.

Ward R. A. and Scanlon J. E., Eds. (1970), *Conference on Anopheline Biology and Malaria Eradication*. Miscellaneous Publ. No. 7. American Entomological Society, Washington DC.

White G. B. (1974), Anopheles gambiae complex and disease transmission in Africa, *Transactions of the Royal Society of Tropical Medicine and Hygiene*. **68**, 278–98.

World Health Organization (1964), *Genetics of Vectors and Insecticide Resistance*. Technical Reports Series No. 268, Geneva.

World Health Organization (1967), *Mosquito Ecology*. Technical Reports Series No. 368, Geneva.

World Health Organization (1968), *Cytogenetics of Vectors of Disease of Man*. Technical Reports Series No. 398, Geneva.

World Health Organization (1972), *Vector Ecology*. Technical Reports Series No. 501, Geneva.

World Health Organization (1975), *Manual on Practical Entomology in Malaria*: Part I – Vector bionomics and organization of antimalaria activities, Part II – Methods and techniques. WHO Offset Publication No. 13, Geneva.

World Health Organization (1975), *Ecology and Control of Vectors in Public Health*. Technical Reports Series No. 561, Geneva.

World Health Organization (1976), *Resistance of Vectors and Reservoirs of Disease to Pesticides*. Technical Reports Series No. 585, Geneva.

Wright J. W. and Pal R. (1967), *Genetics of Insect Vectors of Disease*. Elsevier Publications, Amsterdam.

F. EPIDEMIOLOGY

Black R. H. (1968), *Manual on Epidemiology and Epidemiological Services in Malaria Programmes*. World Health Organization, Geneva.

Bruce-Chwatt L. J. (1965), Palaeogenesis and palaeo-epidemiology of primate malaria. *Bulletin of the World Health Organization*. **32**, 363–87.

Bruce-Chwatt L. J. (1966), Malaria zoonosis in relation to malaria eradication. *Tropical and Geographical Medicine*. **20**, 50–87.

Bruce-Chwatt L. J. (1974), Resurgence of malaria and its control. *Journal of Tropical Medicine and Hygiene*. **77** (Suppl. No. 4), 62–66.

Center for Disease Control (1978), *Malaria surveillance, Annual Summary for 1977*. US Department for Health Education and Welfare, CDC, Atlanta, Georgia.

Christophers S. R., Sinton J. A. and Covell G. (revised by Jaswant Singh and Puri I. M.) (1959), *How to do a Malaria Survey*. Govt. of India Press, Delhi.

Davey T. H. and Gordon R. M. (1933), The estimation of the density of infective anophelines as a method of calculating the relative risk of inoculation with malaria from different species or in different localities. *Annals of Tropical Medicine and Parasitology*. **27**, 27–52.

Draper C. C. and Voller A. (with Carpenter R. G.) (1972), The epidemiological interpretation of serologic data in malaria. *American Journal of Tropical Medicine and Hygiene*. **21**, 696–703.

Garnham P. C. C. (1967), Malaria in mammals excluding man. In *Advances in Parasitology* Vol. 5, Academic Press, London.

Garnham P. C. C. (1971), Malaria as a medical and veterinary zoonosis. In *Progress in Parasitology*. University of London, The Athlone Press, London.

Garrett-Jones C. (1970), Problems of epidemiological entomology as applied to malariology. *Miscellaneous Publications of the Entomological Society of America*. **7**, 168–78.

Gramiccia C. and Hempel Y. (1972), Mortality and morbidity from malaria in countries where malaria eradication is not making satisfactory progress. *Journal of Tropical Medicine and Hygiene*. **75**, 187–192.

Hamon J. and Coz J. (1966), Epidemiologie générale du paludisme humain en Afrique Occidentale. *Bulletin de la Société de Pathologie Exotique* **59**, 466–83.

Johnson D. R. (1973), Recent developments in mosquito borne diseases: malaria. *Mosquito News* **33**, 341–47.

Kligler I. J. (1920), *The epidemiology and control of malaria in Palestine*. University of Chicago Press, Chicago, Ill.

Lysenko A. Y. and Semashko I. N. (1968), Geography of malaria. In *Medical Geography*, Lebedev A. W., Academy of Sciences USSR, Moscow.

Macdonald G. (1957), *The Epidemiology and Control of Malaria*. Oxford University Press, London, New York, Toronto.

Macdonald G. and Goeckel C. W. (1964), The malaria parasite rate and interruption of transmission. *Bulletin of the World Health Organization*. **31**, 365–77.

Macdonald G., Cuellar C. B., and Foll C. V. (1968), The dynamics of malaria. *Bulletin of the World Health Organization*. **37**, 743–55.

Macdonald G. (1973), *Dynamics of tropical disease* (Bruce-Chwatt L. J. and Glanville V., Eds.). Oxford University Press, London.

Moshkowski S. D. (1950), *Basic Laws of Epidemiology of Malaria* (in Russian). Academy of Medical Sciences, Moscow.

Pull J. H. and Grab B. (1974), A simple epidemiological model for evaluating the malaria inoculation rate and the risk of infection in infants. *Bulletin of the World Health Organization*. **51**, 507–16.

Russell P. F. (1956), World wide malaria distribution, prevalence and control. *American Journal of Tropical Medicine and Hygiene*. **5**, 937–65.

Shute P. T. and Maryon M. E. (1969), Imported malaria in the United Kingdom. *British Medical Journal*. **2**, 781–85.

Swaroop S. (1964), *Statistical Methods in Malaria Eradication*. Gilroy A. B. and Uemura K., Eds. Monograph Series No. 51, World Health Organization, Geneva.

Wilson D. B., Garnham P. C. C. and Swellengrebel H. H. (1950), A review of hyperendemic malaria. *Tropical Diseases Bulletin*. **47**, 677–98.

World Health Organization (1961–72), Malaria eradication in – 1960, 1961, 1962, 1963, 1964, 1965, 1966, 1968, 1969, 1970, 1971, 1972. *WHO Chronicle* **15**, 201; **16**, 333; **17**, 335; **18**, 199; **19**, 338; **20**, 286; **21**, 373; **23**, 515; **24**, 395; **25**, 498; **26**, 485.

World Health Organization (1973–76), The malaria situation in – 1973, 1974, 1975, 1976.*WHO Chronicle* **28**, 479–87; **29**, 474–81; **30**, 486–93; **32**, 9–17.

World Health Organization (1978), Information on malaria risk for international travellers. *Weekly Epidemiological Record* No. 25–26, Geneva.

Zulueta J. de, Ramsdale C. W. and Coluzzi M. (1975), Receptivity to malaria in Europe. *Bulletin of the World Health Organization* **52**, 109–11.

G. CONTROL AND ERADICATION

American Mosquito Control Association (1952), *Ground Equipment and Insecticides for Mosquito Control* (Knipling E. F., Ed.). AMCA Bulletin No. 2, Bureau of Entomology, US Department of Agriculture, Washington DC.

Bailey Y. (1977), *Guide to Hygiene and Sanitation in Aviation*, 2nd edition. World Health Organization, Geneva.

Barnes Y. M. (1953), *Toxic Hazards of Certain Pesticides to Man*. Monograph Series No. 16, World Health Organization, Geneva.

Bay, E. C. (1967), Mosquito Control by Fish: A Present Day Appraisal. *WHO Chronicle* **21**, 415–23.

Beklemishev V. N. (1954), *Construction of Water-reservoirs and the Problem of Malaria* (in Russian). Medgiz, Moscow.

Brown, A. W. H. (1951). *Insect Control by Chemicals*. John Wiley & Sons, New York.

Brown A. W. A., Haworth J. and Zahar, A. A. (1976), Malaria eradication and control from a global standpoint. *Journal of Medical Entomology* **13**, 1–25.

Brown A. W. A. (1978), *Ecology of Pesticides*. J. Wiley and Sons, Chichester.

Bruce-Chwatt L. J. (1969), Malaria eradication at the crossroads. *Bulletin of the New York Academy of Medicine* **45**, 999–1012.

Bruce-Chwatt L. J. and Davidson G. (1974), *Malaria and its Control*. Ross Institute Bulletin No. 7, London.

Bruce-Chwatt L. J. and Zulueta J. de (1977), Malaria eradication in Portugal. *Transactions of the Royal Society of Tropical Medicine and Hygiene* **71**, 232–40.

Busvine J. A. (1978), Current problems in the control of mosquitoes. *Nature* **273** (Supplements), 604–7.

Busvine J. A. (1978), The future of insecticidal control of medically important insects. In *Medical Entomology Centenary, Symposium* 106–11. Royal Society of Tropical Medicine and Hygiene, London.

Carmichael G. T. (1972), Anopheline control through water management. *American Journal of Transport Medicine and Hygiene* **21**, 281–6.

Ciuca M., Ed. (1966), *L'éradication du paludisme en Roumanie*. Editions Médicales, Bucarest.

Colbourne M. J. (1962), A review of malaria eradication campaigns in the Western Pacific. *Annals of Tropical Medicine and Parasitology* **56**, 33–43.

Cremlyn R. T. (1978), *Pesticides: Preparation and Mode of Action*. J. Wiley and Sons, Chichester.

Covell G. (1941), *Malaria Control by Antimosquito Measures* (2nd edition). Thacker, Spink Co., Calcutta.

Gabaldon A. (1951), Progress of the malaria campaign in Venezuela, *American Journal of Tropical Medicine and Hygiene* **10**, 124–41.

Gabaldon A. (1969), Global eradication of malaria: Changes of strategy and future outlook. *American Journal of Tropical Medicine and Hygiene* **18**, 641–56.

Gabaldon A. and Berti A. G. (1954), The first large area in the tropical zone to report malaria eradication: North-central Venezuela. *American Journal of Tropical Medicine and Hygiene* **3**, 793–807.

Garcia-Martin G. (1972), Status of malaria eradication in the Americas. *American Journal of Tropical Medicine and Hygiene* **21**, 617–33.

Giglioli, G. (1948), *Malaria, Filariasis and Yellow Fever in British Guiana*. Mosquito Control Service, Medical Department, Georgetown.

Giglioli G. (1951), Eradication of Anopheles darlingi from the inhabited areas of British Guiana by D.D.T. residual spraying. *American Journal of Tropical Medicine and Hygiene* **10**, 142–61.

Gilroy A. B. (1948), *Malaria Control by Coastal Swamp Drainage in West Africa*. Ross Institute of Tropical Hygiene, London.

Gratz N. G. (1977), The importance of chemicals in the control of tropical diseases, pp. 86–180. In *Chemie der Pflanzenschutz – und Schädlings Bekämpfungsmittel*, Vol. III (Wegler R., Ed.). Springer Verlag, Berlin, Heidelberg, New York.

Hayes W. J. (1975), *Toxicology of Pesticides*. Williams & Wilkins, Baltimore.

Herms W. B. and Gray H. F. (1944), *Mosquito Control* (2nd edition). The Commonwealth Fund, New York.

Hildemann W. H. and Walford R. S. (1963), Annual fishes: promising species as biological control agents. *Journal of Tropical Medicine and Hygiene* **66**, 163–6.

Hinman E. H. (1966), *World Eradication of Infectious Diseases*. Charles Thomas, Springfield, Illinois.

Jenkins D. W., Ed. (1960), *Biological Control of Insects of Medical Importance*. Armed Forces Institute of Pathology, Washington DC.

King M. V. (1951), Repellents and insecticides available for use against insects of medical importance. *Journal of Economic Entomology*. **44**, 338–43.

Lepeš T. (1974), Present status of the global malaria eradication programme and prospects for the future. *Journal of Tropical Medicine and Hygiene* **77** (Supplement), 47–53.

Matthews G. A. (1979), *Pesticide Application Methods*. Longman, London and New York.

Magoon E. H. (1945), Drainage for health in the Caribbean area (English and Spanish). *Boletin Oficial de Salubridad y Asistencia Social*, La Habana, Republica de Cuba.

Mellanby K. (1967), *Pesticides and Pollution*. Collins, London.

Ministry of Health, India (1960), *Manual of Malaria Eradication Operations* (2nd edition). Government of India, Delhi.

Mulligan H. W. and Afridi M. K. (1938), The prevention of malaria incidental to engineering construction. *Health Bulletin* No. 25, Government of India Press, New Delhi.

National Malaria Committee (1938), *Malaria Control for Engineers*. US Public Health Service (Cyclostyled), Washington.

Newman P. (1965), *Malaria Eradication and Population Growth*. School of Public Health, University of Michigan, Ann Arbor, Michigan.

Noguer A. (1978), Cost of vector-borne disease control programmes with particular reference to malaria. In *Medical Entomology Centenary Symposium*, 120–6, Royal Society of Tropical Medicine & Hygiene, London.

Pampana E. Y. (1969), *A Textbook of Malaria Eradication* (2nd edition). Oxford University Press, London, New York, Toronto.

Pan-American Health Organization (1972), *Vector Control and the Recrudescence of Vector-borne diseases*. Scientific Publication No. 238, PAHO/WHO, Washington DC.

Perring F. H. and Mellanby K. (1978), *Ecological Effects of Pesticides*. Academic Press, London.

Peters W. (1972), Advances in malariology relating to control and eradication. *British Medical Bulletin* **28**, 28–33.

Pinotti M. (1951), The nation-wide malaria eradication programme in Brazil, *American Journal of Tropical Medicine and Hygiene* **10**, 162–82.

Pull J. H. and Gramiccia G. (1976), Research on malaria control in Africa. *WHO Chronicle* **30**, 286–9. Geneva.

Russell P. F. (1950), Malaria control activities of the World Health Organization. *Journal of the National Malaria Society*. **9**, 1–4.

Service M. W. (1978), Some problems in the control of malaria, pp. 151–64. In *Ecological effects of pesticides* (Perring F. H. and Mellanby K., Eds.). Academic Press, London.

Scharff J. W. (1935), *Antimalarial Drainage*. Criterion Press, Penang.

Schoof H. F. and Taylor R. T. (1972), Recent advances in insecticides for malaria programs. *American Journal of Tropical Medicine & Hygiene*, **21**, 807–12.

Shousha A. T. (1948), Species eradication. The eradication of Anopheles gambiae from Upper Egypt, 1942–45. *Bulletin of the World Health Organization*, **1**, 309–52.

US Public Health Service (1947), *Malaria Control in Impounded Waters* (Bishop E. G., Ed.). US Government Printing Office, Washington DC.

Verdrager J., Mamet R., Roche S. and Klein J. P. (1964), *La Campagne d'Éradication du Paludisme à l'Ile Maurice*. Felix, Imprimeur, Port Louis, Mauritius.

Viswanathan D. K. (1950), *Malaria and its Control in Bombay State*. Poona, India.

Watson M. (1921), *The Prevention of Malaria*. John Murray, London.

Watson D. G. and Brown A. W. A. (1977), *Pesticide Management and Insecticide Resistance*. Academic Press, London, New York, San Francisco.

Wright J. W. (1971), The WHO programme for evaluation and testing of new insecticides. *Bulletin of the World Health Organization*, **44**, 11–22.

Wright J. W., Fritz R. F. and Haworth G. (1972), Changing concepts of vector control in malaria eradication. *Annual Review of Entomology*, **17**, 75–102.

World Health Organization (1956), *Toxic Hazards of Pesticides to Man*. Technical Reports Series No. 114, Geneva.

World Health Organization (1958), *Insect Resistance and Vector Control: Eighth report of the Expert Committee on Insecticides*, Technical Reports Series No. 153, Geneva.

World Health Organization (1960), *Insecticide Resistance and Vector Control: Tenth report of the Expert Committee on Insecticides*, Technical Reports Series No. 191, Geneva.

World Health Organization (1962), *Malaria and Insecticides. Bulletin of the World Health Organization*, **27**, 189–307.

World Health Organization (1962), *Toxic Hazards of Pesticides to Man: Twelfth Report of the Expert Committee on Insecticides*. Technical Reports Series No. 227, Geneva.

World Health Organization (1963), *Insecticide Resistance and Vector Control, Thirteenth Report of the Expert Committee on Insecticides*. Technical Reports Series No. 265, Geneva.

World Health Organization (1963), Vector Control, *Bulletin of the World Health Organization*, Supplement, **29**, 5–186.

World Health Organization (1964), *Application and Dispersal of Pesticides. Fourteenth Report of the Expert Committee on Insecticides*. Technical Reports Series No. 284, Geneva.

World Health Organization (1964), *Equipment for Vector Control*. Geneva.

World Health Organization (1967), *Specifications for Pesticides Used in Public Health*. Geneva.

World Health Organization (1967), *Safe Use of Pesticides in Public Health*. Technical Reports Series No. 356, Geneva.

World Health Organization (1967), *Prevention of the Re-introduction of Malaria*. Technical Reports Series No. 374, Geneva.

World Health Organization (1967), *The Education of Engineers in Environmental Health*. Technical Reports Series No. 376, Geneva.

World Health Organization (1969), *Re-examination of the global stategy of malaria eradication*. Annex 13, Official Records No. 176, 106–26, Geneva.

World Health Organization (1969), *Field Manual for Antilarval Operations in Malaria Eradication Programmes*. Offset Publications, Geneva.

World Health Organization (1970), *Insecticide Resistance and Vector Control*. Technical Reports Series No. 443, Geneva.

World Health Organization (1971). *Application and Dispersal of Pesticides*. Technical Reports Series No. 465, Geneva.

World Health Organization (1972), *Vector Control in International Health*. Geneva.

World Health Organization (1972), *Manual of planning for malaria eradication and malaria control programmes*. WHO Cyclostyled document ME/72.10, Geneva.

World Health Organization (1973), *Specifications for Pesticides Used in Public Health*, 4th edition. World Health Organization, Geneva.

World Health Organization (1973), *Safe Use of Pesticides*. Technical Reports Series No. 513, Geneva.

World Health Organization (1973), *Manual on Larval Control Operations in Malaria Programmes*. WHO Offset Publication No. 1, Geneva.

World Health Organization (1974), *Equipment for Vector Control*, 2nd edition. Geneva.

World Health Organization (1974), *Malaria Control in Countries where Time-limited Eradication is Impracticable at present*. Technical Reports Series No. 537, Geneva.

World Health Organization (1974), *Manual on Personal and Community Protection against Malaria in Development Areas and New Settlements*. Offset Publication No. 10, Geneva.

World Health Organization (1977), *Engineering Aspects of Vector Control Operations*. Technical Report Series No. 603, Geneva.

World Health Organization (1978), *Chemistry and Specifications of Pesticides*. Technical Reports Series No. 620, Geneva.

World Health Organization (1979) *DDT and its Derivatives*, Environmental Health Criteria No. 9, Geneva.

Zulueta de J. (1973), Malaria eradication in Europe: The achievements and difficulties ahead. *Journal of Tropical Medicine and Hygiene*, **76**, 279–82.

Zulueta de J. and Garrett-Jones C. (1965), An investigation on the persistence of malaria transmission in Mexico. *American Journal of Tropical Medicine and Hygiene*, **14**, 63–77.

Zulueta de J. and Muir D. A. (1972), Malaria eradication in the Near East. *Transactions of the Royal Society of Tropical Medicine and Hygiene*. **66**, 679–96.

ANNEX I

International nonproprietary names of antimalarial drugs and some synonyms or proprietary names[1]

Quinine (sulphate, bisulphate, dihydrochloride, hydrochloride)
Quinimax; Quinoforme (formiate)

Acridines

Mepacrine[2] (dihydrochloride)
Acrichin; Acriquine; Atabrin; Erion; Metoquina; Quinacrine

Mepacrine[2] (methanesulfonate)
Atebrine musonate; Quinacrine soluble (For injection)

4-Aminoquinolines

Chloroquine[2] (diphosphate)
Aralen; Avloclor; Bemaphate; Chinamine; Delagil; Gontochin; Imagon; Iroquine; Klorokin; Luprochin; Resochin; Resoquine; Sanoquin; Tanakan; Tresochin; Trochin (and other names)

Chloroquine[2] (sulfate)
Nivaquine; Nivaquine B

Amodiaquine[2] (dihydrochloride)
Cam-aqi; Camoquin; Camoquinal; Flavoquine; Fluroquine; Miaquine

Amodiaquine[2] (base)
Basoquin

Amopyroquine[2] (dihydrochloride)
Propoquin (For injection)

8-Aminoquinolines

Primaquine[2] (diphosphate)
Neo-Quipenyl

Quinocide (dihydrochloride)
Chinocid

---

[1] This list is based on *Chemotherapy of malaria and resistance to antimalarials*, World Health Organization, Technical Reports Series No 529, Geneva, 1973.

[2] International Nonproprietary Name (INN).

Annex I

Dihydrofolate reductase inhibitors (Antifolic compounds)

Proguanil[2] (hydrochloride)
Balusil; Bigumal; Chlorguanide; Chloriguane; Diguanyl; Drinupal; Guanatol; Lepadina; Paludrine; Palusil; Plasin; Proguanide; Tirian

Chlorproguanil[2] (hydrochloride)
Lapudrine

Cycloguanil embonate[2] (For injection)
Camolar; Cycloguanil pamoate

Pyrimethamine[2] (base)
Chloridin; Darapram; Daraprim; Erbaprelina; Malocide; Tindurin (and other names)

Trimethoprim[2]
Syraprim

Quinolinemethanol

Mefloquine[2]

Sulfones

Dapsone[2] (*DDS*)
Avlosulfone; Croysulfone; Damitone; Daphone; Diphenason; Diaphenylsulfone; Diatox; Diphone; Disulone; Eporal; Novophone; Sulfadione; Udolac

Acedapsone[2] (For injection)
Camilan; Hansolar; Rodilone; Sulfadiamine

Sulfonamides

Sulfadiazine[2]
Adiazine; Codiazine; Cremodiazine; Debenal; Diazine; Diazyl; Eskadiazine; Eustral; Keladiazine; Pirimal; Pyrimal; Sterazine; Sulfazine

Sulfadimethoxine[2]
Levisul; Madribon; Madriquid; Sulfadimethoxypyrimidine

Sulfamethoxypyridazine[2]
Davosin; Deposulfal; Depovernil; Kynex; Lederkyn; Midicel; Midikel; Myasul; Spofadiazine; Sulfadurazin; Sulfalex; Sultirène; Unosulf

Sulfadoxine[2]
Fanasil; Fanasulf; Fanzil; Sulformethoxine; Sulforthodimethoxine; Sulforthomidine

Sulfalene[2]
Kelfizina; Kelfizine; Sulfamethoxypyrazine; Sulfametopyrazine

---

[2] International Nonproprietary Name (INN).

Combinations of sulphones or sulphonamides with antifolic compounds (such as pyrimethamine)

Maloprim; Fansidar; Metakelfin; Kelfimet

ANNEX II

Selected list of some common insecticides and their generic and other names[1]

Common name	Chemical name	Other names
Abate	O, O, O', O'-tetramethyl O, O'-thiodi-p-phenylene phosphorothioate	*temephos* OMS-786
allethrin	2, 2-dimethyl-3-(2-methylpropenyl) cyclopropane-carboxylic acid ester with 2-allyl-4-hydroxy-3-methyl-2-cyclopenten-1-one	
Baygon	O-isopropoxyphenyl-N-methyl-carbamate	Arprocarb, Bayer 39007. OMS-33
Baytex	see fenthion	
BHC	mixed isomers of 1, 2, 3, 4, 5, 6-hexa-chlorocyclohexane	HCH, benzene hexachloride, 666
bromophos	O-(4-bromo-2, 5-dichlorophenyl) O, O-dimethyl phosphorothioate	OMS-658
carbaryl	α-naphthyl methylcarbamate	Sevin, OMS-29
carbophenothion	S-(p-chlorophenylthiomethyl) O, O-diethyl phosphorodithioate	
chlordane	1, 2, 4, 5, 6, 7, 10, 10-octachloro-4, 7, 8, 9-tetrahydro-4, 7-methleneindame	chlordan, Velsicol 1068, Octa-Klor, Octachlor

---

[1] Mainly after *Insecticide Resistance and Vector Control*. WHO, Technical Reports Series No. 443; 1970.

Annex II

Common name	Chemical name	Other names
Chlorthion	O,O-dimethyl O-(3-chloro-4-nitrophenyl) phosphorothioate	Bayer 22/190, OMS-217
diazinon	O,O-diethyl O-(2-isopropyl-6-methyl-4-pyrimidyl) phosphorothioate	OMS-469, Basadin
DDT	1,1,1-trichloro-2,2-di (p-chlorophenyl) ethane	Chlorophenothane, dicophane, Gesarol
dichlorvos	2,2-dichlorovinyl dimethyl phosphate	DDVP, Nuvan, Vapona
dieldrin	product containing 85%w/w HEOD	Octalox
chlorpyrifos	O,O-diethyl O-(3,5,6-trichloro-2-pyridyl) phosphorothioate	Dursban
fenchlorphos	O,O-dimethyl O-(2,4,5-trichlorophenyl) phosphorothioate	Ronnel, Dow ET-57, Korlan, Trolene, Etrolene, Nankor
fenitrothion	O,O-dimethyl O-(4-nitro-m-tolyl) phosphorothioate	Sumithion, Folithion, Bayer 41831, OMS-43
fenthion	O,O-dimethyl O-[(4-methylthio)-m-tolyl] phosphorothioate	Baytex, Entex, Bayer 29493, OMS-2, Lebaycid
gamma-HCH	gamma-isomer of 1,2,3,4,5,6-hexachlorocylcohexane	See *lindane*
HCH	1,2,3,4,5,6-hexachlorocyclohexane (mixture of isomers)	BHC, 666
HEOD	1,2,3,4,10,10-hexachloro-6,7-epoxy-1,4,4a,5,6,7,8,8a-octahydro-*endo*-1,4-*exo*-5,8-dimethanonaphthalene	See *dieldrin*
heptachlor	1,4,5,6,7,10,10-heptachloro-4,7,8,9-tetrahydro-4,7-methylene indene a product containing not less than 99% of gamma-HCH	Velsicol 104
lindane		
malathion	O,O-dimethyl S-[1,2-bis (ethoxycarbonyl) ethyl] phosphorodithioate	carbofos, malathon, compound 4049, OMS-1, Cython
methoxychlor	1,1,1-trichloro-2,2-bis (p-methoxyphenyl) ethane	Marlate, DMDT, methoxy DDT
propoxur	O-isopropoxyphenyl methylcarbamate	arprocarb, Baygon OMS-33
*parathion	O,O-diethyl O-(p-nitrophenyl)	
pyrethrum	extract of dried pyrethrum flowers, consisting mainly of pyrethrin I, pyrethrin II, cinerin I and cinerin II	

---

² Insecticide not used in public health.

Common name	Chemical name	Other names
Resmethrin	5-benzyl-3-furylmethyl (±)-*cis, trans*-chrysanthemate	
temephos	O, O, O', O'-tetramethyl-O, O'-thiodi-*p*-phenylene phosphorothioate	Abate, diphenfos
trichlorfon	dimethyl (2, 2, 2-trichloro-1-hydroxyethyl) phosphonate	metriphonate Dipterex, Dylox, Neguvon
tetrachorvinphos	2-chloro-1-(2, 4, 5-trichloro-phenyl) vinyl dimethyl phosphate	Aphoxide, Gardona, SD-8447, Rabon

Note: Common names approved by the International Organization for Standardization (ISO) are used when they exist; they are printed in italic type. Other common names are printed in roman type. Proprietary names (used only when no common name or OMS number exists) are distinguished by an initial capital letter. Letters OMS refer to the WHO list of provisional code designations.

ANNEX III

Information on malaria risk

The major part of this table is based on a document prepared by the US Department of Health, Education and Welfare, Center for Disease Control (Morbidity and Mortality Weekly Report, 1978, vol. 27, No 10 Supplement) and represents a simplified version of the document 'Information on Malaria Risk for International Travellers' issued by the World Health Organization (reprinted from WHO Weekly Epidemiological Record, 1976, No 24, pp. 181–200). Countries which are not listed do not present any risk of malaria, while question marks indicate that no information is available. Information on areas with chloroquine resistance may not be fully up to date. It should be stressed that even in urban areas of tropical countries where the risk of malaria appears to be slight or absent the possibility of infection at the periphery exists. This applies particularly to airports situated usually far from urban centres. Naturally, this annex reflects a transient situation subjected to considerable and often unreported changes.

Annex III

Country	Risk	Areas without risk	Risk exists during (months)	Risk exists below given altitude (metres)	Risk in urban areas	Areas with known chloroquine-resistant *P. falciparum*
AFRICA						
Afars and Issas, Territory	No					
Algeria	Yes	Most of the country except coastal area between Oran and Alger	Jun-Oct	1 200	No	None
Angola	Yes	None	All	All	Yes	None
Botswana	Yes	South-western quarter of country	Nov – May	All	Yes[1]	None
British Indian Ocean Territory	No					
Burundi	Yes	None	All	All	Yes	None
Cameroon, United Republic of	Yes	None	All	All	Yes	None
Cape Verde Islands	Yes	None	All	All		None
Central African Republic	Yes	None	All	All	Yes	None
Chad	Yes	None	Jul-Nov	All	Yes	None
Comoro Islands	Yes	None	All	All	Yes	None
Congo	Yes	None	All	All	Yes	None
Egypt	Yes	Most of the country, except the Nile Delta, El Faiyum area, and part of southern Egypt	Jun – Oct	All	No[2]	None

[1] Except Gaborone and Francistown
[2] No risk except in outskirts

330 *Essential Malariology*

Country	Risk	Areas without risk	Risk exists during (months)	Risk exists below given altitude (metres)	Risk in urban areas	Areas with known chloroquine-resistant *P. falciparum*
AFRICA (cont'd)						
Equatorial Guinea	Yes	None	All	All	Yes	None
Ethiopia	Yes	None	All	2 000	Yes	None
Gabon	Yes	None	All	1 000	Yes	None
Gambia	Yes	None	All	All	Yes	None
Ghana	Yes	None	All	All	Yes	None
Guinea	Yes	None	All	All	Yes	None
Guinea-Bissau	Yes	None	All	All	Yes	None
Ivory Coast	Yes	None	All	All	Yes	None
Kenya	Yes	None	All	2 000	Yes[3]	None
Lesotho	No					
Liberia	Yes	None	All	All	Yes	None
Libyan Arab Republic	Yes	Most country, except south-west quarter	Feb – Aug	All	No	None
Madagascar (Malagasy Republic)	Yes	Antsirabe, Tananarive, and vicinities	Sep – Mar	1 100	Yes	?
Malawi	Yes	None	All	1 700	Yes	None
Mali	Yes	None	All	All	Yes	None
Mauritania	Yes	?	?	?	?	None
Mauritius	No					
Morocco	Yes	Agadir, Casablanca, Rabat-Sale, Tanger, Taza, Tetouan, Tiznit	May – Oct	?	No[4]	None
Mozambique	Yes	None	All	All	Yes	None

Annex III

Country						
Niger	Yes	None	Jul – Nov	All	Yes	None
Nigeria	Yes	None	All	All	Yes	None
Reunion	No					
Rhodesia (Zimbabwe)	Yes	?	?	?	?	None
Rwanda	Yes	None	All	All	Yes	None
St Helena	No					
São Tome and Principe	Yes	?	?	?	?	None
Senegal	Yes	None	All	All	Yes	None
Seychelles	No					
Sierra Leone	Yes	None	All	All	Yes	None
Somali	Yes	None	All	All	Yes	None
South Africa	Yes	Most of country except areas bordering South-West Africa, Botswana	All	1 200	Yes	None
South-West Africa (Namibia)	Yes	?	?	?	?	None
Spanish Sahara	No					
Sudan	Yes	None	All	All	Yes	None
Swaziland	Yes	Most of the country except northern border areas	Dec – Mar	All	Yes	None
Tanzania	Yes	None	All	All	Yes	?
Togo	Yes	None	All	All	Yes	None
Tunisia	Yes	None	May – Nov	All	No	None
Uganda	Yes	None	All	1 800	Yes[5]	None
Upper Volta	Yes	None	All	All	Yes	None
Zaire	Yes	None	All	All	Yes	None
Zambia	Yes	None	Nov – May	All	Yes	?

[3] Risk very low: Nairobi Area
[4] No risk except in outskirts
[5] Little risk in Entebbe, Fort Portal, Jinja, Kampala, or Mbale

Essential Malariology

Country	Risk	Areas without risk	Risk exists during (months)	Risk exists below given altitude (metres)	Risk in urban areas	Areas with known chloroquine-resistant P. falciparum
AMERICAS						
Argentina	Yes	Most of the country except small area in north-west	Sep – May	2 000	No	None
Belize	Yes	None	All	500	Yes	None
Bolivia	Yes	South-western quarter of country	All	2 000	No	None
Brazil	Yes	Brasilia and Distrito Federal; coastal areas from Fortaleza to Salvador and from Rio de Janeiro to Sao Paulo	All	900	No⁶	States in interior of country and Espirito Santo State
Canal Zone	No					
Chile	No					
Colombia	Yes	Bogota and vicinity	All	1 500	No	Malarious areas in northern third of country; some interior provinces
Costa Rica	Yes	Mountainous centre of country	All	500	No	None
Cuba	No					
Ecuador	Yes	Galapagos Islands, Guayaquil and vicinity	All	1 500	Yes	Provinces bordering on Colombia
El Salvador	Yes	None	All	1 000	No	None

Annex III

Country		Area		Altitude (m)		Notes
Falkland Islands	No					None
French Guiana	Yes	Cayenne City	All	All	Yes	None
Guatemala	Yes	Guatemala City and vicinity	Jun – Nov[7]	1 000	No	None
Guyana	Yes	Coastal areas from Georgetown to New Amsterdam; Essequibo River Delta	All	All	No	Areas bordering on Brazil and Guyana
Honduras	Yes	None	All	1 000	No	None
Mexico	Yes	States of Aguascalientes, Baja California Coahuila, Distrito Federal, Guanajuato, Nuevo Leon, and Tlaxcala	All	1 800	No	None
Nicaragua	Yes	None	All	1 000	No	None
Panama (excluding Canal Zone)	Yes	Panama City and Colon City	All	700	No	All malarious areas east of Canal Zone
Paraguay	Yes	Most of country except areas bordering Brazil	Sep – May	All	Yes	None
Peru	Yes	Lima and southern coastal area	All	1 500	No	None
Saint-Pierre and Miquelon	No					
Surinam	Yes	Coastal areas around Paramaribo	All	All	Yes[8]	All malarious areas
Uruguay	No					
Venezuela	Yes	Coastal area between Caracas and Maracaibo	All	600	No	Provinces in interior of country

[6] Except in Amazon River region
[7] North-eastern part of country: risk during all months
[8] Except coastal cities

Country	Risk	Areas without risk	Risk exists during (months)	Risk exists below given altitude (metres)	Risk in urban areas	Areas known known chloroquine-resistant *P. falciparum*
CARIBBEAN						
Dominican Republic	Yes	Most of country except areas bordering Haiti	All	500	No	None
Haiti	Yes	None	Jun – Feb	500	No[9]	None
ASIA						
Afghanistan	Yes	None	May – Nov	2 000	Yes	None
Bahrain	Yes	None	All	All	Yes	None
Bangladesh	Yes	Bogra, Dacca, Jessore, Khulna, Pabna, Rajshahi, and vicinities	All	All	Yes	Areas bordering on Assam State, India, Burma
Bhutan	Yes	None	Mar – Oct	1 600	Yes	None
Brunei	No					
Burma	Yes	Rangoon City and suburbs, Mandalay	Apr – Nov	900	No	All malarious areas
Cambodia	Yes	?	All	All	Yes	Whole country
China	?	?	?	?	?	?
Cyprus	No					
Gaza Strip (Palestine)	Yes	None	Jun – Oct	All	Yes	None
Hong Kong	No					
India	Yes	None	Mar – Oct	1 600	Yes	Assam State
Indonesia	Yes	Djakarta, Surabaya and	All	1 200	Yes	East Kalimantan, Irian Jaya
Iran	Yes	North-western quarter of country (including Teheran and Isfahan)	Jul – Nov	1 500	No	None

Annex III

Country		Area	Months	Altitude		Notes
Iraq	Yes	Most of the country except northern third	May – Nov	1 500	Yes	None
Israel	No					
Japan	No					
Jordan	Yes	Whole country, except Jordan River Valley	Apr – Nov	All	No	None
Korea Democratic People's Republic of N. Korea	No					
Republic of S. Korea	Yes	None	Jun – Sep	All	No	None
Kuwait	No					
Laos	Yes	Vientiane	All	All	Yes	None
Lebanon	No					
Macao	No					
Malaysia	Yes	None	All	1 700	No[10]	All malarious areas of Malaya and Sabah; Sarawak–Sabah border
Maldive Islands	Yes	Male Island	All	All	No	None
Mongolia	No					
Nepal	Yes	None	All	1 200	Yes	None
Oman	Yes	None	All	1 000	Yes	None
Pakistan	Yes	None	Mar – Oct	2 000	Yes	None
Philippines	Yes	Cebu and Leyte Islands, plains areas of Negros and Panay Islands	All	600	No	Luzon, Basilan and Sulu Islands, Mindoro and Palawan
Portuguese Timor	Yes	None	All	All	Yes	None
Qatar	Yes	None	All	All	Yes	None

[9] No risk except in outskirts
[10] Except Sabah

Country	Risk	Areas without risk	Risk exists during (months)	Risk exists below given altitude (metres)	Risk in urban areas	Areas with known chloroquine-resistant P. falciparum
ASIA (cont'd)						
Saudi Arabia	Yes	Urban areas of Jeddah, Mecca, Medina, Riyad	All	?	Yes	None
Singapore	Yes	City District (southern part of island)	All	All	No	None
Sri Lanka (Ceylon)	Yes	Colombo	All	800	Yes	None
Syrian Arab Republic	Yes	Mediterranean Coast, eastern half, and southern half	May – Oct	600	No	None
Thailand	Yes	Most urban areas including Bangkok and suburbs	All	All	No	All malarious areas
Turkey	Yes	Whole country except Adana and surrounding area	Jul – Oct	1 000	No	None
United Arab Emirates	Yes	None	All	All	Yes	None
Viet-Nam, Democratic Republic of	Yes	None	Mar – Nov	1 000	No	All malarious areas in the south
Yemen	Yes	None	Sep – Feb	1 400	Yes	None
Yemen, Democratic	Yes	Aden and airport perimeter	All	All	Yes	None
EUROPE	No					

OCEANIA					
British Solomon Islands	Yes	None	All	400	Yes	None
New Hebrides	Yes	None	All	All	Yes	None
Papua New Guinea	Yes	None	All	2 000	Yes	Some evidence

ANNEX IV

Formulation of suspensions, emulsions, concentrates and sprays for malaria control.
Reproduced from WHO, 1970, Technical Report Series no, 443 *Insecticide Resistance and Vector Control.*

REQUIREMENTS FOR SPRAY FORMULATIONS

Dosage (weight per unit area)	Litres* of spray required per 100 m² (1000 ft²) using following concentrations of technical insecticide :				
	0.25%	0.5%	1.0%	2.5%	5.0%
2 g/m² (200 mg/ft²)	—	—	20	8	4
1 g/m² (100 mg/ft²)	—	20	10	4	2
0.5 g/m² (50 mg/ft²)	20	10	5	2	1
0.2 g/m² (20 mg/ft²)	8	4	2	0.8	0.4

*1 litre is approximately equal to 0.25 USgal or 0.2 UKgal

AMOUNT OF WATER-DISPERSIBLE POWDER (w.d.p.) REQUIRED FOR PREPARATION OF SPRAY SUSPENSIONS

Percentage of toxicant in w.d.p.	Kg (lb) of w.d.p. required for about 380 litres (100 USgal ; 83 UKgal) of finished spray suspension with concentrations of :				
	5%	2.5%	1%	0.5%	0.25%
90	21.0 (46.3)	10.5 (23.1)	4.2 (9.3)	2.1 (4.6)	1.0 (2.3)
75	25.2 (55.6)	12.6 (27.8)	5.0 (11.1)	2.5 (5.6)	1.3 (2.8)
50	37.8 (83.3)	18.9 (41.7)	7.6 (16.7)	3.8 (8.3)	1.9 (4.2)
25	75.6 (166.7)	37.8 (83.3)	15.1 (33.3)	7.6 (16.7)	3.8 (8.3)

Annex IV

PREPARATION OF EMULSION FROM CONCENTRATES OF DIFFERENT STRENGTHS

Percentage of toxicant in emulsion concentrate	Parts of water to be added to 1 part of E.C. when concentration of final form is:				
	5%	2.5%	1%	0.5%	0.25%
80	15	31	79	159	319
60	11	23	50	119	239
50	9	19	49	99	199
25	4	9	24	49	99
10	1	3	9	19	39

PREPARATION OF EMULSION CONCENTRATES FROM TECHNICAL MATERIAL

Concentration desired (%)	Weight of technical material required to make the following volumes of concentrate:[x]		
	100 litres	100 USgal	100 UKgal
35	35 kg	292 lb	350 lb
25	25 kg	208 lb	250 lb
15	15 kg	125 lb	150 lb
12.5	12.5 kg	104 lb	125 lb
6.25	6.25 kg	52 lb	62.5 lb

[x] To every 100 parts of concentrate 2 parts of emulsifier should be added.

ANNEX V

Conversion factors for metric and other units.
1 and 3 reproduced from WHO, 1970, Technical Reports Series No. 443 *Insecticide Resistance and Vector Control*.

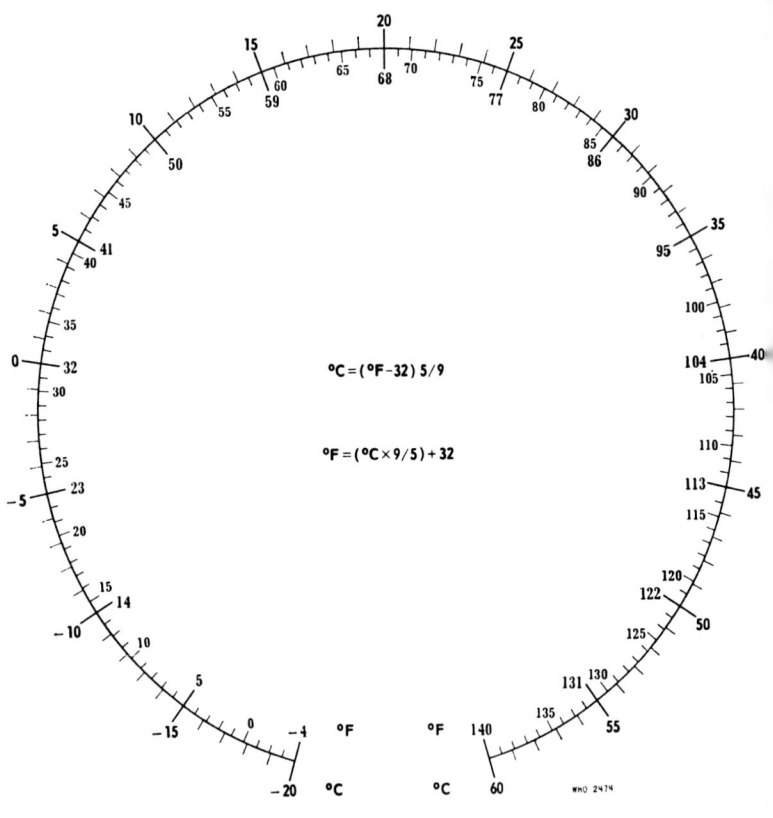

1 Temperature conversion

Annex V

F	C
108°	42·2°
107°	41·7°
106°	41·1°
105°	40·6°
104°	40·0°
103°	39·4°
102°	38·9°
101°	38·3°
100°	37·8°
99°	37·2°
98·4°	36·9°
98°	36·7°
97°	36·1°
96°	35·6°
95°	35·0°
94°	34·4°
93°	33·9°
92°	33·3°
91°	32·8°
90°	32·2°

2 Comparison of selected range of temperatures F° and C°

Length

1600 m	1.6 km	1 mile	1760 yd — 5280 ft
1 10⁵ cm	1000 m	1 kilometre (km)	0.625 mile — 1100 yd
91.4 cm	0.91 m	1 yard (yd)	3 ft — 36 in
1000 mm	100 cm	1 metre (m)	1.093 yd — 3.28 ft — 39.37 in
0.3048 m	30.48 cm	1 foot (ft)	12 in
25.4 mm	2.54 cm	1 inch (in)	1/12 ft
10 000 μ	10 mm	1 centimetre (cm)	0.394 in — 0.033 ft
	1000 μ	1 millimetre (mm)	0.0394 in
0.001 mm	0.0001 cm	1 micron (μ)	0.000039 in (about 1/25 000 in)

Area

	259 ha	1 square mile (sq mile)	640 acres
	100 ha	1 square kilometre (km^2)	0.39 sq mile — 247 acres
10 000 m^2	0.01 km^2	1 hectare (ha)	2.47 acres
4047 m^2	0.405 ha	1 acre	4840 yd^2 — 43 560 ft^2
	10 000 cm^2	1 square metre (m^2)	1.2 yd^2 — 10.76 ft^2 — 1550 in^2
	0.84 m^2	1 square yard (yd^2)	9 ft^2 — 1296 in^2
930 cm^2	0.093 m^2	1 square foot (ft^2)	144 in^2
	6.45 cm^2	1 square inch (in^2)	0.007 ft^2
	100 mm^2	1 square centimetre (cm^2)	0.155 in^2
	93 m^2	1000 square feet (ft^2)	

Volume

1000 litres	1 cubic metre (m^3)	1.307 yd^3 — 35.32 ft^3
2.83 m^3	100 cubic feet (ft^3)	3.7 yd^3
0.77 m^3	1 cubic yard (yd^3)	27 ft^3
28.32 litres	1 cubic foot (ft^3)	0.037 yd^3 — 1728 in^3
16.39 cm^3	1 cubic inch (in^3)	0.000579 ft^3

Liquid capacity

3.79 litres	1 US gallon (USgal)	0.83 UKgal — 231 in^3
4.55 litres	1 UK gallon (UKgal)	1.2 USgal
1000 ml	1 litre	0.26 USgal (0.22 UKgal)
32 USfl oz	1 US quart (qt)	0.9463 litre
Approx. 40 UKfl oz	1 UKqt	1.136 litres
3 teaspoonfuls	1 tablespoonful	0.5 USfl oz

Weight

1000 mg	1 gram (g)	0.0352 oz
28.35 g	1 ounce (oz)	1/16 lb — 437.5 grains
64.8 mg	1 grain	1/7000 lb
453.6 g	1 pound (lb)	16 oz
1000 g	1 kilogram (kg)	2.2 lb — 35.27 oz
1000 kg	1 metric ton	2204 lb
907 kg	1 US short ton	2000 lb — 0.893 UK ton
1018 kg	1 UK ton (1 US long ton)	2240 lb — 1.12 US short tons

3 Conversion factors: metric and English units

Annex V

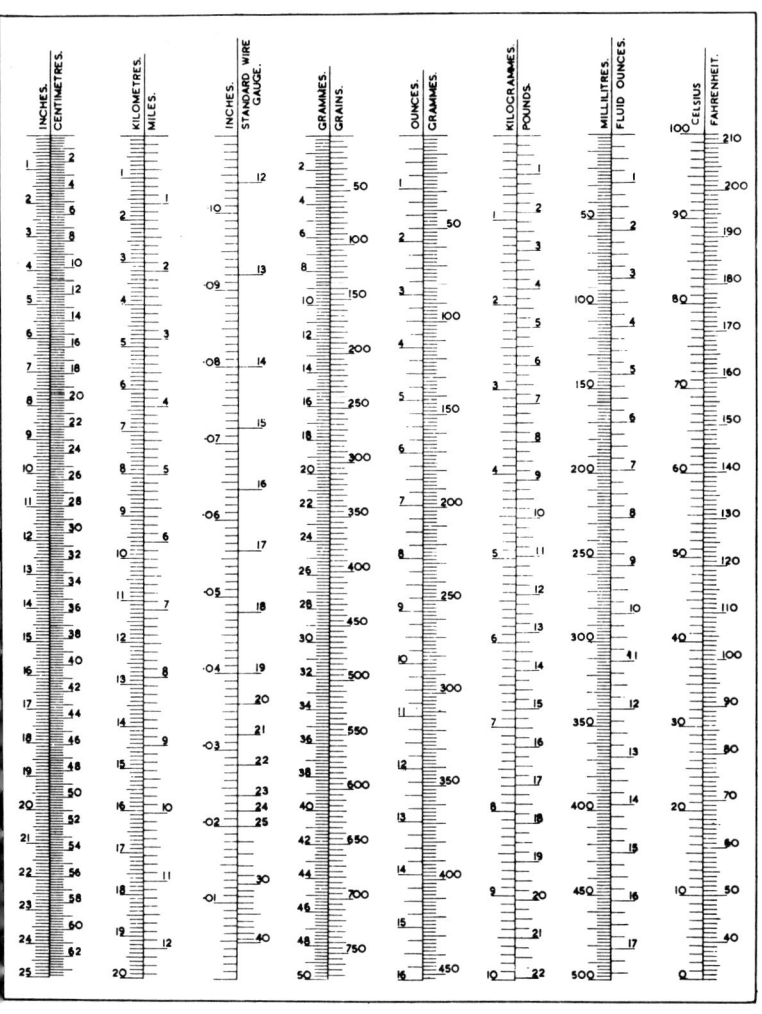

4 Useful conversion scales

Index

Abate, 242
Acquired immunity, 59
Acridines, 324
Acute malaria, treatment of, 192–5
Adrenaline, 77
Aedes, 98
Aerosols, 244, 245, 250, 276
Aestivation, 120
Africa, 165, 286
　equatorial, 209, 211
　north, 211
　north-west, 209
Age-grading methods, 105
Agent factors, 131–2
Aircraft spraying techniques, 252
Albumin, 74
Algid malaria, 38
Alkylating agents, 231
Allethrin, 236
Americas, 287
4-Aminoquinoline, 196, 198, 203, 206, 275, 289, 324
8-Aminoquinoline, 74, 201, 324
Amodiaquine, 3, 174, 176, 179, 186, 192, 193, 195, 196, 199, 203, 275
Amopyroquine, 179
Anaemia, 52, 56, 65, 72
Anopheles, 3, 4, 97–128, 130, 151–3, 158, 159, 210
　adult, 101
　age-grading, 105
　anatomy and physiology, 99–106
　anthropophilic, 121
　behaviour characteristics, 121
　behaviour pattern, 120–2
　classification of, 110
　collection of larvae and adults, 125–7
　comparison with other tribes, 98, 101
　density, 126, 152
　dissection of midgut, 127–8
　dissection of salivary glands, 128
　distribution, 99, 106–14
　domestic, 121
　eggs, 99
　entomological methods, 125–8
　exophilic, 121
　feeding habits, 120
　female, 115
　flight range, 122
　genetic compatibility, 123
　identification of species, 106–9
　internal anatomy, 103–6
　larvae, 99, 101, 106
　larval habitats, 117–19
　malaria infection in, 127–8
　male, 115
　natural history of, 115–24
　proboscis, 102
　pupa, 101
　seasonal fluctuations, 119–20
　sibling species and species complexes, 110
　species complexes, 122–4
　species of importance, 106–9
　sub-genera, 97
　zoological classification, 97
　zoophilic, 121, 138
A. aconitus, 164
A. albimanus, 118, 167, 168, 265
A. albitarsis, 167
A. annularis, 160, 161
A. aquasalis, 122, 166, 167
A. atroparvus, 50, 131, 159
A. barbirostris, 110
A. bellator, 167
A. campestris, 163
A. claviger, 120, 160
A. cruzi, 167
A. culicifacies, 120, 152, 161, 162, 265
A. darlingi, 167
A. dureni, 31

A. fluviatilis, 122, 161, 162
A. freeborni, 167
A. funestus, 165, 166
A. gambiae, 102, 110, 115, 118, 120, 123, 129, 133, 135, 165, 166, 265
A. hyrcanus, 164
A. labranchiae, 159–60
A. letifer, 163
A. leucosphyrus, 160, 164
A. litoralis, 163
A. maculatus, 160, 163, 164
A. maculipennis, 123, 159
A. mangyanus, 163
A. melas, 123, 165
A. merus, 123
A. messeae, 159
A. minimus, 160, 162
A. minimus flavirostris, 163
A. moucheti, 106
A. nili, 166
A. nuñez-tovari, 167
A. pharoensis, 166
A. philippinensis, 160, 161
A. pseudopunctipennis, 167
A. punctimacula, 167
A. punctulatus, 110, 164
A. quadrimaculatus, 50, 167
A. sacharovi, 120, 160, 265
A. sergenti, 160
A. stephensi, 50, 119, 135, 161, 265
A. sundaicus, 161, 163, 164
A. superpictus, 160
A. umbrosus, 110, 163, 164
A. varuna, 161
Antibodies, 60, 62, 64
Antifolic compounds, 325
Antigen-antibody complexes, 66
Antigen fractions, 64
Antigens, 91
Antilles, 166
Antimalarial drugs, 169, 184, 278, 292, 324
   action of, 169, 172, 184
   chemical formulae, 175
   clearance from the body, 185
   clinical uses, 177–83
   collective protection, 204–7
   combinations of compounds, 190, 207
   curative (therapeutic) use, 171
   dosage, 186–7, 202, 206
   frequency of administration, 186, 206
   in common use, 188
   individual protection, 201–3
   intravenous injections, 193–4
   long-term effects, 205
   mass administration, 174, 207–8
   method of distribution, 206
   new compounds, 183–4
   nomenclature, 187–92
   pharmacological considerations, 184–6
   presumptive treatment, 171
   properties of, 176
   protective (prophylactic) use, 170
   protective value, 200
   radical treatment, 174
   repository, 183
   resistance, 195–9
   selection for collective protection, 205
   structure and relationship, 174–84
   suppressive (clinical prophylactic), 171
   toxic effects, 199–201
   transmission prevention, 171
   uses of, 170–4
Antimetabolites, 231
Aotus, 34
Aotus trivirgatus, 33, 51, 197
Arprocarb, 242
Asia, South-East, 163, 209, 210, 288
Assam, 160, 209, 229
Atebrin, 3
Atomisers, 252
Australasia, 164
Australia, 164
Autochthonous malaria, 135
Average enlarged spleen (AES), 143–4
Avian plasmodia, 30

Bali, 164
Band forms, 27
Basic reproduction rate, 158

Index

Bastianelli, Giuseppe, 3
Baytex, 241
B-cells, 61, 62
Behaviouristic resistance, 260
Bengal, 160, 161
Benzene hexachloride (BHC), 4, 238
Bibliography, 294
Big spleen disease, 66
Bignami, Amico, 3
Bigumal, 187
Bilirubin, 71
Biological control methods, 228–32
Biological modification, 275
Birds, malaria parasites of, 30–1
Black, R. H., 154
Blackwater fever, 69–75
    classical researches, 69
    clinical picture, 73–5
    diagnosis, 74
    epidemiology, 70
    pathogenesis, 70
    pathology, 69, 71–3
    treatment, 75
Blood circulation, 57
Blood collection, 96
Blood culture, 91
Blood donors, 91
Blood examination, 77–91, 141, 144–6
Blood feeds, 151–2
Blood films
    examination of, 84–91
    preparation of, 77–91
Blood slides, 282
Blood transfusion, 46–9, 75
Blood urea, 194
Bombay, 161
Bone-marrow, 56
Bone-marrow stem cells, 62
Borneo, 164
Borrow-pits, 219
Brain, 54, 55
Bruce, David, 2
Bucket-sprayers, 253
Burkitt's lymphoma, 66

Capture stations, 219
Carbamates, 242, 267, 272

Carbaryl, 242
Caribbean, 166
Central America, 167
Central nervous system, 53–5
Cercopithecus aethiops, 32
Cerebral malaria, 38, 57
Chemical control methods, 232–44
Chemoprophylaxis, 169–208
Chemosterilant compounds, 231
Chemotherapy, 169–208, 292
Children, malaria in, 42–4
Chlorguanide, 174, 187
Chlorinated hydrocarbons, 237, 261, 262, 267, 271, 289
Chloroquine, 3, 174–9, 186, 192–6, 199, 201, 203, 208, 275–8
Chlorproguanil, 180
Chlorpromazine, 194
Cholinesterase, 272
Chronic malaria, 44
Clindamycin, 184
Clinical course, 35–51
    in children, 42–4
Clinical pathology, 56–8
Cold stage, 37
Complications, 44
Compression sprayer, 253
Confidence intervals, 149
Congenital (or neo-natal) immunity, 60
Conversion factors, 340, 342
Conversion scales, 343
Corticosteroids, 194
Crescents, 26
Cross resistance, 262
Crude parasite density index, 146
Crude parasite rate, 146
Culex, 98
Culverts, placement, 119
Cycloguanil embonate, 183
Cytostome, 22

Dapsone (diamino diphenyl sulphone), 176, 181, 198
Data recording, 147–9
DDT, 4, 164, 216, 234, 237–8, 247, 248, 261, 262, 271–3, 276–80

348 Essential Malariology

De Meillon, 3
Decamethrin, 237
Delhi, 161
Diacetylsulphone, 183
Diagnosis, 76–96
  blackwater fever, 74–5
  differentiation, 76
Diamino-diphenyl sulphone (DDS), 176, 181
Diapause, 116
Diazepam, 194
Dibutyl phthalate (DBP), 214
Dichlorvos (DDVP), 241
Dieldrin, 4, 164, 239–40, 261, 262, 271
Diethyl-toluamide (DET), 214
Dihydrofolate reductase inhibitors, 325
Dimethrin, 237
Dimethyl phthalate (DMP), 214
Dimilin, 268
DNA, 13
Double gel diffusion tests, 91
Drainage systems, 220–6, 275
Drying measures, 228

Electrolyte estimation, 194
ELISA test, 94
Endemic malaria 139–40
  of high epidemic potential, 210
  of low epidemic potential, 209
Endemicity, 135
  classification of, 147
Endocytosis, 22
Endophagy, 122
Environmental contamination, 272
Environmental factors, 132–5
Enzyme-linked immuno-sorbent method, 95
Epidemic malaria, 45, 135
Epidemic wave, 138
Epidemics, 129, 204
  causes, 137–8
  regional, 138
  seasonal, 139
  use of term, 137

Epidemiology, 129–8, 209–11, 280
  characteristics of selected areas, 159–68
  milestones in, 8
  quantitative, 149–59
  zones of malaria, 110–14
Epstein-Barr virus, 66
Eradication, 280–93
  aim of, 159
  and control compared, 281
  cost of, 277
  epidemiological principles, 280–1
  future of, 290–3
  global, 283–93
  global strategy, 291
  organisation, 282
  phases, 282–3
  progress of, 285
  technical problems, 286
Erythrocyte sedimentation rate, 56
Erythrocytes
  differential characteristics of, 90
  morphological characteristics of, 93
Erythrocytic cycle of schizogony, 20
Erythrocytic phase, 19
Erythrocytic schizogony, 26
Europe, 288
  Northern and Central, 159
Exflagellation, 14
Exo-erythrocytic schizogony, 13, 19
Exophagy, 122

Fanasil, 183
Fansidar, 198
Fenitrothion, 241
Fenthion, 241
Fever, pathogenesis of, 52–3
Field's stain, 83, 84
Filariasis, 97
Filling measures, 220
Fish for malaria control, 229–31
Flagellum, 14
Flushing methods, 228
Freund's complete adjuvant, 68

Index

G6PD, 59, 74
Gametes, 14, 152
Gametocytes, 14, 20, 28, 29, 137
Gametocytocidal drugs, 169
Gastro-intestinal symptoms, 39
Gastro-intestinal tract, 56
Genetic control, 231
Geographical reconnaissance, 257
Giemsa stain, 79, 80, 82, 85
Glomerulonephritis, 56, 65
Glucose-6-phosphate
   dehydrogenase (G6PD), 59, 74
Gonotrophic cycle, 152, 154
Gonotrophic dissociation, 116
Gorgas, William Crawford, 3
Grassi, Battista, 3
Guyana, 167

Hackett's method, 143
Haematin, 19
Haematological changes, 53
Haemoglobin, 58–9, 71
Haemoglobin S, 58
Haemoglobinuria, 74
Haemolysis, 73
Haemozoin, 19
Health services, xi
Hepatocystes kochi, 32
Heterologous antigens, 91
Hexachlorocyclohexane (HCH), 4, 238–9, 248, 261, 262, 271
Hexachloro-octahydro-epoxy-dimethano-naphthalene (HEOD), 239
Hibernation, 120
Hill malaria, 210
History of malaria, 1–9
   milestones in, 5–9
Holoendemic malaria, 147
Holoendemicity, 140
Homologous antigen, 91
Horton Hospital, 50
Host factors, 130–1
Hot stage, 37
Human blood index, 121, 152
Human plasmodia. *See* Plasmodia
Hyperendemic malaria, 147

Hyperendemicity, 139
Hypoendemic malaria, 147
Hypoendemicity, 139

Idiopathic splenomegaly, 66
Imagicidal measures, 247
Imagicidal methods, 249
Immune responses, 58–64, 66, 67
Immunisation, 67–9
Immunity, 170
Immunofluorescence, 95
Immunoglobulins, 62–4, 91
Immuno-haemagglutination, 95
Immunopathology, 65–7
Immuno-precipitation techniques, 91, 95
Immunosuppression, 66
Imported malaria, 45–7, 135
Incidence, 136
Incubation period, 19, 35, 38, 49
Indalone, 214
Index
   of stability, 155
   use of term, 136
India, 209, 210
   north-east, 160
   north-west, 211
   peninsular, 161
   plains of, 161
   southern, 229
Indigenous malaria, 135
Indirect fluorescent antibody (IFA) test, 91, 96
Indirect haemagglutination (HA) test, 91
Indonesia, 164
Induced malaria, 135
Infection risk, 46–7
Inoculation rate, 153
Insecticide resistance, 260–8
   causal factors, 265
   counteracting, 265
   determination of, 263–4
   general considerations, 260
   geographical distribution, 265
   nature and cause of, 261–3
   present state of, 265–8

Insecticides, 3, 4, 121, 216, 217, 219, 247, 276, 278, 280, 289, 292, 326
  avoidance of, 260
  classification, 232–3
  degree of hazard, 268
  emergency treatment of poisoning by, 270–2
  equipment for application of, 244–5
  formulations of, 243–4
  potential toxicity, 268
  precautions to be observed, 269
  protective equipment, 269
  safe use of, 268–73
  types of, 232–43
International Code of Zoological Nomenclature, 109
Intestinal leishmaniasis, 142
Introduced malaria, 135
Irrigation works, 119

Jaundice, 74
Java, 164
Jesuit's powder, 2
Joss sticks, 214, 247

Kala azar, 142
Kalimantan, 164
Kallikreins, 57
Karachi, 161
Kenya, 210
Kerala, 161
Khmer Republic, 163
Kidney, 56, 57, 71
Kikuth, 3
Krebs cycle, 29

Labour forces, malaria of, 211, 275
Landrin, 242
Larval control, 217
Larvicides, 245–7, 275, 278
Larvivorous fish, 229
Laveran, Alphonse, 2

Laverania, 10
Laverania falcipara, 10
Leucocytosis, 56
Leucopenia, 56
Lidos, construction of, 227
Lincomycin, 184
Liver, 56, 72, 75
Long-term relapse, 40

M 4888, 187
Macaca irus, 32, 33
Macdonald, George, 151, 153, 154
Macrogametocyte, 20, 24
Maegraith, B. G., 57
Malaria
  assessment of infection, 135–6
  classification, 135
  deliberate transmission of, 130
  epidemic, 135
  epidemiological zones of, 110–14
  geographical distribution, 129–30
  history of, 1–9
    milestones in, 5–9
  man-made, 119, 218, 274
  natural transmission of infection, 130
  prevention of, 212
  resurgence of, xi
  treatment of. *See* Treatment
  use of term, 11
Malaria control, 209–79
  and eradication compared, 281
  antilarval measures, 217
  classification of control measures, 274
  cost of, 277–9
  formulation of sprays, 338
  in development projects, 275–7
  milestones in, 8–9
  planning, 273
  principles of, 212
  selection of methods of, 273–7
Malaria parasites, 5, 10–34
  diagnostic characteristics in blood film, 87
  differentiation of strains of, 13
  in mosquito host, 13–17

Index

Malaria parasites *cont.*
  in vertebrate host, 17
  life cycle of, 13–22
  mixed infections, 29
  morphology, 13–22
  of animals, 30–4
  of birds, 30–1
  of monkeys, 32
  ultrastructure, 20–2
  See also under specific names
Malaria Reference Laboratory, 50
Malaria survey, 140–9
  recording of data and their statistical significance, 147–9
Malarial granuloma, 55
Malarial haemoglobinuria. *See* Blackwater fever
Malariogenic potential, 139
Malariometric surveys, 147–9
Malariometry, 140
Malathion, 240–1, 269, 278
Man-made malaria, 119, 218, 274
Manson, Patrick, 2, 3
Manson's schistosomiasis, 142
Maurer's dots, 26
Mauss, 3
Mediterranean area, 159, 289
Mefloquine, 176, 184, 196
Mepacrine, 3, 174, 176, 177, 199, 201
Merozoites, 17, 20
Mesoendemic malaria, 147
Mesoendemicity, 139
Metakelfin, 182
Methoprene, 268
Microgamete, 14
Microgametocyte, 20, 24
Middle East, 159, 211
Mietzsch, 3
Mist-blowers, 250
Monkeys, malaria parasites of, 32
Monocytosis, 56
Morbidity rate, 136, 137
Mosquito boots, 213
Mosquito coils, 214
Mosquito control, 216–17, 265
Mosquito nets, 212–15
Mosquitos, classification of, 97
Muller, Paul, 4

Natural immunity, 58
Naturalistic measures, 228
Nephropathies, 65
Nephrotic syndrome, 56, 65
Net reproduction rate, 155
Neurosyphilis, therapy, 130
New Guinea, 164
New Hebrides, 164
North America, 168
Nozzle spray patterns, 254
Nutrition effects, 137

Oöcyst, 15, 22, 24, 127, 128, 153
Oökinete, 14, 15, 22, 153
Organophosphorus compounds, 240, 248, 262, 267, 271, 272
Orissa, 161
Ovale malaria, 41
Owl monkey, 51
Oxyhaemoglobin, 73

Pacific, Western, 290
Pakistan, 211
  plains of, 161
Paludrine, 187
Pamaquine, 3
Para-amino-benzoic acid (PABA), 29
Parasite count, 85–7, 145
Parasite density index, 145, 146
Parasite rate, 144, 145
Parasites. *See* Malaria parasites
Parathion, 269
Paris green, 235–7, 246
Paroxysms, 37
Passive immunity, 59
Pathogenesis of fever, 52–3
Pathological conditions, 65
Pathology, 52–8
Period prevalence, 136
Permethrin, 237
Pernicious malaria, 38
Petroleum oils, 233–5
Philippines, 163
Physiological resistance, 260, 261

Pigment, 19, 55
Pinotti's method, 207, 208
Placenta, 56
Plasmodium, 10, 11, 127, 130, 152
  animal, 30–4
  antigens, 61
  avian, 30
  detection of, 77
  evolutionary history of, 1
  human, 22–30
    characteristics of infection, 23
    physiology of, 29–30
  rodent, 31–2
  simian, 32
P. berghei, 10, 31, 67
P. berghei yoelii, 32
P. brasilianum, 33
P. cynomolgi, 32, 33
P. cynomolgi bastianellii, 33
P. falciparum, 1, 10, 11, 17, 18, 20, 24–7, 38–9, 44–59, 64–70, 75, 86, 87, 91–3, 129–32, 138, 139, 154, 164, 171, 176–84, 193–8, 201, 203, 204, 281, 287–90
P. inui, 33
P. knowlesi, 32, 33, 50, 68
P. kochi, 32
P. malariae, 1, 10, 11, 18, 19, 27–8, 37, 41–2, 47–53, 56, 65, 85, 92, 93, 130, 178, 179
P. ovale, 11, 18, 19, 28, 41, 47, 50, 52, 85, 90, 92, 93, 130, 178, 179
P. relictum, 30
P. rodhaini, 10, 27
P. simium, 33
P. tenue, 25
P. vivax, 1, 11, 15, 18, 19, 21–4, 35, 36, 40–1, 47–52, 58, 68, 85, 92, 93, 129, 131, 132, 138, 139, 154, 178–83, 203, 204
P. vivax hibernans, 35, 41
P. vivax North Korean strain, 51
Poikilocytosis, 56
Point prevalence, 136
Polychromasia, 56
Post-epidemic period, 138
Precipitin tests, 121
Prednisolone, 194
Prednisolone phosphate, 75

Pre-erythrocytic schizogony, 13, 17
Pregnancy, 39, 44–5
Premunition, 60
Pre-patent period, 19, 35
Prevalence, 136
Primaquine, 3, 174, 179, 186, 201
Primary attack, 35, 37
Proguanil, 3, 174, 180, 186, 187, 195, 196, 199, 201, 204, 206, 275, 276
Propoquine, 179
Propoxur, 242
Protective clothing, 213
Provocation, method, 77
Punjab, 161, 211
Pyrethrins, 236
Pyrethrum, 3, 216, 236, 247, 249, 276
Pyrimethamine, 3, 174, 181, 182, 186, 195–201, 204, 206, 275, 276

Quartan malaria, 41–2
Quartan malaria nephrosis, 65
Quinine, 174, 176, 177, 192, 196, 198, 199, 203
Quinolinemethanol, 176, 325

Rainfall effects, 132–3
Rate, use of term, 136
Receptivity, 139, 283
Recrudescence, 35, 37, 40
Recurrence, 35, 37, 40
Red blood cells, 19, 20, 30, 52, 53, 55, 56, 75, 85, 91, 92
Relapses, 35, 37, 40, 41
Relapsing malaria, 193
Renal dysfunction, 57
Renal failure, 65, 75
Renal insufficiency, 44
Repellents, 214
Residual immunity, 60
Resmethrin, 237
Resting places, 121
Rieckmann, K. H., 197, 198
Ring forms, 19

Index

Risk areas, 328
Rodent malaria, 58
Rodent plasmodia, 31–2
Rosette, 28
Ross, Ronald, 3, 151, 155
Russell, P. F., 126, 212
Rutgers-612, 214

Schizogonic periodicity, 20
Schizogony, 13, 20, 22
Schizont, 20, 28, 29
Schizontocidal drugs, 169, 203
Schüffner's stippling, 24, 28, 85
Schulemann, W., 3
Screening, 215
Seasonal fluctuations, 119–20
Serological tests, 91–6
  appraisal of, 95–6
  details of, 94
Sevin, 242
Short-term relapse, 37, 40
Sickle cell haemoglobin, 58
Simian malaria, 58
Simian plasmodia, 32
Sind, 211
Site selection for malaria protection, 215
Sludging process, 53
Sluicing, 228
Smokes, 250
Socio-economic advance, xi
Source reduction, 216, 219–28
South America, 167, 209, 210
South Pacific, 164
Species infection rate, 146
Species parasite density index, 146
Spleen, 55, 66
  average enlarged, 143–4
Spleen examination, 141–4
Spleen rate, 141, 143, 147
Sporogonic cycle, 153
Sporontocidal drugs, 169
Sporozoite, 4, 15, 16, 67, 127, 128, 153
Sporozoite rate, 128, 141, 153
Spray formulations, 338

Spraying, 248, 269, 276, 277, 278, 280
Spraying cycle, 259
Spraying equipment, 249–53
Spraying round, 259
Spraying squad, 257
Spraying technique, 257–60
Sri Lanka, 162, 209, 210
Stable malaria, 135
Stippling, 24, 28, 85
Stirrup-pumps, 253
Sub-tropical seasonal malaria, 211
Sulphadimethoxine, 182
Sulphadoxine, 183, 198
Sulphalene (sulphamethoxy-pyridazine), 182, 198
Sulphamethoxypyridazine (sulphalene), 182, 198
Sulphonamides, 176, 182, 196, 201, 275, 325
Sulphones, 74, 176, 181, 201, 275, 325
Sulphorthomidine, 183
Sweating stage, 37
Systemic manifestations, 39

Tamil Nadu, 161
T-cells, 61, 62
Temephos, 242
Temperature conversion, 340
Temperature curves, 36
Tennessee Valley Authority, 228
Tetramethrin, 237
Thamnomys surdaster, 31
Therapeutic malaria, 49–51
Thomson, J. J., 151
Tile pipes, 226
Tissue schizont, 17
Tissue schizontocide, 169
Tissue stage, 13, 17
Toxaemia of pregnancy, 39, 45
Toxonemes, 22
Training, 292, 293
Transfusion malaria, 46–9
Treatment
  of acute malaria, 192–5
  of falciparum malaria, 193
  milestones in, 7–8

Treponema pallidum, 49
Trimethoprim, 176, 198
Trinidad, 166
Trophozoites, 19, 27, 28
Tropical splenomegaly syndrome (T.S.S.), 66

Ultra low volume (ULV) technique, 251–2
Unstable malaria, 135
Urine, 73, 74
Urine tests, 57
USA, 167

Vaccination, 68
Vaccine, 67, 292
Valium, 194
Vascular failure, 73, 75
Vasculomyelinopathy, 55

Venezuela, 167
Viet-Nam, 163
Viral diseases, 97
Vulnerability, 139, 283

Water management, 228
Watson, Malcolm, 3
Western Ghats, 161
World Health Organization, 196, 278, 280, 283, 292
WR 142490, 184

Young's formula, 186

Ziemann's stippling, 28
Zygote, 14